# Contemporary Debates and Controversies in Cardiac Electrophysiology, Part I

*Guest Editors*

RANJAN K. THAKUR, MD, MPH, MBA, FHRS
ANDREA NATALE, MD, FACC, FHRS

# CARDIAC ELECTROPHYSIOLOGY CLINICS

www.cardiacEP.theclinics.com

*Consulting Editors*
RANJAN K. THAKUR, MD, MPH, MBA, FHRS
ANDREA NATALE, MD, FACC, FHRS

December 2011 • Volume 3 • Number 4

SAUNDERS an imprint of ELSEVIER, Inc.

**W.B. SAUNDERS COMPANY**
*A Division of Elsevier Inc.*

1600 John F. Kennedy Boulevard • Suite 1800 • Philadelphia, Pennsylvania 19103-2899

http://www.theclinics.com

**CARDIAC ELECTROPHYSIOLOGY CLINICS Volume 3, Number 4**
**December 2011 ISSN 1877-9182, ISBN-13: 978-1-4557-1090-4**

Editor: Barbara Cohen-Kligerman
Developmental Editor: Teia Stone

*Cardiac Electrophysiology Clinics* (ISSN 1877-9182) is published quarterly by Elsevier Inc., 360 Park Avenue South, New York, NY 10010-1710. Months of issue are March, June, September, and December. Subscription prices are $180.00 per year for US individuals, $266.00 per year for US institutions, $95.00 per year for US students and residents, $202.00 per year for Canadian individuals, $297.00 per year for Canadian institutions, $258.00 per year for international individuals, $318.00 per year for international institutions and $136.00 per year for Canadian and foreign students/residents. To receive student/resident rate, orders must be accompanied by name of affilliated institution, date of term, and the signature of program/residency coordinator on institution letterhead. Orders will be billed at individual rate until proof of status is received. Foreign air speed delivery is included in all Clinics subscription prices. All prices are subject to change without notice. **POSTMASTER:** Send address changes to Cardiac Electrophysiology Clinics, Elsevier Health Sciences Division, Subscription Customer Service, 3251 Riverport Lane, Maryland Heights, MO 63043. **Customer Service: 1-800-654-2452 (US and Canada). From outside of the US and Canada, call 314-477-8871. Fax: 314-447-8029. E-mail: JournalsCustomerService-usa@elsevier.com (for print support); JournalsOnlineSupport-usa@elsevier.com (for online support).**

*Reprints.* For copies of 100 or more of articles in this publication, please contact the Commercial Reprints Department, Elsevier Inc., 360 Park Avenue South, New York, NY 10010-1710. Tel.: 212-633-3812; Fax: 212-462-1935; E-mail: reprints@elsevier.com.

Opened ICD pocket demonstrating tremendous lead burden in a 53-year-old man with ischemic cardiomyopathy status-post single chamber ICD implant complicated by repeated high voltage lead fracture with lead replacement and abandonment. The extraction procedure was made challenging by the intense lead-lead binding, particularly at the level of the superior vena cava coil. See "Should Every Broken Lead Be Extracted?" by Melanie Maytin, MD, and Laurence M. Epstein, MD, for further details.

Printed and bound by CPI Group (UK) Ltd, Croydon, CR0 4YY

Transferred to Digital Print 2011

# Contributors

## CONSULTING EDITORS

**RANJAN K. THAKUR, MD, MPH, MBA, FHRS**
Professor of Medicine, and Director,
Arrhythmia Service, Thoracic and
Cardiovascular Institute, Sparrow Health
System, Michigan State University,
Lansing, Michigan

**ANDREA NATALE, MD, FACC, FHRS**
Executive Medical Director of the Texas
Cardiac Arrhythmia Institute at St David's
Medical Center, Austin, Texas; Consulting
Professor, Division of Cardiology, Stanford
University, Palo Alto, California; Clinical
Associate Professor of Medicine, Case
Western Reserve University, Cleveland, Ohio;
Senior Clinical Director, EP Services, California
Pacific Medical Center, San Francisco,
California; Department of Biomedical
Engineering, University of Texas, Austin, Texas

## AUTHORS

**AMIN AL-AHMAD, MD, FHRS**
Assistant Professor, Department of Medicine,
Stanford University School of Medicine, Palo
Alto, California

**SANA M. AL-KHATIB, MD**
Associate Professor of Medicine, Division
of Cardiology, Department of Medicine,
Duke University, Durham, North Carolina

**RONG BAI, MD**
Texas Cardiac Arrhythmia Institute, St David's
Medical Center, Austin, Texas

**ULRIKA BIRGERSDOTTER-GREEN, MD**
University of California San Diego, San Diego,
California

**J. DAVID BURKHARDT, MD, FHRS**
Texas Cardiac Arrhythmia Institute, St David's
Medical Center, Austin, Texas

**DANIEL J. CANTILLON, MD**
Department of Cardiovascular Medicine,
Cardiac Electrophysiology and Pacing, Heart
and Vascular Institute, Cleveland Clinic,
Cleveland, Ohio

**CORRADO CARBUCICCHIO, MD**
Cardiac Arrhythmia Research Center, Centro
Cardiologico Monzino, IRCCS, Milan, Italy

**MICHELA CASELLA, MD, PhD**
Cardiac Arrhythmia Research Centre, Centro
Cardiologico Monzino, IRCCS, Milan, Italy

**STUART J. CONNOLLY, MD, FRCPC**
Professor and Chair, Division of Cardiology,
Department of Medicine, Population Health
Research Institute and Hamilton Health
Sciences, McMaster University, Hamilton,
Ontario, Canada

**TAHMEED CONTRACTOR, MD**
Department of Cardiology, Lehigh Valley
Health Network, Allentown, Pennsylvania

**ANTONIO DELLO RUSSO, MD, PhD**
Cardiac Arrhythmia Research Centre, Centro
Cardiologico Monzino, IRCCS, Milan, Italy

**NICOLAS DERVAL, MD**
Hôpital Haut Lévêque and Université
Bordeaux II, Bordeaux, France

**LUIGI DI BIASE, MD, PhD, FHRS**
Texas Cardiac Arrhythmia Institute, St David's
Medical Center; Department of Biomedical

Engineering, University of Texas, Austin, Texas; Department of Cardiology, University of Foggia, Foggia, Italy

**SYAMKUMAR M. DIVAKARAMENON, MBBS, MD, DM**
Assistant Professor, Division of Cardiology, Department of Medicine, McMaster University and Hamilton Health Sciences, Hamilton, Ontario, Canada

**LAURENCE M. EPSTEIN, MD**
Division of Cardiovascular Medicine, Brigham and Women's Hospital, Boston, Massachusetts

**LORNE J. GULA, MD**
Division of Cardiology, University of Western Ontario, London, Ontario, Canada

**MICHEL HAISSAGUERRE, MD**
Hôpital Haut Lévêque and Université Bordeaux II, Bordeaux, France

**JONATHAN L. HALPERIN, MD**
Robert and Harriett Heilbrunn Professor of Medicine, The Cardiovascular Institute, Mount Sinai School of Medicine, Mount Sinai Medical Center, New York, New York

**STEPHEN C. HAMMILL, MD**
Professor of Medicine, Division of Cardiovascular Diseases, Mayo Clinic, Rochester, Minnesota

**JEFFREY S. HEALEY, MD, MSc, FRCPC**
Associate Professor, Division of Cardiology, Department of Medicine, Population Health Research Institute and Hamilton Health Sciences, McMaster University, Hamilton, Ontario, Canada

**SWAPNIL HIREMATH, MD, MPH**
Division of Nephrology, The Ottawa Hospital, Ottawa, Ontario, Canada

**MELEZE HOCINI, MD**
Hôpital Haut Lévêque and Université Bordeaux II, Bordeaux, France

**HENRY HSIA, MD, FACC, FHRS**
Division of Cardiology, Stanford University, Palo Alto, California

**JOHN H. IP, MD**
Associate Professor of Medicine, Ingham Regional Medical Center, Michigan State University, Lansing, Michigan

**AMIR S. JADIDI, MD**
Hôpital Haut Lévêque and Université Bordeaux II, Bordeaux, France

**PIERRE JAIS, MD**
Hôpital Haut Lévêque and Université Bordeaux II, Bordeaux, France

**MARK E. JOSEPHSON, MD**
Herman Dana Professor of Medicine, Harvard Medical School; Chief, Cardiovascular Division and Director, Harvard-Thorndike Electrophysiology Institute and Arrhythmia Service, Beth Israel Deaconess Medical Center, Boston, Massachusetts

**GEORGE J. KLEIN, MD**
Division of Cardiology, University of Western Ontario, London, Ontario, Canada

**SEBASTIEN KNECHT, MD, PhD**
Hôpital Haut Lévêque and Université Bordeaux II, Bordeaux, France

**ANDREW D. KRAHN, MD**
Division of Cardiology, University of Western Ontario, London, Ontario, Canada

**DANIEL B. KRAMER, MD**
Clinical Fellow in Medicine, Cardiovascular Division, Department of Medicine, Beth Israel Deaconess Medical Center, Harvard Medical School, Boston, Massachusetts

**MARK S. KREMERS, MD**
Clinical Electrophysiologist, MidCarolina Cardiology, Charlotte, North Carolina

**DOUGLAS S. LEE, MD, PhD**
Associate Professor of Medicine, Division of Cardiology, Peter Munk Cardiac Centre, University Health Network, University of Toronto; Scientist, Institute for Clinical Evaluative Sciences, Toronto, Canada

**PETER LEONG-SIT, MD**
Division of Cardiology, University of Western Ontario, London, Ontario, Canada

**STEVEN M. MARKOWITZ, MD**
Division of Cardiology, Department of Medicine, Cornell University Medical Center, New York, New York

**MELANIE MAYTIN, MD**
Brigham and Women's Hospital, Boston, Massachusetts

**SHINSUKE MIYAZAKI, MD**
Hôpital Haut Lévêque and Université Bordeaux II, Bordeaux, France

**CARLOS A. MORILLO, MD, FRCPC**
Professor and Director of the Arrhythmia Service, Division of Cardiology, Department of Medicine, Population Health Research Institute and Hamilton Health Sciences, McMaster University, Hamilton, Ontario, Canada

**GIRISH M. NAIR, MBBS, FRCPC**
Associate Professor, Division of Cardiology, Department of Medicine, Population Health Research Institute and Hamilton Health Sciences, McMaster University, Hamilton, Ontario, Canada

**KRISHNAKUMAR NAIR, MD**
Assistant Professor of Medicine, Division of Cardiology, University Health Network, Peter Munk Cardiac Centre, University of Toronto, Toronto, Canada

**ANDREA NATALE, MD, FACC, FHRS**
Executive Medical Director of the Texas Cardiac Arrhythmia Institute at St David's Medical Center, Austin, Texas; Consulting Professor, Division of Cardiology, Stanford University, Palo Alto, California; Clinical Associate Professor of Medicine, Case Western Reserve University, Cleveland, Ohio; Senior Clinical Director, EP Services, California Pacific Medical Center, San Francisco, California; Department of Biomedical Engineering, University of Texas, Austin, Texas

**BRIAN OLSHANSKY, MD**
Professor of Medicine, Department of Internal Medicine, University of Iowa Hospital and Clinics, Iowa City, Iowa

**LUIGI PADELETTI, MD**
Department of Heart and Vessels, University of Florence, Florence, Italy

**PATRIZIO PASCALE, MD**
Hôpital Haut Lévêque and Université Bordeaux II, Bordeaux, France

**MEHUL B. PATEL, MD**
Department of Clinical Cardiac Electrophysiology, The Bay Pines Veterans Affairs Health Care System, University of South Florida, Tampa, Florida

**MICHALA PEDERSEN, MD**
Hôpital Haut Lévêque and Université Bordeaux II, Bordeaux, France

**LAURA PERROTTA, MD**
Department of Heart and Vessels, University of Florence, Florence, Italy

**PAOLO PIERAGNOLI, MD**
Department of Heart and Vessels, University of Florence, Florence, Italy

**GIUSEPPE RICCIARDI, MD**
Department of Heart and Vessels, University of Florence, Florence, Italy

**LAURENT ROTEN, MD**
Hôpital Haut Lévêque and Université Bordeaux II, Bordeaux, France

**FREDERIC SACHER, MD**
Hôpital Haut Lévêque and Université Bordeaux II, Bordeaux, France

**JAVIER SANCHEZ, MD**
Texas Cardiac Arrhythmia Institute, St David's Medical Center, Austin, Texas

**PASQUALE SANTANGELI, MD**
Texas Cardiac Arrhythmia Institute, St David's Medical Center, Austin, Texas

**DANIEL SCHERR, MD**
Hôpital Haut Lévêque and Université Bordeaux II, Bordeaux, France

**ASHOK J. SHAH, MD**
Hôpital Haut Lévêque and Université Bordeaux II, Bordeaux, France

**ALLAN C. SKANES, MD**
Division of Cardiology, University of Western Ontario, London, Ontario, Canada

**S. ADAM STRICKBERGER, MD**
Washington Electrophysiology, and
Cardiovascular Research Institute,
Washington Hospital Center,
Washington, DC

**RAJESH N. SUBBIAH, MBBS, PhD**
Department of Cardiology, St Vincent's
Hospital, Darlinghurst; University of
New South Wales, Sydney, New South
Wales, Australia

**RENEE M. SULLIVAN, MD**
Electrophysiology Fellow, University of Iowa
Hospital and Clinics, Iowa City, Iowa

**CHARLES D. SWERDLOW, MD**
Cedars Sinai Heart Center, Cedars-Sinai
Medical Center, Los Angeles, California

**RANJAN K. THAKUR, MD, MPH, MBA, FHRS**
Professor of Medicine, and Director,
Arrhythmia Service, Thoracic and
Cardiovascular Institute, Sparrow Health
System, Michigan State University,
Lansing, Michigan

**CLAUDIO TONDO, MD, PhD**
Cardiac Arrhythmia Research Centre, Centro
Cardiologico Monzino, IRCCS, Milan, Italy

**JACK V. TU, MD, PhD**
Professor of Medicine, Division of Cardiology,
Schulich Heart Centre, Sunnybrook Health
Sciences Centre, University of Toronto;
Scientist, Institute for Clinical Evaluative
Sciences, Toronto, Canada

**GANESH VENKATARAMAN, MD**
Washington Electrophysiology, and
Cardiovascular Research Institute,
Washington Hospital Center,
Washington, DC

**JAMES A. WHITE, MD**
Division of Cardiology, University of Western
Ontario, London, Ontario, Canada

**STEPHEN B. WILTON, MD, PhD**
Hôpital Haut Lévêque and Université
Bordeaux II, Bordeaux, France

**RAYMOND YEE, MD**
Division of Cardiology, University of Western
Ontario, London, Ontario, Canada

# Contents

Data from implantable cardioverter-defibrillator (ICD) registries offer access to information about the real-world patient as opposed to randomized control data, which tend to study selected patients in ideal care environments. This article discusses similarities and differences between registries and randomized control trials on ICDs. Registries in the United States, Canada, and elsewhere are discussed. The role of registry data for evaluation of complications and for examining accessibility and patterns of ICD care delivery are examined. In addition, the article discusses data from registries for monitoring quality and appropriateness of ICD care.

The registry was developed through a partnership of the Heart Rhythm Society and American College of Cardiology Foundation using the expertise of the National Cardiovascular Data Registry. All hospitals in the United States that implant implantable cardioverter–defibrillators (ICDs) in Medicare beneficiaries participate in the registry, with 1497 hospitals involved and over 750,000 procedures entered. The registry is being used to assess the ICD's performance. The registry is being combined with Medicare claims data to serve as a risk-adjusted performance measure. This article reviews lessons learned from the registry to date.

Recent studies have examined the use of cardiac resynchronization therapy (CRT) specifically in patients with mild or absent clinical heart failure. Expanding use of CRT to these populations would be a marked change in cardiovascular medicine with broad implications for already-strained budgets. This article examines the evidence for and against this expansion and suggests specific unresolved questions that require cautious consideration.

Sudden cardiac death (SCD) still represents the most challenging and controversial issue in cardiology. Even though implementation of implantable cardioverter-defibrillators in high-risk patients is effective in reducing SCD, the occurrence of life-threatening arrhythmias in the general population is disproportionately high as an expression of latent cardiac disease. Substrate myocardial analysis seems to be of pivotal importance to detect anatomic abnormalities underlying clinical conditions predisposing to major arrhythmic events. High-density electroanatomic mapping may be considered an effective technique to identify myocardial substrate abnormalities and to improve the identification of markers of increased arrhythmic risk in patients with ventricular arrhythmic disorders.

Although modern implantable cardioverter defibrillators (ICDs) can sense malignant ventricular arrhythmias, sudden death may occur from shock failure. Risk factors for high defibrillation thresholds (DFTs) have been identified. Patients may be at risk for ineffective defibrillation unless system modifications lower the DFT. The most common implant criterion (limited testing 10J below the maximal output of the device) is imprecise in measuring the safety margin of ICDs and may not predict clinical outcomes. This article suggests preservation of DFT testing, particularly in patients at risk for high DFTs, and investigation into safe testing protocols that improve prediction of clinical outcomes.

Implantable defibrillator (ICD) therapy improves survival of patients at risk for sudden cardiac death. Defibrillation efficacy (DE) testing is routinely performed at the time of ICD implantation. The evaluation of DE has small but finite risks. Advances in ICD technology have greatly enhanced DE. The available data suggest that the evaluation of DE during ICD implantation does not improve first shock efficacy or survival, and may not be necessary.

There are two methods for assessing defibrillation efficacy at implantable cardioverter defibrillator implantation. The direct, defibrillation method requires one or more sequences of induced ventricular fibrillation followed by defibrillation shocks. The pattern of success and failure of these shocks is used to estimate the defibrillation safety margin or the defibrillation threshold. The indirect vulnerability method relies on close correlation between the upper limit of vulnerability, determined by delivering shocks in regular rhythm, and the minimum shock strength that defibrillates reliably. The vulnerability method is less intuitive than the defibrillation method but can determine defibrillation safety margin without inducing ventricular fibrillation. Which method is better?

Dual-chamber implantable cardioverter defibrillators (ICDs) offer specific advantages and programming flexibility that single-chamber ICDs cannot. The ICD of choice for the patient who has an indication for an ICD but does not need cardiac resynchronization therapy is a dual-chamber ICD in most cases.

There is prognostic, therapeutic, and psychological importance in identifying the cause of ventricular fibrillation. Although the majority of cardiac arrests conform to stereotypical patterns of structural coronary and myocardial diseases, a minority re-main elusive to standard testing and require further testing and advanced imaging. A significant proportion of these remain undiagnosed. Until understanding of these causes leads to definitive disease-specific treatment, protection with an implantable cardioverter defibrillator is generally warranted. Ongoing studies are needed in genetic and electrophysiologic fields to expand understanding in this area, ideally leading to optimal therapy and prevention strategies.

Daniel J. Cantillon

Sudden deaths among cardiac transplant recipients are most commonly related to bradyarrhythmias, yet most bradyarrhythmias in this population are benign. This paradox makes indications for cardiac implantable devices challenging and requires understanding of the unique considerations in this population. Lethal events are typically late onset and often associated with allograft vasculopathy or rejection. Early identification and permanent pacemaker implantation have been associated with favorable outcomes. Discerning appropriate treatment of arrhythmias in the transplant population requires a systematic approach using preoperative data, operative considerations, and acquired posttransplant conditions.

Laura Perrotta, Giuseppe Ricciardi, Paolo Pieragnoli, and Luigi Padeletti

Management of alerts and advisories involving implantable cardiac defibrillators has become part of current clinical practice. The competing risks of device failure and complications associated with device replacement must be carefully assessed. Media greatly influence how physicians and patients perceive a recall, and therefore efforts must be made to avoid decisions based on perceived risks. Awareness of the potential risk of malfunction could increase patient anxiety. Health care professionals should be adequately informed of all aspects related to a device recall, trained in recall management, and able to inform patients and involve them in an accurate and transparent decision-making process.

Tahmeed Contractor, Mehul B. Patel, and Ranjan K. Thakur

Stroke and thromboembolism are catastrophic complications of atrial fibrillation (AF). Implantable heart rhythm devices can reliably detect atrial high rate events (AHREs), which are supposedly tantamount to having AF or flutter. The critical duration, frequency, or overall burden of AHRE that increases stroke risk is still unknown, and thus the threshold level of AHREs (duration and frequency) that warrants anticoagulation in patients with device-detected AHREs is still unclear. This article reviews the current literature on the risk of stroke with device-detected AHREs and raises questions that need further clarification.

John H. Ip and Jonathan L. Halperin

Atrial fibrillation (AF) is the most common arrhythmia requiring medical treatment. Atrial fibrillation and atrial flutter (AFl) are common cardiac arrhythmias associated with an increased incidence of stroke in patients with additional risk factors. The focus of this article, oral anticoagulation (OAC) therapy, reduces the risk of stroke. However, it is usually initiated after AF is documented on an electrocardiogram or after an ischemic event occurs.

Cardiovascular disease accounts for 41% of all-cause mortality in end-stage renal disease (ESRD), with sudden cardiac death (SCD) accounting for two-thirds of these patients. Although implantable cardioverter-defibrillators (ICDs) prevent SCD, little is known about their efficacy in ESRD because such patients have been excluded from major randomized controlled trials (RCTs). Some small, single-center retrospective analyses suggest that ESRD patients may not benefit as much as normal renal function patients whereas other studies suggest the opposite. Given the gaps in our understanding of SCD in ESRD and the clinical equipoise regarding ICD efficacy, an RCT is the next logical step.

Implantable cardioverter defibrillators (ICDs) have been firmly established as the treatment of choice in patients at high risk of sudden cardiac death. However, a majority of patients will invariably develop recurrent ventricular arrhythmia and receive shocks at some point after ICD implantation. Ventricular arrhythmia and ICD therapy are poor prognostic markers in such patients, and are associated with an increased risk of mortality and morbidity. Antiarrhythmic drug (AAD) therapy should be initiated in patients with ventricular arrhythmia and ICD shocks. Amiodarone is the most effective AAD available, with sotalol being the next best alternative.

With expanded indications for device therapy, the use of cardiovascular implantable electronic devices (CIEDs) has greatly increased over the past decade. There has been a similar increase in device complications. Clinicians increasingly are faced with the challenging choice of extraction or abandonment of sterile, superfluous CIED leads. As with any intervention, the decision to proceed with lead extraction for the management of lead malfunctions mandates a comparison of the risks of extraction with the risks of lead abandonment. Decisions regarding lead extraction must be made on an individual case-by-case basis, integrating various patient and lead characteristics and operator-related variables.

Catheter ablation of ventricular tachycardia (VT) has improved arrhythmia-free survival in patients with multiple VT episodes refractory to antiarrhythmic drugs. Recent studies have evaluated the role of early intervention with catheter ablation in patients experiencing a single episode of life-threatening ventricular arrhythmias and undergoing secondary prevention defibrillator implantation. Such "primary VT ablation" strategy has proven effective in reducing the VT recurrence rate compared with standard medical therapy (no antiarrhythmic drug). This article summarizes the evidence on primary VT ablation and discusses its clinical indications and outcomes compared with standard catheter ablation of drug-refractory recurrent VT (ie, secondary VT ablation).

Ablation data are currently limited to a small, select population of patients with refractory ventricular fibrillation (VF) storm with medium duration of follow-up. It might be too early to recommend against the implantation of implantable cardioverter-defibrillators in patients with successfully ablated medically refractory index VF storm. Further study is needed to define the role of ablation in cases that are not medically refractory.

# Cardiac Electrophysiology Clinics

## ACCESS THE CLINICS ONLINE!

Available at:
**www.theclinics.com**

# Foreword
# On the Front Lines

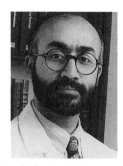
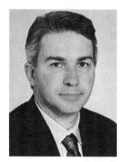

Ranjan K. Thakur, MD, MPH, MBA, FHRS     Andrea Natale, MD, FHRS

*Consulting Editors*

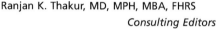

*It is better to debate a question without settling it than to settle a question without debating it.*
> —From Joseph Joubert, French moralist and essayist, 1754–1824

Debates and controversies clarify and spur human understanding and are the essential fuel for scientific progress. So, it is fitting to mark the second anniversary of the *Cardiac Electrophysiology Clinics* with an issue devoted to Contemporary Debates and Controversies. In fact, because of the myriad contemporary issues worthy of discussion, this issue of the *Clinics* focuses on some of the contemporary controversies around device therapy for ventricular arrhythmias and the June 2012 issue will highlight issues surrounding ablative therapy.

The implantable cardioverter defibrillator (ICD) was FDA approved over a quarter century ago, in 1985. Understanding defibrillation and proving the utility of the ICD for preventing sudden cardiac death (SCD) for various arrhythmic substrates were the focus of some of the initial research efforts. In the intervening years, we have also witnessed the development of cardiac resynchronization therapy (CRT) for refractory heart failure. While many landmark studies have established the utility of these therapies, many new questions have arisen. We have selected a few of these to highlight in the present issue of the *Clinics*. Some examples include the following:

- The survival advantage of ICDs over conventional therapy seen in randomized clinical trials is usually not seen in the community once the devices become widely utilized for the given indication. The first article by Nair and colleagues explores this issue in depth.
- ICD registries have collected enormous amounts of data on implant indication, timing, complications, etc. We are beginning to see new research from these data that will impact device therapy in the coming decades. Dr Hammill has outlined the important lessons we have learned from registries and additional insights we may gain by examining these data further.
- Cardiac electrophysiology has grown in leaps and bounds over the last four decades. This success has been due to and has fueled further development of therapies that have enhanced the duration and quality of patients' lives. As we push these boundaries, we must critically examine which patients benefit the most from these expensive interventions. Drs Kramer and Josephson point out some cautionary notes as we expand CRT indications to patients

Card Electrophysiol Clin 3 (2011) xiii–xiv
doi:10.1016/j.ccep.2011.09.001
1877-9182/11/$ – see front matter

cardiacEP.theclinics.com

with narrower QRS complexes as well as to disease states, such as patients with end-stage renal disease, where the efficacy of ICD and CRT devices is unproven.

- While the primary prevention strategy clearly works, cost pressures on health care systems demands a higher yield of appropriate ICD discharges while at the same time reducing inappropriate therapies. To shed light on this, Dr Dello Russo and colleagues report on the utility of scar mapping as a risk-stratifying tool to identify truly high-risk patients for SCD, thereby making ICD therapy more cost-effective.

These examples illustrate some of the contemporary issues that our field is grappling with. The reader will get a better idea by examining the full table of contents. We endeavored to select topics that are germane to today's practice and contributors who are thought leaders in the respective areas. We have learned much from our contributors and we hope that the readership will also benefit from their wisdom in these pages.

Ranjan K. Thakur, MD, MPH, MBA, FHRS
Thoracic and Cardiovascular Institute
405 West Greenlawn, Suite 400
Lansing, MI 48910, USA

Andrea Natale, MD, FHRS
Texas Cardiac Arrhythmia Institute
Center for Atrial Fibrillation at
St. David's Medical Center
1015 East 32nd Street, Suite 516
Austin, TX 78705, USA

E-mail addresses:
Thakur@msu.edu (R.K. Thakur)
Andrea.natale@stdavids.com (A. Natale)

# Why Are Implantable Cardioverter Defibrillator Outcomes in Practice Different from Clinical Trials?

Krishnakumar Nair, MD[a], Jack V. Tu, MD, PhD[b,c],
Douglas S. Lee, MD, PhD[c,*]

## KEYWORDS

- Implantable defibrillators • Registry • Trials
- Population-based studies

The risk of sudden cardiac death (SCD) is increased after myocardial infarction (MI), especially in patients with left ventricular ejection fraction (LVEF) less than or equal to 35%.[1–3] The mortality benefit of implantable cardioverter defibrillators (ICDs) in SCD has been shown in randomized primary and secondary prevention trials.[4–9] Reduced LVEF is also an important risk parameter that predicts both all-cause mortality and sudden arrhythmic death.[10,11] ICD therapy led to a 31% reduction of all-cause mortality in patients with LVEF less than or equal to 30% and remote MI in the landmark Multicenter Automatic Defibrillator Implantation Trial II (MADIT-II).[7] The Sudden Cardiac Death in Heart Failure Trial (SCD-HeFT) gave additional support to these findings in patients with heart failure with ischemic or non-ischemic cardiomyopathy and with LVEF less than or equal to 35%.[9,10]

As with most other conditions, information about the real-world use and effectiveness of implantable defibrillators can be obtained only from registries. Clinical registries and randomized controlled trials have congruent populations; however, they can differ substantially in many other aspects including device indications, access, and outcomes after ICD implantation.

## SIMILARITIES AND DIFFERENCES BETWEEN RANDOMIZED TRIAL AND REGISTRY POPULATIONS
### Coherence Between Trial and Registry Populations

It is often desired to compare patients who are enrolled into randomized controlled trials with real-world populations to determine how well the

Disclosure: The Institute for Clinical Evaluative Sciences (ICES) is supported in part by a grant from the Ontario Ministry of Health and Long-Term Care. The opinions, results, and conclusions are those of the authors and no endorsement by the Ministry of Health and Long-Term Care or by the ICES is intended or should be inferred. This work was supported by operating grant no. MOP 111150 from the Canadian Institutes of Health Research. Dr Tu is supported by a Canada Research Chair in Health Services Research and is a career investigator of the Heart and Stroke Foundation. Dr Lee is supported by a clinician-scientist award from the Canadian Institutes of Health Research. The authors have nothing else to disclose.

[a] Peter Munk Cardiac Centre and the Division of Cardiology, University Health Network, University of Toronto, 200 Elizabeth Street, Gerrard Wing, Toronto, ON M5G 2C4, Canada
[b] Division of Cardiology, Schulich Heart Centre, Sunnybrook Health Sciences Centre, University of Toronto, 2075 Bayview Avenue, Toronto, ON M4N 3M5, Canada
[c] Institute for Clinical Evaluative Sciences, Room G-106, 2075 Bayview Avenue, Toronto, ON M4N 3M5, Canada
* Corresponding author.
E-mail address: dlee@ices.on.ca

Card Electrophysiol Clin 3 (2011) 511–520
doi:10.1016/j.ccep.2011.07.002
1877-9182/11/$ – see front matter © 2011 Elsevier Inc. All rights reserved.

former reflect patients with the disease or condition in the population. Coherence has been documented among patients with ICDs enrolled in registries and those who have been recruited into randomized trials.[12] In the European Survey to Evaluate Arrhythmia Rate in So-Called High-Risk Myocardial Infarction (SEARCH-MI) registry, Santini and colleagues[12] reported that "routine clinical practice in European patients can replicate the results of therapeutic interventions observed in more selected MADIT-II trial populations." At 1 year, 21% of patients in the registry had an arrhythmic event appropriately terminated, compared with 17% of patients from the MADIT-II study. At 2 years, the results were similar, with 31% of SEARCH-MI patients and 27% of the MADIT-II patients having had an arrhythmic event terminated by the ICD. Overall mortality or SCD were comparable at 1 and 2 years. However, the parallels between registries and trials are dependent on several factors including physician, patient, and health system factors as well as the diffusion of technology with time.

### Population-Based Studies of ICD Recipients and How They Differ From Randomized Controlled Trial Populations

Randomized clinical trials often have highly selected patients in comparison with community studies, and therefore interventions may have attenuated effects in population-based studies,[13] as has been reported from studies of community-based patients with heart failure and MI.[14] These differences have been attributed, in part, to differences in age and comorbidity burden, because the elderly and those with noncardiac comorbidities are often excluded from randomized trials.[15]

### EXAMPLES OF REGISTRIES
#### US National ICD Registry

The Center for Medicare and Medicaid Services (CMS) selected the National ICD Registry[16] as the sole repository for ICD implantation data for Medicare beneficiaries in 2006.[17–20] The registry was developed through a partnership of the Heart Rhythm Society (HRS; www.HRSonline.org) and the American College of Cardiology Foundation (ACCF; ww.acc.org) using the expertise of the National Cardiovascular Data Registry (NCDR; www.accncdr.com).

#### Ontario ICD Registry

The Ontario ICD Database is a prospective registry of all patients who are referred for consideration of an ICD to a cardiac electrophysiologist.[21] The Ontario Ministry of Health and Long-Term Care has mandated that all recipients of ICDs in Ontario, Canada, must have their data entered into the database, and therefore this registry captures all patients undergoing this procedure on a province-wide level. The study population of the Ontario ICD Database includes all patients aged 18 years or older who are referred for consideration of an ICD implant to a hospital in Ontario where defibrillators are implanted. The registry is broadly inclusive of patients who are referred for primary or secondary prevention indications, and all types of underlying cardiac conditions are included.

### EXAMINATION OF COMPLICATIONS
#### US National ICD Registry

The Yale Center for Outcomes Research and Evaluation has worked with HRS, ACCF, and the NCDR under contract with the Center for Medicare and Medicaid Services (CMS) to develop a performance measure for ICD complications using the US National ICD Registry for the initial clinical data to allow risk adjustment and Medicare claims data for 30-day and 90-day adverse events. The adverse events include[16]:

- Pneumothorax or hemothorax requiring a chest tube within 30 days
- Hematoma requiring transfusion or surgical evacuation within 30 days
- Pericardial tamponade or pericardiocentesis within 30 days
- Mechanical complications with system or lead revision within 90 days
- Device-related infection within 90 days
- ICD replacement within 90 days
- Death within 30 days.

Initial analysis using this performance measure identified the median complication rate for hospitals as 7% with the lowest decile being 4% and the highest decile 13%.[16] This wide range of complications provides an opportunity for improvement by moving hospitals with the highest rate of complications closer to the median and moving the median closer to the lowest decile group.[16] The average age of patients was 68 years with 74% men and 83% white. The average LVEF was 29% and 82% were New York Heart Association (NYHA) class II to III. Complications at the time of device implantation and before hospital discharge for new implants (replacement procedures excluded) occurred in 3.2% and included procedure-related, in-laboratory death (0.02%), hematoma (0.89%), and lead dislodgement (1.05%). The NCDR ICD Registry has reported in-hospital complication rates of 1.3% for major complications and 3.6% for any complication, although reporting was not mandatory from all hospitals and lead complications were not included.[22]

### Ontario ICD Database

Investigators of the Ontario ICD Database studied predictors of procedural complications among 3340 patients (mean age 63.8 ± 12.5 years, 78.5% men).[23] Major complications occurred in 4.1% of de novo procedures. Complications after de novo defibrillator implantation were strongly associated with device type. Compared with those undergoing a single-chamber device, implantation of a cardiac resynchronization defibrillator (adjusted hazard ratio [HR] 2.17, 95% confidence interval [CI] 1.38–3.43, $P<.001$) or dual-chamber device (adjusted HR 1.82, 95% CI 1.19–2.79, $P = .006$) was associated with increased risk of major complications. Major complications were increased in women (adjusted HR 1.49, 95% CI 1.02–2.16, $P = .037$) and when left ventricular end-systolic dimension exceeded 45 mm (adjusted HR 1.54, 95% CI 1.08–2.20, $P = .018$). Major complications (excluding death) occurring early after defibrillator implantation were associated with increased adjusted risk of subsequent death up to 180 days after defibrillator implant (adjusted HR 3.70, 95% CI 1.64–8.33, $P = .002$). Direct implant-related (surgical) complications were associated with increased risk of early death with an adjusted HR of 24.89 ($P = .01$). Indirect (underlying disease-related) clinical complications also conferred an increased risk of near-term death with an adjusted HR of 12.35 ($P = .001$) after defibrillator implantation.

Krahn and colleagues[24] studied predictors of short-term complications after ICD replacement from the Ontario ICD Database. In 1081 patients undergoing ICD replacement, 47 patients (4.3%) experienced 88 complications within 45 days, with 47 major complications occurring in 28 patients (2.6%). The most common complications included infection (n = 23), lead revision (n = 35), electrical storm (n = 14), and pulmonary edema (n = 13). Risk factors associated with complications after ICD replacement included the presence of angina, antiarrhythmic therapy, increased number of previous procedures, and low implanter volume. Major complications were also associated with increased risk of subsequent mortality.

### Other Registries

The importance of lead-related complications has been highlighted in several other ICD registries. Pocket hematoma, chronic pain, and lead and device dislodgements leading to operative revisions and reoperation in 3.0% were the most common complications in a voluntary German ICD Registry of new implants.[25] Another study reported that lead-related and pocket-related complications occurred in 2.1% and 1.8%, respectively.[26] The prospective REPLACE registry reported that ICDs and particularly cardiac resynchronization therapy (CRT) ICDs were associated with a greater risk of complications. The registry reported a 4.0% complication rate in 1031 patients undergoing generator replacement, and a higher rate of 15.3% in 713 patients with both generator replacement and a lead addition.[27]

In ICD replacements for advisory indications reported by the Canadian Heart Rhythm Society, the overall complication rate in a retrospective series of 533 ICD replacements was higher than expected at 8.1%,[28] with major complications (including death) occurring in 2.0% of patients. Subsequent analysis showed that the number of previous pocket procedures and combined operators (consultant and trainee) were risk factors associated with this high complication rate.[29]

### Procedural Volume and Complications

Freeman and colleagues[30] examined initial ICD implantations between January 2006 and December 2008 at hospitals participating in the NCDR ICD Registry and reported that the rate of adverse events declined progressively with increasing procedure volume ($P$ trend <.0001). This relationship remained significant ($P$ trend <.0001) after adjustment for patient, operator, and hospital characteristics. The volume-outcome relationship was evident for all ICD subtypes, including single-chamber ($P$ trend = .004), dual-chamber ($P$ trend <.0001), and biventricular ICDs ($P$ trend = .02). Hospitals in the lowest volume quartile had 26% higher odds of any adverse event than the highest volume hospitals. This effect of higher procedure volume on lower adverse events was confirmed in other studies including that of Al-Khatib and colleagues,[31] who examined mechanical complications and infections after ICD implantation in Medicare beneficiaries.

## REGISTRIES EXAMINING ACCESSIBILITY AND PATTERNS OF ICD CARE DELIVERY
### Why are Evaluations of Access and Patterns of Care Important?

Translation of evidence from landmark randomized trials is often reflected in practice guidelines.[7,32–34] However, translation of new knowledge into real-world practice is influenced by several factors and entails several intermediate steps. Variations in ICD implantation rates are likely complex and multifactorial. Although there were few differences between the ACC/AHA/HRS[35] and ESC/EHRA[36] updates to the 2006 common European and American guidelines,[37] there were significant disparities in implantation rates both within Europe and in intercontinental comparisons.

Potential explanations for these disparities include differences in the number of implanting centers and implanting electrophysiologists per capita, physicians' lack of awareness about evidence for ICDs, and reimbursement resource constraints in many countries. The use of ICDs is likely further influenced by the high cost of these devices and barriers to access including organizational and cultural factors.[38–40] However, the factors that explain the wide geographic heterogeneity in device implant rates have not been definitively identified.[38,41]

## Accessibility and Patterns of ICD Care

### Variations in ICD access by geography

i) Regional variation in the national cardiovascular data registry. The indications and rates of ICD implantation may vary depending on the sex, race, hospital,[42–44] and geographic region. This information on variations in use is critical for planning and can be provided by registry data. Variations in ICD care have been shown even in well-resourced regions. In the Get With The Guidelines registry, implantation rates of ICDs varied markedly with some hospitals implanting ICDs in 80% of eligible patients, whereas other hospitals did not implant any ICDs in any eligible patient.[42] A cross-sectional analysis[45] among the Medicare, fee-for-service population from the National Cardiovascular Data Registry showed substantial variation in the rate ratios of ICD implantation, ranging from 0.39 to 1.77 (compared with the national average of 1.0). This ratio was not explained by the supply of cardiologists, electrophysiologists, or by the proportion of patients meeting trial inclusion criteria. The investigators concluded that marked geographic variation (greater than fourfold) in the use of primary prevention ICDs existed across the United States, and that it was not correlated with physician supply, disease prevalence, or rural-urban differences.[45]

ii) Barriers in access to ICD care. Although no official statistics are reported in Europe, the similar cardiovascular risk profile and cardiovascular mortality of Western Europeans and North Americans may suggest that SCD prevalence and risk should also be similar.[46] An analysis conducted in 2005[46] found that a minority of patients (8%) meeting criteria for ICDs underwent the procedure. A potentially important reason for the major differences in ICD

use between continents is that Europe, on a per capita basis, has a far smaller number of implanting centers and electrophysiologists.

Udell and colleagues[47] conducted a population-based retrospective cohort study examining the province of Ontario, Canada. Patients were eligible if they had been previously hospitalized for heart failure or an acute coronary syndrome within 5 years. Exclusion criteria included an existing ICD or prior cardiac arrest. Of 48,426 patients, 440 received an ICD, with a gradual 30-fold increase in implantation rates in the study period (0.12%–3.9%). ICD recipients were more likely to be men (odds ratio [OR] 4.14, 95% CI 3.24–5.30), were younger than 75 years of age (OR 3.19, 95% CI 2.57–3.96), were residents of a metropolitan area (OR 1.42, 95% CI 1.04–1.90), and were of higher socioeconomic status (OR 1.32, 95% CI 1.08–1.61). Thus, there were geographic and sociodemographic access barriers to ICD implantation.

In a Web-based registry[38] in Emilia-Romagna, an Italian region with approximately 4.3 million inhabitants, data from all consecutive patients resident in the 9 provinces in this region who underwent first implant of an ICD or a biventricular ICD between January 2006 and December 2008 were collected. Within the province, ICD implantation rates were approximately twofold higher than the region with the lowest rate, despite similar access to health care and geographic similarity. A national survey of ICD implants conducted in the United Kingdom from 1998 to 2002[48] reported a more than fourfold ratio in ICD implant rates when the regions with the highest and lowest implant rates were compared. Although these differences were initially attributed to differential strategies for screening and referral, subsequent evaluations continued to show disparities in ICD access even after accounting for indication, variations in service provision, and socioeconomic deprivation.[49] Additional barriers to ICD access may also include variability in how guidelines are applied in clinical practice, differential allocation of financial resources, and absence of a common strategy for sudden death prevention. Other factors may also be identified in the future.[41,50]

### Variations in access by hospital

A large United States registry of hospitalized patients with heart failure found that the proportion of patients implanted with, or planned for ICD implantation was only 20% of eligible patients, ranging from 0% to 80%.[42] At the hospital level, the variability in ICD use in eligible patients was substantial, with a 35-fold variation between the hospitals with the highest and lowest implant rates.[42] A prominent factor associated with hospital-level variation may relate to the ability to implant electrical devices, as well as the distribution of age, sex, ethnicity, and insurance status of its patients.[42,50]

In a registry from a regional center in the United Kingdom, Scott and colleagues[51] found that implantation rates of ICDs and CRT devices was higher at hospitals with device specialists among the staff members, and higher in centers that were able to perform device implantation. Greater variations, up to threefold higher, were found when only ICDs implanted for primary prevention in patients with coronary artery disease were examined.

### Variations in access by patient characteristics

Several studies have provided evidence suggesting that sex and race are also important factors in the implantation of ICDs, with women and African Americans having lower rates of implantation.[43,44,47,52,53] MacFadden and colleagues[54] examined sex disparities and sex-specific trends in ICD implantation according to indication in patients with cardiac arrest (1998–2007) in Ontario, Canada. Among 9246 eligible secondary prevention patients (age 66.3 ± 14.3 years; 3577 women [39%]) with cardiac arrest, men were more likely to undergo ICD implantation, with an HR adjusted for age, comorbidity, and arrhythmia of 1.92 (95% CI 1.66–2.23). Among 105,516 patients with MI (age 68.3 ± 12.7 years; 42,987 women [41%]), men were 3 times more likely to undergo ICD implantation, with an adjusted HR of 3.00 (95% CI 2.53–3.55). Among 61,160 patients with heart failure (age 76.2 ± 12.0 years; 31,575 women [52%]), ICD implantation was more likely in men, with an adjusted HR of 3.01 (95% CI 2.59–3.50). Although it has been believed that the later age at presentation with cardiac disease in women, the greater burden of comorbidities with increasing age, and sex differences in LVEF may be contributing factors, these influences did not explain the differences in ICD implantation between men and women.[43,53]

The odds of ICD implant for secondary prevention increased with time by 21% (95% CI 13%–30%) in women and by 6% (95% CI 2%–11%) in men, but rates of ICD use in men for primary prevention indications remained persistently higher. Although sex differences in secondary prevention are declining with time, disparities in primary prevention persist.

### MONITORING QUALITY AND APPROPRIATENESS OF ICD CARE

Registries can provide complementary information on the quality and appropriateness of care related to ICD implantation. Thus, patients who could be implanted with a device and have evidence to support such an intervention but were not implanted may be identified. Conversely, patients who did not meet criteria for an ICD according to evidentiary standards, but did undergo device implantation, may also be identified. The former may die of SCD that may have been prevented by ICD implantation, whereas the latter may experience complications, unnecessary procedures, and inappropriate shocks, which may impair quality of life. Both of these aspects of care are of importance to patients and to the health care system, and greater efforts to redirect care to those who may benefit from ICDs would optimize outcomes.

### Further Opportunities to Reduce the Occurrence of SCD in Potential Patients at Risk

The Prevention of Sudden Cardiac Death (PreSCD II) registry showed that many patients with guideline-based ICD indications did not undergo defibrillator implantation.[55] This registry included a large cohort of post-MI patients who were predominantly referred to cardiac rehabilitation centers within 4 to 8 weeks after an acute MI (9512 patients) and an additional 1100 patients (10.7% of the total patient cohort) who were admitted for inpatient cardiac rehabilitation and whose index MI occurred more than 1 year before cardiac rehabilitation. In the PreSCD II registry, ICD implantation occurred in 47% of all patients within 1 year after myocardial infarction, whereas 68% of patients received their ICD more than 6 months after their MI.[55] Hence, in this registry, ICD implantations occurred in a wide range of post-MI-to-ICD implantation times, covering a range that extended from that of the Immediate Risk Stratification Improves Survival (IRIS) trial,[56] Defibrillator in Acute Myocardial Infarction Trial (DINAMIT),[8] and the MADIT-II[7] studies. Most patients in PreSCD II were enrolled later in their post-MI course than the DINAMIT or IRIS trials, but earlier than the MADIT-II trial, in which only 12% of the patients were recruited within the first 6 months after their myocardial infarction.

In PreSCD II, patients who received an ICD had an adjusted 44% lower mortality (HR 0.56, 95% CI 0.32–1.01; $P$ = .053) than comparable patients without ICD therapy. All-cause mortality was significantly reduced only when the ICD was implanted late (more than 11 months) after MI ($P<.001$). Only 9.7% of patients after MI in this registry had an ejection fraction of less than 40%. This finding is relevant in the era of primary PCI for acute MI, where it has been observed that less than 5% of patients have an LVEF less than 30%.[57,58]

### Non–Evidence-Based ICD Implantations

Survival benefit from ICD therapy could not be shown in patients recovering from an acute MI and in patients who received an ICD at the time of coronary artery bypass graft surgery.[8,56,59] The 2006[37] and 2008[35] practice guidelines for ICD therapy mandate at least a 40-day period following an MI before an ICD is implanted for a primary prevention indication. These guidelines also emphasize that ICD therapy is not indicated for patients with NYHA class IV symptoms, who are not candidates for cardiac resynchronization therapy. These guidelines specify that recommendations for primary prevention ICDs apply only to patients whose LVEF is low despite receiving optimal medical therapy and imply that ICD therapy is not recommended for patients with a new diagnosis of heart failure.[35,37] The degree to which physicians in routine clinical practice follow these evidence-based recommendations is not clear from trials and requires registry data to assess.

After examining data submitted to the NCDR ICD Registry between January 1, 2006, and June 30, 2009, Al-Khatib and colleagues[60] found that 22.5% of implanted ICDs were non–evidence-based (ie, patients who were either excluded from the major primary prevention clinical trials of ICD therapy or shown not to benefit from an ICD in other studies). These patients who received a non–evidence-based ICD were classified into 4 subgroups: (1) ICD implantation within 40 days of an acute MI, (2) within 3 months of coronary artery bypass graft surgery, (3) recent diagnosis of congestive heart failure, and (4) presence of NYHA class IV symptoms. Patients who received a non–evidence-based ICD were significantly older, had more comorbid disease in the form of heart failure, atrial fibrillation or flutter, ischemic heart disease, cerebrovascular disease, chronic lung disease, diabetes, and end-stage renal disease. They were also at higher risk of postprocedural complications and worse intermediate and long-term outcomes including death. It was estimated that 1 excess complication occurred for every 121 non–evidence-based ICD implantations.

In the subgroup of patients with NYHA class IV symptoms, patients were more likely to have non-ischemic dilated cardiomyopathy than ischemic cardiomyopathy. Adjusting for potential confounders, the occurrence of any adverse event and death was significantly higher in patients who received a non–evidence-based device (P<.001).

There was a nonsignificantly increased risk of hematoma in the non–evidence-based ICD group (P = .07), and the median length of hospital stay was significantly longer for patients who received a non–evidence-based ICD compared with patients who received an evidence-based ICD (3 days vs 1 day; P<.001). When the analyses were repeated after excluding patients with NYHA class IV symptoms, the rates of any postprocedure complication, death, and hematoma were significantly higher in patients who received a non–evidence-based ICD.

There was significant variation in the distribution of non–evidence-based ICD implants across sites, with no clustering of such implants by site. The rate of non–evidence-based ICD implants was 20.8% for electrophysiologists (95% CI 20.5%, 21.1%), and this was significantly lower than the rate for nonelectrophysiologists. The rates of non–evidence-based ICD implants were 24.8% (95% CI 24.2%, 25.3%) for nonelectrophysiologist cardiologists, 36.1% (95% CI 34.3%, 38.0%) for thoracic surgeons, and 24.9% (95% CI 23.8%, 25.9%) for other specialties (P<.001 for all comparisons). Another study from the ICD Registry suggested better outcomes when ICDs are implanted by physicians who have had extensive training in electrophysiology.[61] In this study,[61] board-certified electrophysiologists or those who had undergone electrophysiology training had lower complication rates from ICD implantation than other physician groups. Taken together, these 2 studies suggest that intensive training may improve the preoperative evaluation of patients, as well as the operative and immediate postoperative care of patients undergoing ICD implantation. Potential reasons for these subspecialty effects include better knowledge of the data on primary prevention ICDs on the part of electrophysiologists, and their commitment to adhere to practice guidelines.

### Caveats of Assessing Appropriateness from ICD Registries

There are several caveats for the assessment of appropriateness of defibrillator care from large ICD registries. The first is rigorous attention to data quality for some important emerging variables in particular. Although the NCDR ICD Registry was a well-audited tool with robust data and a large number of patients,[62] the accuracy of the onset of heart failure has been questioned, which is particularly cogent because the largest group of patients who received non–evidence-based ICDs in the report by Al-Khatib and colleagues[60] were those with a recent diagnosis of congestive heart failure. Secondly, care provided by an electrophysiologist was an important marker of care quality. However, more physicians self-reported that they were board-certified electrophysiologists in the ICD Registry than have been board certified.[62]

Although registries provide useful clinical data, it may be unreasonable to expect that all ICD implants should be appropriate based on retrospective review of a large dataset. Only a small number of sites in the NCDR ICD Registry had a non–evidence-based ICD implantation rate of less than 6%, suggesting that this threshold might be a reasonable lower bound. Further data are needed to determine the acceptable upper bounds for non–evidence-based ICD implants. Although cardiac electrophysiologists were found to have a rate of 21%, the target should be less than this threshold. As registries continue to monitor metrics, such as those discussed earlier, attention to data quality and accuracy will become even more important.

## SUMMARY

Studies on evidence-based therapies[63] suggest that the barriers to device therapy are complex.[39] Registry data focusing on the number of potentially eligible patients in the real world[64] as well as on actual implant rates[42,50,51,63] are useful for assessing the appropriateness of ICD use and for assessing the effectiveness of guideline implementation. Although there is some coherence between trial and registry data, the availability of registries allows for examination of an array of potential outcomes that cannot be examined in randomized trials. Registry data give operators and auditors access to real-world complication rates, with some registries revealing unexpectedly high complication rates. Risk factors for complications after procedures, such as procedural volume and type of device implanted, have become clear through registries.

Heterogeneity in ICD implant rates is multifactorial and may be related to geography, patient characteristics, provider-related variability, temporal effects, and variations in access related to care networks and barriers to referral.[38] Registries can also identify patients who needed a device but did not undergo the procedure, and conversely they can also identify patients who were inappropriately implanted with a device. It is increasingly important to assess hospital performance and to provide feedback to hospitals about their outcomes and compliance with clinical guideline recommendations. Providing such feedback to

hospitals has the potential to improve adherence to practice guidelines and eventually patient outcomes. Ultimately, data from registries provide physicians with feedback from audits, and provide health authorities with information needed to generate and refine health care policies related to ICD implantation. In the future, registries that examine longitudinal outcomes may also provide useful information on risk stratification, to better determine patient risks and potentially improve patient selection for ICDs.

## REFERENCES

1. Huikuri HV, Tapanainen JM, Lindgren K, et al. Prediction of sudden cardiac death after myocardial infarction in the beta-blocking era. J Am Coll Cardiol 2003;42:652–8.
2. Yap YG, Duong T, Bland M, et al. Temporal trends on the risk of arrhythmic vs non-arrhythmic deaths in high-risk patients after myocardial infarction: a combined analysis from multicentre trials. Eur Heart J 2005;26:1385–93.
3. Solomon SD, Zelenkofske S, McMurray JJ, et al. Sudden death in patients with myocardial infarction and left ventricular dysfunction, heart failure, or both. N Engl J Med 2005;352:2581–8.
4. A comparison of antiarrhythmic-drug therapy with implantable defibrillators in patients resuscitated from near-fatal ventricular arrhythmias. The Antiarrhythmics Versus Implantable Defibrillators (AVID) investigators. N Engl J Med 1997;337:1576–83.
5. Kuck KH, Cappato R, Siebels J, et al. Randomized comparison of antiarrhythmic drug therapy with implantable defibrillators in patients resuscitated from cardiac arrest: the Cardiac Arrest Study Hamburg (CASH). Circulation 2000;102:748–54.
6. Buxton AE, Lee KL, Fisher JD, et al. A randomized study of the prevention of sudden death in patients with coronary artery disease. Multicenter Unsustained Tachycardia Trial investigators. N Engl J Med 1999;341:1882–90.
7. Moss AJ, Zareba W, Hall WJ, et al. Prophylactic implantation of a defibrillator in patients with myocardial infarction and reduced ejection fraction. N Engl J Med 2002;346:877–83.
8. Hohnloser SH, Kuck KH, Dorian P, et al. Prophylactic use of an implantable cardioverter-defibrillator after acute myocardial infarction. N Engl J Med 2004;351:2481–8.
9. Bardy GH, Lee KL, Mark DB, et al. Amiodarone or an implantable cardioverter-defibrillator for congestive heart failure. N Engl J Med 2005;352:225–37.
10. Myerburg RJ. Implantable cardioverter-defibrillators after myocardial infarction. N Engl J Med 2008;359:2245–53.

11. Moss AJ. Implantable cardioverter defibrillator therapy: the sickest patients benefit the most. Circulation 2000;101:1638–40.

12. Santini M, Russo M, Botto G, et al. Clinical and arrhythmic outcomes after implantation of a defibrillator for primary prevention of sudden death in patients with post-myocardial infarction cardiomyopathy: the survey to evaluate arrhythmia rate in high-risk MI patients (SEARCH-MI). Europace 2009;11:476–82.

13. Lee DS, Tu JV, Austin PC, et al. Effect of cardiac and noncardiac conditions on survival after defibrillator implantation. J Am Coll Cardiol 2007;49:2408–15.

14. Braunstein JB, Anderson GF, Gerstenblith G, et al. Noncardiac comorbidity increases preventable hospitalizations and mortality among Medicare beneficiaries with chronic heart failure. J Am Coll Cardiol 2003;42:1226–33.

15. Jong P, Vowinckel E, Liu PP, et al. Prognosis and determinants of survival in patients newly hospitalized for heart failure: a population-based study. Arch Intern Med 2002;162:1689–94.

16. Hammill SC, Kremers MS, Stevenson LW, et al. Review of the registry's fourth year, incorporating lead data and pediatric ICD procedures, and use as a national performance measure. Heart Rhythm 2010;7:1340–5.

17. Hammill S, Phurrough S, Brindis R. The national nistry: now and into the future. Heart Rhythm 2006;3: 470–3.

18. Hammill SC, Stevenson LW, Kadish AH, et al. Review of the registry's first year, data collected, and future plans. Heart Rhythm 2007;4:1260–3.

19. Hammill SC, Kremers MS, Kadish AH, et al. Review of the ICD Registry's third year, expansion to include lead data and pediatric ICD procedures, and role for measuring performance. Heart Rhythm 2009;6: 1397–401.

20. Hammill SC, Kremers MS, Stevenson LW, et al. Review of the registry's second year, data collected, and plans to add lead and pediatric ICD procedures. Heart Rhythm 2008;5:1359–63.

21. Lee DS, Birnie D, Cameron D, et al. Design and implementation of a population-based registry of implantable cardioverter defibrillators (ICDs) in Ontario. Heart Rhythm 2008;5:1250–6.

22. Peterson PN, Daugherty SL, Wang Y, et al. Gender differences in procedure-related adverse events in patients receiving implantable cardioverter-defibrillator therapy. Circulation 2009;119:1078–84.

23. Lee DS, Krahn AD, Healey JS, et al. Evaluation of early complications related to de novo cardioverter defibrillator implantation insights from the Ontario ICD Database. J Am Coll Cardiol 2010;55:774–82.

24. Krahn AD, Lee DS, Birnie D, et al. Predictors of short term complications after ICD replacement: results from the Ontario ICD Database. Circ Arrhythm Electrophysiol 2011;4(2):136–42.

25. Gradaus R, Block M, Brachmann J, et al. Mortality, morbidity, and complications in 3344 patients with implantable cardioverter defibrillators: results from the German ICD registry EURID. Pacing Clin Electrophysiol 2003;26:1511–8.

26. Gold MR, Peters RW, Johnson JW, et al. Complications associated with pectoral cardioverter-defibrillator implantation: comparison of subcutaneous and submuscular approaches. Worldwide Jewel investigators. J Am Coll Cardiol 1996;28:1278–82.

27. Poole JE, Gleva MJ, Mela T, et al. Complication rates associated with pacemaker or implantable cardioverter-defibrillator generator replacements and upgrade procedures: results from the REPLACE registry. Circulation 2010;122:1553–61.

28. Gould PA, Krahn AD. Complications associated with implantable cardioverter-defibrillator replacement in response to device advisories. JAMA 2006;295: 1907–11.

29. Gould PA, Gula LJ, Champagne J, et al. Outcome of advisory implantable cardioverter-defibrillator replacement: one-year follow-up. Heart Rhythm 2008;5:1675–81.

30. Freeman JV, Wang Y, Curtis JP, et al. The relation between hospital procedure volume and complications of cardioverter-defibrillator implantation from the implantable cardioverter-defibrillator registry. J Am Coll Cardiol 2010;56:1133–9.

31. Al-Khatib SM, Lucas FL, Jollis JG, et al. The relation between patients' outcomes and the volume of cardioverter-defibrillator implantation procedures performed by physicians treating Medicare beneficiaries. J Am Coll Cardiol 2005;46:1536–40.

32. Chrysostomakis SI, Vardas PE. 'Shocking' discrepancies. Europace 2010;12:1055–6.

33. Kadish A, Dyer A, Daubert JP, et al. Prophylactic defibrillator implantation in patients with nonischemic dilated cardiomyopathy. N Engl J Med 2004; 350:2151–8.

34. Mark DB, Nelson CL, Anstrom KJ, et al. Cost-effectiveness of defibrillator therapy or amiodarone in chronic stable heart failure: results from the sudden cardiac death in heart failure trial (SCD-HEFT). Circulation 2006;114:135–42.

35. Epstein AE, DiMarco JP, Ellenbogen KA, et al. ACC/AHA/HRS 2008 guidelines for device-based therapy of cardiac rhythm abnormalities: a report of the American College of Cardiology/American Heart Association Task Force on Practice Guidelines (Writing Committee to revise the ACC/AHA/NASPE 2002 guideline update for implantation of cardiac pacemakers and antiarrhythmia devices): developed in collaboration with the American Association for Thoracic Surgery and Society of Thoracic Surgeons. Circulation 2008;117:e350–408.

36. Vardas PE, Auricchio A, Blanc JJ, et al. Guidelines for cardiac pacing and cardiac resynchronization

therapy: the Task Force for Cardiac Pacing and Cardiac Resynchronization Therapy of the European Society of Cardiology. Developed in collaboration with the European Heart Rhythm Association. Eur Heart J 2007;28:2256–95.

37. Zipes DP, Camm AJ, Borggrefe M, et al. ACC/AHA/ESC 2006 guidelines for management of patients with ventricular arrhythmias and the prevention of sudden cardiac death: a report of the American College of Cardiology/American Heart Association Task Force and the European Society of Cardiology Committee for Practice Guidelines (writing committee to develop guidelines for management of patients with ventricular arrhythmias and the prevention of sudden cardiac death): developed in collaboration with the European Heart Rhythm Association and the Heart Rhythm Society. Circulation 2006;114:e385–484.

38. Boriani G, Berti E, Biffi M, et al. Implantable electrical devices for prevention of sudden cardiac death: data on implant rates from a 'real world' regional registry. Europace 2010;12:1224–30.

39. Al-Khatib SM, Sanders GD, Carlson M, et al. Preventing tomorrow's sudden cardiac death today: dissemination of effective therapies for sudden cardiac death prevention. Am Heart J 2008;156:613–22.

40. McHale B, Harding SA, Lever NA, et al. A national survey of clinician's knowledge of and attitudes towards implantable cardioverter defibrillators. Europace 2009;11:1313–6.

41. Greenberg SM, Epstein AE, Deering T, et al. A comparison of ICD implantations in the United States versus Italy. Pacing Clin Electrophysiol 2007;30(Suppl 1):S143–6.

42. Shah B, Hernandez AF, Liang L, et al. Hospital variation and characteristics of implantable cardioverter-defibrillator use in patients with heart failure: data from the GWTG-HF (Get With the Guidelines-Heart Failure) registry. J Am Coll Cardiol 2009;53:416–22.

43. Hernandez AF, Fonarow GC, Liang L, et al. Sex and racial differences in the use of implantable cardioverter-defibrillators among patients hospitalized with heart failure. JAMA 2007;298:1525–32.

44. Curtis LH, Al-Khatib SM, Shea AM, et al. Sex differences in the use of implantable cardioverter-defibrillators for primary and secondary prevention of sudden cardiac death. JAMA 2007;298:1517–24.

45. Matlock DD, Peterson PN, Heidenreich PA, et al. Regional variation in the use of implantable cardioverter-defibrillators for primary prevention: results from the National Cardiovascular Data Registry. Circ Cardiovasc Qual Outcomes 2011;4:114–21.

46. John Camm A, Nisam S. European utilization of the implantable defibrillator: has 10 years changed the 'enigma'? Europace 2010;12:1063–9.

47. Udell JA, Juurlink DN, Kopp A, et al. Inequitable distribution of implantable cardioverter defibrillators in Ontario. Int J Technol Assess Health Care 2007;23:354–61.

48. Cunningham AD, Plummer CJ, McComb JM, et al. The implantable cardioverter-defibrillator: postcode prescribing in the UK 1998-2002. Heart 2005;91:1280–3.

49. McComb JM, Plummer CJ, Cunningham MW, et al. Inequity of access to implantable cardioverter defibrillator therapy in England: possible causes of geographical variation in implantation rates. Europace 2009;11:1308–12.

50. Mehra MR, Yancy CW, Albert NM, et al. Evidence of clinical practice heterogeneity in the use of implantable cardioverter-defibrillators in heart failure and post-myocardial infarction left ventricular dysfunction: findings from improve HF. Heart Rhythm 2009;6:1727–34.

51. Scott PA, Turner NG, Chungh A, et al. Varying implantable cardioverter defibrillator referral patterns from implanting and non-implanting hospitals. Europace 2009;11:1048–51.

52. Gauri AJ, Davis A, Hong T, et al. Disparities in the use of primary prevention and defibrillator therapy among blacks and women. Am J Med 2006;119(167):e117–21.

53. El-Chami MF, Hanna IR, Bush H, et al. Impact of race and gender on cardiac device implantations. Heart Rhythm 2007;4:1420–6.

54. MacFadden DR, Tu JV, Chong A, et al. Evaluating sex differences in population-based utilization of implantable cardioverter-defibrillators: role of cardiac conditions and noncardiac comorbidities. Heart Rhythm 2009;6:1289–96.

55. Voller H, Kamke W, Klein HU, et al. Clinical practice of defibrillator implantation after myocardial infarction: impact of implant time: results from the PRESCD II registry. Europace 2011;13(4):499–508.

56. Steinbeck G, Andresen D, Seidl K, et al. Defibrillator implantation early after myocardial infarction. N Engl J Med 2009;361:1427–36.

57. Shiga T, Hagiwara N, Ogawa H, et al. Sudden cardiac death and left ventricular ejection fraction during long-term follow-up after acute myocardial infarction in the primary percutaneous coronary intervention era: results from the HIJAMI-II registry. Heart 2009;95:216–20.

58. Zaman S, Sivagangabalan G, Narayan A, et al. Outcomes of early risk stratification and targeted implantable cardioverter-defibrillator implantation after St-elevation myocardial infarction treated with primary percutaneous coronary intervention. Circulation 2009;120:194–200.

59. Bigger JT Jr. Prophylactic use of implanted cardiac defibrillators in patients at high risk for ventricular arrhythmias after coronary-artery bypass graft

surgery. Coronary artery bypass graft (CABG) patch trial investigators. N Engl J Med 1997;337:1569–75.

60. Al-Khatib SM, Hellkamp A, Curtis J, et al. Non-evidence-based ICD implantations in the United States. JAMA 2011;305:43–9.

61. Curtis JP, Luebbert JJ, Wang Y, et al. Association of physician certification and outcomes among patients receiving an implantable cardioverter-defibrillator. JAMA 2009;301:1661–70.

62. Kadish A, Goldberger J. Selecting patients for ICD implantation: are clinicians choosing appropriately? JAMA 2011;305:91–2.

63. Fonarow GC, Yancy CW, Albert NM, et al. Heart failure care in the outpatient cardiology practice setting: findings from improve HF. Circ Heart Fail 2008;1:98–106.

64. Israel CW. Do some implant too many defibrillators or others too few? Europace 2009;11:982–4.

# Implantable Cardioverter–Defibrillator Registries—What Have We Learned?

Stephen C. Hammill, MD[a],*, Mark S. Kremers, MD[b], Sana M. Al-Khatib, MD[c]

## KEYWORDS

- Implantable cardioverter defibrillator • Registry
- Outcomes research

*"The National ICD Registry is a milestone in the history of ICD therapy that should improve the care of patients. It is also likely to be the focal point of scrutiny of ICD outcomes, as well as physician performance and reimbursement."[1]*

Implantable cardioverter–defibrillator (ICD) coverage was expanded by the Center for Medicare and Medicaid Services (CMS) on Jan. 27, 2005, based on the results of the Sudden Cardiac Death and Heart Failure Trial (SCD-HeFT).[2–7] A requirement of expanded coverage included use of a registry to track ICD's implanted for primary prevention of sudden cardiac death in Medicare beneficiaries. CMS selected the National ICD Registry as the sole repository for ICD implantation data for Medicare beneficiaries April 1, 2006.[2–4] The registry was developed through a partnership of the Heart Rhythm Society (HRS) and American College of Cardiology Foundation (ACCF) using the expertise of the National Cardiovascular Data Registry (NCDR). The registry has made substantial progress toward several predefined goals, which will be discussed in this review [2]:

Reveal the degree to which clinicians are managing ICD therapy in accordance with evidence-based medicine

Enable clinicians to compare the in-hospital outcomes with those of other physicians

Provide insights for clinical investigation

Highlight the ICD's performance outside of clinical trial constraints

Provide a detailed view of the morbidity, mortality, and resource use associated with ICD therapy

Perform local hospital needs for quality assurance and quality improvement

Serve as a hospital and physician response to performance measures initiatives.

The registry is currently collecting data from 1497 hospitals in the United States and has data from over 750,000 ICD implants and 75,000 lead procedures as of Dec. 31, 2010. Although the CMS requirement is to only enter patients receiving an ICD for primary prevention of sudden cardiac death, to their credit, 84% of hospitals have chosen to submit data on all device recipients, regardless of age or device indication, which accounts for

The authors have nothing to disclose.
a Division of Cardiovascular Diseases, Mayo Clinic, 200 First Street Southwest, Rochester, MN 55905, USA
b MidCarolina Cardiology, 1718 East 4th Street, Suite 501, Charlotte, NC 28204, USA
c Division of Cardiology, Department of Medicine, Duke University, 2400 Pratt Street, Durham, NC 27705, USA
* Corresponding author.
*E-mail address:* hammill.stephen@mayo.edu

Card Electrophysiol Clin 3 (2011) 521–527
doi:10.1016/j.ccep.2011.08.008

92% of implants entered into the registry. Approximately 95% of all ICDs implanted in the United States are entered into the National ICD Registry based upon NCDR estimates. This extensive reporting provides the most comprehensive characterization of contemporary ICD practice and permits meaningful comparison with published randomized controlled trials such as SCD-HeFT[7] and the Multicenter Automatic Defibrillator Implantation Trial II (MADIT-II).[8] **Table 1** lists the characteristics of patients enrolled in SCD-HeFT and MADIT-II compared with patients in the National ICD Registry, indicating that the registry has a greater proportion of women and patients with atrial fibrillation, hypertension, and diabetes. The National ICD Registry better depicts the type of patients receiving ICDs in the real world, in contrast to randomized–controlled trials of primary prevention, where patient entry was restricted.

A key aspect of the registry is to improve quality performance at hospitals implanting ICDs, which is achieved, in part, through benchmarking reports provided to hospitals on a quarterly basis detailing the outcome for all data elements plus an executive summary that includes performance metrics. Each hospital is compared with hospitals of similar procedure volume and the national aggregate. Reviews of the annual data reports published by the National ICD Registry Steering Committee[3–6] have demonstrated gradual trends in improvement of outcomes during the first 4 years of registry activity. Total adverse procedure-related events have decreased from 3.77% in 2006 to 2.87% in 2009.

The importance of entering data on all patients and not just Medicare beneficiaries has been stressed, as metrics for hospitals that elect to enter only Medicare beneficiaries may be difficult to compare with those of hospitals of similar procedure volume that enter all patients. The more complete recording by entering all patients encompasses a broader population with a lower mean age and less comorbidity with anticipated lower rates of procedure-related complications. Payers including CMS are increasingly interested in reporting valid measures of patient outcomes to improve performance. Unfortunately, many payers are turning to their own administrative databases to assess physician performance. Such databases have significant limitations,[9–14] including:

> Data definitions are often imprecise.
> Final coding might not be supported by the clinical record in a substantial proportion of cases.[10]
> It is difficult to distinguish comorbidities from complications.
> Important clinical risk data (eg, left ventricular ejection fraction [LVEF] and New York Heart Association (NYHA) symptom classification) are not available.[9]

Prospective clinical registries maintained by professional societies such as the National ICD Registry eliminate these inherent deficiencies of administrative data.[9] Clinical registries have the advantage of providing more detailed and accurate data than administrative data, allowing for risk-adjusted outcomes,[11] but they are often limited by the lack of long-term follow-up information. Unfortunately, obtaining reliable follow-up information using chart-level data or subsequent patient contact is too resource-intensive and expensive to collect in a representative national sample such as that included in the National ICD Registry. A hybrid approach that is being employed to develop reliable performance measures combines the NCDR clinical data with Medicare claims data for follow-up that capitalizes on the strengths of both data resources.[9] The Yale Center for Outcomes Research and Evaluation under the direction of Krumholz and colleagues has worked with, ACCF, and the NCDR under contract with CMS to develop a performance measure for ICD complications using the National ICD Registry for the initial clinical data to allow risk adjustment and Medicare claims data for 30- and 90-day adverse events. The adverse events include[15]:

> Pneumothorax or hemothorax requiring a chest tube at 30 days
> Hematoma requiring transfusion or surgical evacuation at 30 days
> Pericardial tamponade or pericardiocentesis at 30 days

**Table 1**
**Characteristics of patients entered into SCD-HeFT, MADIT II, and the National ICD Registry; differences between randomized-controlled trials and the general population**

|  | MADIT-II | SCD-HeFT | ICD Registry |
|---|---|---|---|
| Age (years) | 64.5 | 60 | 68.1 |
| Male gender (%) | 85 | 76 | 74 |
| Diabetes (%) | 35 | 30 | 37 |
| Atrial fibrillation (%) | 9 | 16 | 31 |
| Hypertension (%) | 53 | 56 | 75 |

*Abbreviations:* ICD, implantable cardioverter–defibrillator; MADIT-II, Multicenter Automatic Defibrillator Implantation Trial II; SCD-HeFT, Sudden Cardiac–Death in Heart Failure Trial.

Mechanical complications with system revision (lead revision) at 90 days

Device-related infection at 90 days

ICD replacement at 90 days

Death at 30 days.

The initial analysis using the performance measure identified that the median complication rate for hospitals was 7%, with the lowest decile being 4% and the highest decile 13%. This wide range of complications provides an opportunity for improvement by moving hospitals with the highest rate of complication closer to the median and moving the median closer to the lowest decile group. The ICD complication measure was endorsed by the National Quality Forum in the fall of 2010. NCDR registries such as the National ICD Registry will have increasing value with respect to obtaining risk-adjusted data for performance measures and quality improvement. This has the potential to translate into increased reimbursement, as providers start being paid for performance and value.[16] The ACCF has been contracted by CMS through a sole-source 5-year contract "to build upon, implement, and maintain" risk-adjusted outcome measures, including the "Hospital Risk-Standardized Complication Rate following Implantation of ICD Measure" using the National ICD Registry.[17]

The National ICD Registry has evolved to version 2.0, which corrects and expands the original data collection form. The new version, which has been used by hospitals since April 2010, was developed over 2 years by a working group comprised of clinical electrophysiology and heart failure physicians, nurses, abstractors, and registry experts, enhancing the ICD registry data form, eliminating data elements that were not used, better defining data elements that were confusing, and adding data fields to allow entry of pediatric patients and lead information. The working group made efforts to ensure that data will be collected to cover ICD and cardiac resynchronization therapy (CRT)-D indications included in the ACC/American Heart Association (AHA)/HRS 2008 Guidelines for Device-Based Therapies.[18] The registry has been enhanced to include data on atrial, ventricular, defibrillation, epicardial, and left heart leads implanted at the time of generator placement, or if at another procedure, the lead is revised, replaced, extracted, or surgically abandoned. This provides follow-up of lead performance and will be a measure of long-term lead-related complication that requires a full lead procedure for correction such as dislodgement, perforation, removal for infection, and lead failure. The group worked

closely with the US Food and Drug Administration (FDA) to allow version 2.0 enhancements to serve as a postmarket surveillance tool to assess lead performance as part of the FDA sentinel network. The recently published recommendations from HRS on lead performance policies and guidelines emphasized that "the National ICD Registry offers great promise as a postmarket surveillance tool. Because of the large numbers of leads in the registry, it may be possible to identify infrequent but important lead performance issues, determine lead reliability rates, and compare the performance of various lead models."[19] Recently, Boston Scientific and the FDA have reported that the National ICD Registry will be used for a postapproval study in a MADIT-CRT population.[20]

## LESSONS LEARNED FROM ICD RESEARCH PUBLICATIONS

The Agency for Health care Research and Quality (AHRQ) made the following observation focusing on the National ICD Registry: "Observational registries can quickly accumulate large amounts of data on real-world practice and effectiveness of new treatments and procedures. Physicians and hospitals can use these data to further quality improvement efforts at a local level, and physician associations can evaluate data to determine the effectiveness of existing clinical guidelines."[21] The National ICD Registry is accruing ICD implants at the rate of 10,000 per month, providing a wealth of information on ICD implantation and outcomes on patients outside the constraints of randomized–controlled trials. The information allows for assessment of ICD implantation at small hospitals and large tertiary referral centers; urban, suburban, and rural hospitals; and by physicians with different levels of experience and training. A rigorous data quality recording process is in place to improve data accuracy, and a direct audit of a sample of clinical records is performed annually to evaluate the data entered into the registry compared with the original source data in the patient's record.

Despite vigorous efforts to ensure data quality, the data have important limitations. The quality of the data is dependent upon how carefully it is entered and how accurately supporting information such as measurement of ejection fraction and duration of heart failure is documented by the treating physician. The individual entering the data needs to be experienced with the nuances of ICD implantation and issues surrounding patients with ischemic and nonischemic cardiomyopathies. The registry data do not have the rigor of data from controlled clinical trials because of the lack of a dedicated study nurse or data abstractor and the goal to keep the registry data form short enough to be manageable in the setting of a busy clinical practice. Individuals entering data into the registry need to enter accurate data, since a portion of registry data is submitted to CMS to support payment.

The National ICD Registry Research and Publication Subcommittee has reviewed 22 abstracts that have been presented at the HRS, ACC, and AHA annual scientific sessions. Fourteen manuscripts have been published, and 13 manuscripts are in progress. Data from the National ICD Registry are being used to better understand the application of ICD therapy in the general population, including gender differences and procedure-related adverse events[22]; association of physician certification and outcomes and appropriate use of CRT-D[23]; racial and ethnic differences in patients receiving cardiac resynchronization therapy with a defibrillator (CRT-D)[24]; gender differences in ICD use according to randomized trial enrollment criteria[25]; and ICD outcomes in patients with end-stage renal disease.[26]

The association between physician certification and outcomes[23] was evaluated using ICD registry data between January 2006 and January 2007; 111, 293 ICD implantations were reported, with electrophysiologists performing 71%, nonelectrophysiology cardiovascular physicians implanting 22%, and thoracic surgeons implanting 2%. The complication rate was 3.5% for electrophysiologists, 4% for nonelectrophysiology cardiovascular physicians, and 5.8% for thoracic surgeons. This study also identified that of 35,841 patients who met criteria for CRT-D, 83% received a CRT-D if their implantation was performed by an electrophysiologist, 76% if implanted by nonelectrophysiology cardiovascular physician, and 58% if implanted by a thoracic surgeon. This study suggested that board-certified electrophysiologists had fewer complications and more appropriate device selection for a CRT-D. This was the first study that reported a relationship between the extent of training as measured by board certification and procedure-related outcomes. A study by Cheng and associates[27] evaluated the risk of acute lead dislodgement and in-hospital mortality in patients enrolled in the National ICD Registry and identified that dislodgements occurred more often in patients with more comorbidities and in patients undergoing implantation by nonelectrophysiology-trained implanters. This study supports the publication by Curtis.[22] This publication also identified that ICD implantations by trained electrophysiologists were associated with fewer complications. In the study by Cheng,[27] acute lead dislodgement was significantly associated with an increased length of stay, hematoma, infection, cardiac arrest, cardiac perforation, pneumothorax, and in-hospital death. The adjusted odds ratio of the effect of acute lead dislodgement on the development of serious adverse events (cardiac arrest, tamponade, pneumothorax, infection) was 5.62 (95% confidence interval [CI] 4.76–6.6, $P<.00001$), and in-hospital death had an odds ratio of 2.66 (95% CI 1.98–3.57, $P<.00001$). Physicians who had completed an electrophysiology fellowship had fewer dislodged leads. This finding was not related to implantation volume but "more likely represents inherent differences in the way the training is performed." The only two factors associated with a lower likelihood of acute lead dislodgment were board certification and board eligibility in electrophysiology.

A study by Freeman and colleagues[28] evaluated the relationship between hospital procedure volume and complications of ICD implantation using data from the National ICD Registry and reported that patients who had an ICD implanted at a high-volume hospital were less likely to have an adverse event associated with the procedure than patients who had an ICD implanted at a low-volume hospital. Hospitals in the lowest quartile of annual ICD volume had a 3.82% risk of complication including 0.6% in-hospital death compared with hospitals in the highest quartile, demonstrating a 3.08% risk of complication and 0.4% risk of death. This finding was most significant for placement of a dual-chamber ICD, where the complication rate in the lowest quartile of annual ICD volume was 3.97% with 0.59% risk of in-hospital death, compared with hospitals in the highest quartile, showing a 2.85% complication and 0.37% risk of in-hospital death.

A report by Fein and associates[29] reviewed the prevalence and predictors of off-label use of CRT-D therapy in patients in the National ICD Registry between January 2006 and June 2008. Of 45,392 patients who received a CRT-D, 23.7% were placed without meeting standard CRT implantation criteria (ejection fraction 35% or less, NYHA functional Class 3–4, and QRS interval duration 120 ms or greater). Patients who had a CRT-D placed outside of the guidelines most often had either class 1 or 2 heart failure or QRS interval duration under 120 milliseconds. Closer adherence to published guidelines may improve the cost–benefit ratio for CRT-D therapy.

Al-Khatib and colleagues[30] recently published data from the National ICD Registry on nonevidence-based primary prevention ICD implantations, reporting that a substantial proportion of ICD implants were nonevidence-based, and the risk of in-hospital death and procedure-related complication was significantly higher in patients who received a nonevidence-based ICD. Patients were classified as receiving a nonevidence-based implant if they had a myocardial infarction within 40 days before ICD implantation, coronary artery bypass grafting within 3 months before ICD implantation, NYHA class 4 symptoms, or newly diagnosed heart failure at the time of ICD implantation. Of 111,707 primary prevention ICD implants, 22.5% were for nonevidence-based indications, with 8.3% implanted within 40 days of myocardial infarction, 0.73% implanted within 3 months of coronary artery bypass grafting, 2.7% in patients with NYHA class 4 symptoms, and 14% in patients with newly diagnosed heart failure (patients may have met more than 1 criteria). The National ICD Registry specifically asks in the data form if a history of congestive heart failure (CHF) has been present and, if so, was the duration "within the past 3 months, 3 to 9 months, greater than 9 months." This is in the background of the guidelines recommending patients be on maximal medical therapy before receiving the ICD, and it is assumed to be unlikely that maximal medical therapy can be achieved in the group with symptomatic CHF receiving less than 3 months of treatment. The risk of both in-hospital death and procedure-related complication was significantly higher in the nonevidence-based ICD group (0.6% vs 0.2% for in-hospital death, and 3.2% vs 2.4% for postprocedure complication). The rate of nonevidence-based implants was significantly lower for electrophysiologists (20.8%) than for nonelectrophysiology cardiologists (24.8%) and thoracic surgeons (36.1%). There was a wide variation among hospitals, with some hospitals implanting only 5% of ICDs outside guidelines and other hospitals implanting 55% of ICDs outside guidelines (**Fig. 1**). Ralph Brindis, president of the ACCF, stated "when we see that level of variation, there is no way even a skeptic could say that we don't have room for improvement in the way that we apply ICD technology."[31]

It is important to note that many patients appropriately receive ICDs outside guidelines based upon the physician's clinical judgment. This includes patients who have an established cardiomyopathy and present to the hospital with a small "troponin leak" subsequently coded as a myocardial infarction. In addition, patients may require coronary revascularization and have either a pre-existing cardiomyopathy or develop an indication for a permanent pacemaker. In such patients, it may be elected to implant the ICD due to their increased risk of sudden death and need for a pacing device.

In summary, the National ICD Registry has proven to be a successful partnership between HRS and ACCF, collecting data from 486,025 ICD implantations from 1434 hospitals and 5246 implanting physicians from 2006 to 2009.[6] The quarterly benchmarking reports have offered hospitals the opportunity to assess outcomes related to ICD implantation and improve quality. A risk-adjusted performance measure has been developed using the ICD registry, approved by the National Quality Forum, and supported by CMS. Version 2.0 of the registry is collecting data at the time of lead procedures, and multiple research papers have evaluated the use of the ICD in patients outside randomized–controlled trials and have reported the advantage of lower procedure-related complications and improved device selection when the procedure is done by a trained electrophysiologist. The increasing emphasis on outcome measures in all specialties

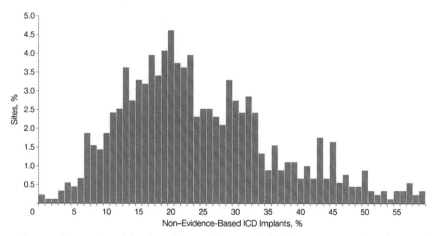

**Fig. 1.** Rates of nonevidence-based implantable cardioverter–defibrillators across sites. (*From* Al-Khatib SM, Hellkamp A, Curtis J, et al. Nonevidence-based ICD implantations in the United States. JAMA 2011;305:43–9; with permission.)

of medicine by CMS and other payers has the risk of inappropriate conclusions when based upon flawed administrative databases maintained by the payers. Fortunately, the National ICD Registry provides an important source of patient data that can more reliably be used to assess risk-adjusted patient outcomes.

## REFERENCES

1. Anderson KP. Estimates of implantable cardioverter defibrillator complications. Circulation 2009;119:1069–71.

2. Hammill S, Phurrough S, Brindis R. The National ICD Registry: now and into the future. Heart Rhythm 2006;3:470–3.

3. Hammill SC, Stevenson LW, Kadish AH, et al. National ICD registry annual report 2006. Review of the registry's first year, data collected, and future plans. Heart Rhythm 2007;4:1260–3.

4. Hammill SC, Kremers MS, Stevenson LW, et al. National ICD registry annual report 2008. Heart Rhythm 2008;5:1359–63.

5. Hammill SC, Kremers MS, Kadish AH, et al. Review of the ICD registry's third year, expansion to include lead data and pediatric ICD procedures, and role for measuring performance. Heart Rhythm 2009;6(9):1397–401.

6. Hammill SC, Kremers MS, Stevenson LW, et al. National ICD Registry Annual Report 2009. Review of the registry's fourth year, incorporating lead data and pediatric ICD procedures, and use as a national performance measure. Heart Rhythm 2010;7:1340–5.

7. Bardy GH, Lee KL, Mark DB, et al. Sudden Cardiac–Death in Heart Failure Trial (SCD-HeFT) investigators. Defibrillator for congestive heart failure. N Engl J Med 2005;352:225–37.

8. Moss AJ, Zareba W, Hall WJ, et al. Multicenter Automatic Defibrillator Implantation Trial II Investigators. Prophylactic implantation of a defibrillator in patients with myocardial infarction and reduced ejection fraction. N Engl J Med 2002;346(12):877–83.

9. Hammill SC, Curtis J. Publicly reporting ICD outcomes. Grading the report card. Circ Arrhythm Electrophysiol 2008;1:235–7.

10. Fisher ES, Whaley FS, Krushat, et al. The accuracy of Medicare Hospital Claims Data: progress has been made but problems remain. Am J Public Health 1992;82:243–8.

11. Shahian DM, Silverstein T, Lovett AF, et al. Comparison of clinical and administrative data sources for hospital coronary artery bypass graft surgery report cards. Circulation 2007;115:1518–27.

12. Al-Khatib SM, Greiner MA, Peterson ED, et al. Patient and implanting physician factors associated with mortality and complications following implantable cardioverter defibrillator implantation 2002-2005. Circ Arrhythm Electrophysiol 2008;1:240–9.

13. Krumholz HM, Brindis RG, Brush JE, et al. Standards for statistical models used for public reporting of health outcomes: an American Heart Association Scientific Statement from the quality of care and outcomes research interdisciplinary writing group: co-sponsored by the council on epidemiology and prevention and the stroke council: endorsed by the American College of Cardiology Foundation. Circulation 2006;113:456–62.

14. Krumholz HM, Wang Y, Mattera JA, et al. An administrative claims model suitable for profiling hospital performance based on thirty-day mortality rate among patients with an acute myocardial infarction. Circulation 2006;113:1683–92.

15. Available at: http://www.qualitymeasures.ahrq.gov. Accessed August 19, 2011.

16. Medicare program; proposed changes to the hospital inpatient prospective payment systems for acute care hospitals and the long-term care hospital prospective payment system and proposed fiscal year 2011. Federal Register 2010;75(85). Proposed rules. CMS-1498-P. 23852–24332.

17. Available at: https://www.fbo.gov/index. Accessed August 19, 2011.

18. Epstein AE, DiMarco JP, Ellenbogen KA, et al. ACC/AHA/HRS 2008 guidelines for device-based therapy of cardiac rhythm abnormalities. J Am Coll Cardiol 2008;51:1–62.

19. Maisel WH, Hauser RG, Hammill SC, et al. Recommendations from the Heart Rhythm Society Task Force on Lead Performance Policies and Guidelines. Developed in collaboration with the American College of Cardiology and the American Heart Association. Heart Rhythm 2009;6:869–85.

20. Available at: www.accessdata.fda.gov/scripts/cdrh/cfdocs/cfPMA/pma_pas.cfm?t_id=439786&;c_id=380. Accessed August 19, 2011.

21. Effective health care. registries for evaluating patient outcomes: a user's guide. Agency for Healthcare Research and Quality; 2007. p. 17–9. Available at: www.ahrq.gov. Accessed August 19, 2011.

22. Peterson PN, Daugherty SL, Wang Y, et al. Gender differences in procedure related adverse events in patients receiving implantable cardioverter–defibrillator therapy. Circulation 2009;119:1078–84.

23. Curtis JP, Luebbert JJ, Wang Y, et al. Association of physician certification and outcomes among patients receiving an implantable cardioverter–defibrillator. JAMA 2009;301:1661–70.

24. Farmer SA, Kirkpatrick JN, Heidenreich PA, et al. Ethnic and racial disparities in cardiac resynchronization therapy. Heart Rhythm 2009;6:325–31.

25. Daugherty SL, Peterson PN, Wang Y, et al. Use of implantable cardioverter defibrillators for primary

prevention in the community; do women and men equally meet trial enrollment criteria? Am Heart J 2009;158:224–9.

26. Aggarwal A, Wang Y, Rumsfeld JS, et al. Clinical characteristics and in-hospital outcome of patients with end-stage renal disease on dialysis referred for implantable cardioverter-defibrillator implantation. Heart Rhythm 2009;6:1565–71.

27. Cheng A, Wang Y, Curtis JP, et al. Acute lead dislodgements and in-hospital mortality in patients enrolled in the national cardiovascular data registry implantable cardioverter defibrillator registry. J Am Coll Cardiol 2010;56:1651–6.

28. Freeman JV, Wang Y, Curtis JP, et al. The relation between hospital procedure volume and complications of cardioverter–defibrillator implantation from the implantable cardioverter–defibrillator registry. J Am Coll Cardiol 2010;56:1133–9.

29. Fein AS, Wang Y, Curtis JP, et al. Prevalence and predictors of off-label use of cardiac resynchronization therapy in patients enrolled in the national cardiovascular data registry implantable cardiac defibrillator registry. J Am Coll Cardiol 2010;56: 766–73.

30. Al-Khatib SM, Hellkamp A, Curtis J, et al. Nonevidence-based ICD implantations in the United States. JAMA 2011;305:43–9.

31. Brindis R. Wide Variations Found in use of Heart Implants. Healthcare Business News. 2011; 12:01ET. [Tags: Systems, The Week in Healthcare].

# Expanding the Use of Cardiac Resynchronization Therapy: Words of Caution

Daniel B. Kramer, MD[a,b,*], Mark E. Josephson, MD[b,c]

## KEYWORDS

- Cardiac resynchronization therapy • Congestive heart failure
- Left ventricular systolic dysfunction

In a world of diminishing returns, where clinically and statistically significant benefits become increasingly elusive, pharmacologic and device-based therapies for systolic heart failure (HF) have consistently provided incremental improvement. In the past 20 years, serial clinical trials have demonstrated mortality benefits for beta-blockers,[1] angiotensin-converting enzyme inhibitors,[2,3] aldosterone antagonists,[4,5] implantable cardioverter-defibrillators (ICDs),[6,7] and cardiac resynchronization therapy (CRT)[8,9] for selected patients with clinical HF caused by left ventricular (LV) systolic dysfunction against a background of gradually improving medical therapy. There is no question that millions of patients have benefited from these breakthroughs, and likely many millions more are eligible for these therapies but do not receive them in accordance with consensus guidelines.[10,11]

However, these interventions bear significant costs. Device-based therapy in particular places a substantial and growing financial burden on health care systems, and the devices themselves place patients at risk for serious adverse events at implantation and throughout the experience of living with these permanent devices.[12,13] At the same time, there are powerful financial incentives for both physicians and industry to increase use and broaden the eligible population for device implantation.

Recent studies have examined the use of CRT specifically in patients with mild or absent clinical HF.[14–16] Expanding use of CRT to these populations would be a marked change in cardiovascular medicine with broad implications for already-strained budgets. This article examines the evidence for and against this expansion and suggests specific unresolved questions that require cautious consideration.

## EVIDENCE FOR CRT IN SEVERE HEART FAILURE

Several pioneering trials demonstrated functional and morphologic improvements with CRT with or without defibrillator back-up (CRT-D or CRT-P, respectively) in symptomatic HF (defined here as New York Heart Association [NYHA] II or higher).[17,18] More recent studies established improvements in clinical outcomes, albeit with slightly

Disclosures: Dr Kramer has no financial conflicts of interest to disclose. Dr Josephson is a consultant for Biosense Webster and has received honoraria for educational programs from Medtronic.

[a] Cardiovascular Division, Department of Medicine, Beth Israel Deaconess Medical Center, Harvard Medical School, West Campus, Baker 4, 185 Pilgrim Road, Boston, MA 02215, USA

[b] Harvard Medical School, USA

[c] Cardiovascular Division, Harvard-Thorndike Electrophysiology Institute and Arrhythmia Service, Beth Israel Deaconess Medical Center, West Campus, Baker 4, 185 Pilgrim Road, Boston, MA 02215, USA

* Corresponding author.

*E-mail address:* dkramer@bidmc.harvard.edu

different trial designs in each. All studies used a composite end point of death plus either HF or cardiovascular hospitalization or worsening NYHA class. Although the combined end points produced more events and greater statistical power for the primary analyses, the studies were largely underpowered to tease apart the impact of CRT or the ICD functions on the individual components.[19]

The Comparison of Medical Therapy, Pacing, and Defibrillation in Chronic Heart Failure (COMPANION) study randomized 1520 patients with NYHA Class III (n = 1302) or IV (n = 218) HF, QRS greater than 120 ms, in a 1:2:2 fashion to optimal medical therapy, CRT-P, or CRT-D.[8] The primary composite end point was the time to death from or hospitalization for any cause. CRT-P and CRT-D both reduced the primary end point compared with optimal medical therapy (hazard ratio [HR] 0.81 and 0.80, respectively), an approximate 12% absolute and 20% relative risk reduction for either device. The hazard ratios for death alone were 0.76 for CRT-P and 0.64 for CRT-D, with the latter reaching statistical significance.

The Cardiac Resynchronization in Heart Failure (CARE-HF) study randomized 813 patients with NYHA Class III (n = 763) or IV (n = 50) HF to CRT-P or optimal medical therapy followed for 29.4 months, with a primary end point of time to death from any cause or an unplanned cardiovascular hospitalization.[9] Again, the combined end point was markedly reduced by CRT-P with a hazard ratio of 0.63, with a similar reduction (20% vs 30%) in mortality alone. Interestingly, the improvement in sudden cardiac death seen in CARE-HF was more dramatic than has been seen in studies of ICDs alone, perhaps speaking to the severity of HF in the treated population.

Last, the Resynchronization-Defibrillation for Ambulatory Heart Failure Trial (RAFT) evaluated the added benefits for CRT versus ICD therapy alone in 1798 patients with LV systolic dysfunction and a wide QRS and symptoms consistent with NYHA Class II (n = 1438) or III (n = 360) to an ICD or CRT-D implant.[20] CRT-D reduced the primary end point of death or HF hospitalization more than 40 months with a hazard ratio of 0.75, with a similar relative risk reduction for mortality alone, despite more than twice as many adverse events.

## EVIDENCE FOR CRT IN MILD HEART FAILURE

The Multicenter Automatic Defibrillator Implantation Trial-Cardiac Resynchronization Therapy (MADIT-CRT) and Resynchronization Reverses Remodeling in Systolic Left Ventricular Dysfunction (REVERSE) trials provide most of the data for expanding CRT beyond the severe HF populations.[21,22] Each included both NYHA I and II patients; the evidence for the symptomatic patients (NYHA Class II) is summarized briefly here in support of the applicability of CRT to these patients. MADIT-CRT randomized 1820 patients with left ventricular ejection fraction (LVEF) of less than 30%, QRS greater than 130 ms, and either ischemic or nonischemic cardiomyopathy to CRT-D or ICD alone (in 3:2 ratio) with a background of optimal medical therapy.[14] The NYHA Class II cohort included 821 nonischemic subjects and 734 ischemic subjects. (The remaining 265 subjects were ischemic patients in NYHA Class I.) The primary end point of the study was a composite of death or an HF "event," defined as an episode with "signs and symptoms consistent with congestive heart failure that was responsive to intravenous decongestive therapy on an outpatient basis or an augmented decongestive regimen with oral or parenteral medications during an in-hospital stay." Over an average follow-up of 2.4 years, CRT-D reduced the primary end point from 25.3% in the ICD group to 17.2% in the CRT-D group, for a hazard ratio of 0.66 (P = .001). Mortality alone was similar in the 2 groups (7.3 and 6.8, respectively), and the overall study results were driven largely by the reduction in HF events. The subgroup analyses evaluating treatment effect by both etiology and NYHA class suggest that the benefits were seen only in the NYHA Class II population, however.

REVERSE implanted 610 patients with CRT-D and randomized them in a 2:1 fashion to CRT-on (419) or CRT-off (191). The primary end point assessed at 12 months was an intricate "HF clinical composite response" in which patients were adjudicated to be worse, unchanged, or improved according to the described study protocol:

"Patients were judged to be worsened if they died, were hospitalized (at any time during the 12 months) because of or associated with worsening HF, crossed over or permanently discontinued double-blind treatment because of worsening HF at any time during the 12 months, demonstrated worsening in NYHA functional class at their 12-month visit, or reported moderately or markedly worse heart failure symptoms compared with before CRT implant (Patient Global Assessment) when asked at the 12-month follow-up. Patients were judged to be improved if they had not worsened and had demonstrated improvement in NYHA functional class at 12 months and/or reported moderately or markedly improved heart failure symptoms at the 12-month follow-up. Patients who were not worsened or improved were classified as unchanged. Hospitalizations and crossovers only contributed to the end point if the AEAC verified their relatedness to HF. Because asymptomatic patients (NYHA functional class I) were included in the study and their NYHA status could not improve, the percent of patients worsened was used to compare the efficacy of CRT between study groups."[15]

Interestingly, despite its complexity and an appealing trend, the difference in this primary end point was not statistically significant between the 2 groups (16% vs 21%, $P = .10$). However, the CRT-on group experienced greater reductions in LV end-systolic volume and time to first hospitalization, leading to an overall positive conclusion from the investigators. These benefits, notably, were limited to the NYHA Class II (n = 503) subcohort. Only 107 study subjects had NYHA Class I HF, and although the study was not powered to evaluate these groups separately, the hazard ratios for the Class I group suggest a more limited impact (HR 0.87, 95% confidence interval [CI] 0.37–2.03 vs HR 0.60, 95% CI 0.35–1.01).

## LIMITATIONS IN SYMPTOMATIC PATIENTS

Together, these trials provide support for CRT in *symptomatic* HF. Importantly, these studies variously described the negative features of device therapy ranging from implant-related complications to inappropriate shocks, infections requiring explantation, or possibly proarrhythmia from pacing alone. Additionally, the relatively small number of NYHA Class IV patients illustrates one of the important barriers in interpreting studies whose populations (and subsequent conclusions) may seem wider than they really are. On the basis of COMPANION, CRT was approved for use in the United States by the Food and Drug Administration (FDA) in NYHA Class III or IV, for example, even though fewer than 15% of the study patients were in Class IV. This theme—entry criteria compared with exit characteristics of study patients—is a recurrent and vexing problem in cardiovascular device studies and challenges rapid extrapolation of new data to widely defined populations.[19,23–25] Several other problems with these CRT studies have limited enthusiasm for implantation, however, and these will remain important when considering exposing asymptomatic patients to the risks of therapy.

## INCONSISTENT RESPONSE TO CRT

One problem is the inconsistent response to CRT. Although estimates vary, approximately 30% of patients do not respond to therapy even under clinical trial settings.[26,27] There are many proposed

explanations for this suboptimal response rate, including lead position, interaction of leads with nonviable myocardium, and imperfect overlap between QRS width and true ventricular dyssynchrony. These possibilities have each been explored in attempts to refine patient selection, without any consistently demonstrated ability to predict response using current measures of dyssynchrony.[28–33] Similarly, refinement of CRT settings for nonresponders remains investigational, with one recent study showing no added benefit from an optimization strategy.[34,35] As realizing the benefits of CRT in asymptomatic patients will likely require a much longer time horizon, possibly including multiple generators, it seems prudent to strive for more precise patient selection and optimization before widespread use. Thus, symptomatic patients would seem to offer more opportunities for demonstrating and refining strategies for patient selection.

## SUBGROUP ANALYSES

A related problem with CRT in advanced HF is the persistent suggestion of important subgroups that fail to achieve meaningful improvement. Interpreting subgroups from large clinical trials is difficult and subject to bias and confounding that may exaggerate or obscure benefits.[36–38] Nevertheless, not all subgroups are the same, and those that are prespecified, physiologically plausible, and indicative of particularly powerful interactions may merit particular attention, even if only in a "hypothesis-generating" way from a purist's perspective. Indeed, it is not uncommon for significant public health decisions, including recommendations for cardiac devices, to weigh subgroups heavily in decision making. For example, QRS width in MADIT-II[7] was initially adopted by the Centers for Medicare and Medicaid Services as a limiting factor for reimbursement in ICD implantation. Dogmatic adherence to clinical trial precepts would question this quite reasonable limitation on device therapy, or at least demand a separate prospective study validating the signal, an unlikely prospect given the current incentives for clinical trial design. Nevertheless, recent expansion of the labeling for CRT was specifically restricted to patients with left bundle branch block (LBBB), given the strength of the signal difference, physiology of the intervention, and consistency with prior studies illustrating the same limited benefits in patients with non-LBBB conduction delay.[39]

Other than patients with LBBB versus non-LBBB, are there important subgroups in advanced HF that seem not to benefit from CRT, and thus merit particular attention in the asymptomatic population? We would highlight 3 subgroups that are consistently prespecified, biologically compelling, and illustrative of marked differences in treatment outcome: (1) QRS width, (2) etiology of heart failure, and (3) chronic kidney disease.

## QRS Width

QRS width, as noted previously, is an imperfect but durable marker of interventricular and intraventricular conduction delay. But even this characterization is an oversimplification, as there are important physiologic differences between "wide-QRS" patients with delayed activation to the posterolateral left ventricular compared with patients with normal endocardial activation but delay from endocardium to epicardium.[27] Preexciting the left ventricle would be expected to improve ventricular coordination only in the former group.

Even if QRS duration alone is taken at face value, how delayed is delayed enough? COMPANION, CARE-HF, and RAFT all required minimum QRS widths of 120 ms for inclusion, a standard that has been incorporated into current guidelines for patient selection.[10,40] But the average QRS in all 3 was closer to *150 ms to 160 ms*, a substantial difference that plays out importantly in the subgroup analyses of all 3 studies. Markedly more treatment benefits were seen in the patients with QRS greater than 160 ms in CARE-HF, QRS greater than 148 ms in COMPANION, and QRS greater than 150 ms in RAFT. The latter 2 suggested *no* benefit at all in patients with narrower QRS complexes, consistent with the largest randomized study evaluating narrow QRS patients specifically.[41] This highlights the difference between entry and exit criteria in clinical trials, a contentious but persistent problem in interpreting mega-trials in particular.[19,23–25,42] Although the inclusion criteria are the starting point for study design and interpretation, blindly extrapolating these to real-world patients defies common sense. Consider again the "NYHA Class III or IV HF" entry criteria for COMPANION and CARE-HF. Surely appropriate extrapolation to real-world patients demands recognition that the vast majority of patients actually studied in both trials were NYHA Class III. Similarly, caution should be used when the differences between entry and exit criteria are stark, as with QRS width in these 3 trials, a clinically important and physiologically sound discrepancy.

One concrete way in which cautious skepticism could, but typically does not, translate into clinical practice would be withholding the strongest level (Class IA) of recommendation in society guidelines for cases in which this discrepancy is particularly dramatic. For CRT, however, the Class IA recommendation has been applied to patients with a QRS of 120 ms or greater, despite the demonstration of benefit only in those patients with QRS of 150 ms or greater. Given the recent labeling expansion based on MADIT-CRT, this is likely to remain true moving forward. It is important to recognize the downstream effects of treatment recommendations, even if their stated goals are restricted to guiding clinicians and patients toward sensible therapies.[43]

Having already achieved the most robust endorsement, there is little reason to expect manufacturers—the driving force behind most device-based trials in electrophysiology—to dedicate resources toward exploring different QRS subgroups prospectively. Further, guidelines have become increasingly potent in defining care as "high quality," "appropriate," or "evidence based."[44,45] This may be problematic for producing future studies, as investigators and institutional review boards may not consider it feasible or ethical to randomize patients away from "evidence-based" therapies, thus trapping the clinical community in the constraints of the original, broad inclusion criteria of pivotal studies. It is chilling, then, to consider rapidly expanding the eligible CRT population within these same wide, yet binding, parameters.

## Renal Function

A similar pattern is seen with renal function, which has emerged as a potent mitigating factor for ICD therapy by itself.[46–48] There are similar studies in CRT populations illustrating that renal function may limit response. One prospective study of 490 patients found that those with a glomerular filtration rate (GFR) less than 60 had higher mortality than those with a GFR higher than 60, and responders (defined in this study by decrease in LV systolic volume) were more common in patients with higher GFR.[49] This suggests that renal function may limit CRT's effectiveness both through competing causes of mortality but also through more direct physiologic interference. Another single-center series of 482 patients found chronic kidney disease (again defined as GFR <60) to be a risk factor for mortality after adjustment.[50] In CARE-HF, interestingly, unadjusted subgroup analysis suggested that more benefit was seen in patients with GFR higher than 60, whereas the reverse was true in RAFT.

Again, these subgroups would ideally serve to guide additional studies refining patient selection, and yet these trials have not been done in advance of expanding this same trial design to healthier (and larger) populations.[51]

### Etiology of HF

Renal function and QRS width are continuous variables treated as categorical for both entry criteria and subgroup analyses, with the associated challenges described previously. But CRT outcomes also vary dramatically based on etiology of heart failure, another factor that limits our enthusiasm for prompt extrapolation to healthier patients. Etiology of underlying cardiomyopathy interacts both in theory and possibly in practice with CRT effectiveness, and certainly influences the usefulness of ICDs.[52–54] Even those patients with "ischemic heart disease" are broadly heterogeneous, with substantial and physiologically significant differences in site of infarction and scar.

The CARE-HF investigators noted less of a morphologic impact of CRT in patients with ischemic heart disease although a similar impact on mortality.[55] A similar impact on echocardiographic parameters was seen in MADIT-CRT.[56] There did not appear to be important differences in clinical effect based on etiology in RAFT or COMPANION. However, as much of the proposed benefits of "preventative" CRT implantation stems from reversal or prevention of preclinical adverse remodeling, the possibility of etiology-specific effects merits careful consideration.

## EVIDENCE AND PROBLEMS FOR CRT IN ASYMPTOMATIC PATIENTS

The reservations noted previously regarding CRT in even severe symptomatic heart failure—QRS width, important comorbidities, such as renal function, and etiology of heart failure—limit our enthusiasm for device implantation. At our institution, we consider CRT more useful for nonischemic versus ischemic patients, and generally consider therapy in either group only for those patients with QRS durations that approach 140 to 150 ms. It is not clear whether or not these same problems would affect the usefulness of CRT in asymptomatic patients; however, event rates would certainly be lower overall and thus any factors that mitigate benefits, and bias a theoretical study of just this population toward the null, would be magnified in importance. There are no studies evaluating NYHA Class I patients alone, and so expanding CRT to this group requires a charitable view of their inclusion in the trials of mild HF.

We noted earlier that the largest studies of CRT in mild heart failure included relatively few asymptomatic patients: 107 of 610 in REVERSE, and 265 of 1820 in MADIT-CRT. In both of these smaller cohorts, the overall study findings appeared to be muted at best or possibly neutral. Although neither study was powered to evaluate NYHA Class I patients independently, this did not stop the manufacturer from seeking their inclusion in the expanded labeling for CRT, which was approved by the FDA and is likely destined to become integrated into updated guidelines for devices and HF. This reflects the same pattern seen with the use of ICDs in non–infarct-related cardiomyopathy: no single study in this population has demonstrated a statistically significant mortality benefit, a pattern reproduced by the (underpowered) subgroup in the Sudden Cardiac Death in Heart Failure Trial (SCD-HeFT), and yet this population retains the American Heart Association/American College of Cardiology Class IB recommendation for implantation.[57] Does a similar fate await asymptomatic patients with HF, represented with only 372 (15%) patients of 2430 of the pivotal studies?

Asymptomatic patients, in sum, do not appear to have improved mortality and may or may not have improvements in HF hospitalizations. Although functional and morphologic benefits may persist in this group, these surrogate outcomes alone were not sufficient for FDA approval in more severe heart failure, and larger studies with hard outcomes were performed.

### Blinding

There are additional problems specific to the asymptomatic patients that warrant consideration. For purists who consider the inclusion of NYHA Class I patients in MADIT-CRT and REVERSE to be sufficiently persuasive, it bears mention that only REVERSE was double-blinded. That is, the patients in MADIT-CRT knew which device they had received, and (if even lightly informed of the point of the study) surely were aware of the purported benefits of CRT compared with background therapy. Although the HF events in MADIT-CRT were blindly adjudicated, in the absence of patient blinding one wonders whether or not the placebo effect might sufficiently influence patient perceptions of their illness, and therefore influence their own disease management, report of symptoms, and need for escalation of therapy. Choice of follow-up treatment of patients was not blinding, and it would not be surprising if physicians unwittingly treated ICD-only patients more aggressively and thus accrued "HF events" more briskly.

### What Does "Asymptomatic" Mean?

A related problem with regard to physician blinding is the characterization of patients as "asymptomatic." Some 10% of the MADIT-CRT population was assessed as having NYHA Class III or even IV symptoms at least 3 months before randomization.[26] It is not known how many of these ended up in the "asymptomatic" cohort, but one wonders if a more objective measure of cardiac function (such as V02 max or more crudely with biomarkers, such as N-terminal pro-B-type natriuretic peptide) is needed to validate patient assignments. At the bedside, patients who carry a diagnosis of HF commonly have competing explanations for fatigue or dyspnea on exertion: pulmonary disease, anemia, obesity, simple deconditioning, and so forth.[58] Separating these out from mild HF is not trivial, but ascribing symptoms to these conditions and rendering a patient's HF status as "asymptomatic" may be misleading in the absence of objective criteria.

### Special Circumstances: CRT in the Elderly and Off-Label Use

Endorsing CRT for asymptomatic patients, or even those with mild HF, necessarily involves consideration of its application to populations even farther afield from these groups. Data from the National Cardiovascular Device Registry (NCDR) showed that, in a time where only NYHA Class III or IV with LVEF less than 35% and QRS width greater than 120 ms were considered eligible for implantation based on guidelines and FDA labeling, 23.7% of patients receiving devices did not meet these criteria.[59] Of these, 13% were in NYHA Class I or II and 12% had a QRS less than 120 ms. Off-label usage may well be appropriate in many circumstances, but in this case indicates the liberties physicians may take with the published evidence. If a similar pattern were seen with expansion of CRT to asymptomatic patients, would indications creep even farther afield? Would patients with more mild LV systolic dysfunction suddenly seem to be attractive candidates?

A concrete example of this phenomenon is the use of ICDs and CRT in elderly individuals. The benefits of either therapy in this population are controversial.[60–63] Meta-analyses have found no benefit in patients older than 65 for ICDs in primary prevention or those older than 75 in secondary prevention.[64,65] Despite this, data from the NCDR show that 42% of all ICD recipients in the United States were older than 70 and 12% were older than 80. In this oldest group, nearly 40% of implants were CRT-D.[62] We view this extensive use of ICDs and CRT-D, in particular in the elderly,

with great skepticism, and with trepidation about further exposure of elderly patients with asymptomatic heart failure to device implantation and the attendant risks in the absence of compelling evidence for short-term benefits.

### SUMMARY

Before expanding CRT to asymptomatic patients, we would caution clinicians and patients to consider closely the complexities outlined here. Only by advocating for definitive clinical trials aimed at targeted refinement for device therapy will we be able to extend the use of CRT wisely.

CRT improves morbidity and mortality in selected patients with symptomatic HF caused by LV systolic dysfunction despite optimal medical therapy, although at great financial cost and with important risks to patients. Recent studies have examined the use of CRT specifically in patients with mild or absent clinical HF; however, even in symptomatic patients, the response to CRT is inconsistent and raises questions about important subgroups in need of further study. Truly asymptomatic patients are not well represented in studies of "mild" heart failure, and the same questions on patient selection would apply even more forcefully to a group that would need many more years to manifest the benefits of therapy. Elderly asymptomatic patients in particular may be particularly prone to overtreatment in this context. The clinical community should call for more compelling evidence before expanding guidelines and practice to include CRT in asymptomatic heart failure.

### REFERENCES

1. Effect of metoprolol CR/XL in chronic heart failure: Metoprolol CR/XL Randomised Intervention Trial in Congestive Heart Failure (MERIT-HF). Lancet 1999; 353(9169):2001–7.

2. Effects of enalapril on mortality in severe congestive heart failure. Results of the Cooperative North Scandinavian Enalapril Survival Study (CONSENSUS). The CONSENSUS Trial Study Group. N Engl J Med 1987;316(23):1429–35.

3. Effect of enalapril on survival in patients with reduced left ventricular ejection fractions and congestive heart failure. The SOLVD Investigators. N Engl J Med 1991;325(5):293–302.

4. Pitt B, Zannad F, Remme WJ, et al. The effect of spironolactone on morbidity and mortality in patients with severe heart failure. Randomized Aldactone Evaluation Study Investigators. N Engl J Med 1999;341(10):709–17.

5. Pitt B, Remme W, Zannad F, et al. Eplerenone, a selective aldosterone blocker, in patients with left

ventricular dysfunction after myocardial infarction. N Engl J Med 2003;348(14):1309–21.

6. Moss AJ, Hall WJ, Cannom DS, et al. Improved survival with an implanted defibrillator in patients with coronary disease at high risk for ventricular arrhythmia. Multi-center Automatic Defibrillator Implantation Trial Investigators. N Engl J Med 1996;335(26):1933–40.

7. Moss AJ, Zareba W, Hall WJ, et al. Prophylactic implantation of a defibrillator in patients with myocardial infarction and reduced ejection fraction. N Engl J Med 2002;346(12):877–83.

8. Bristow MR, Saxon LA, Boehmer J, et al. Cardiac-resynchronization therapy with or without an implantable defibrillator in advanced chronic heart failure. N Engl J Med 2004;350(21):2140–50.

9. Cleland JG, Daubert JC, Erdmann E, et al. The effect of cardiac resynchronization on morbidity and mortality in heart failure. N Engl J Med 2005;352(15):1539–49.

10. Hunt SA, Abraham WT, Chin MH, et al. 2009 focused update incorporated into the ACC/AHA 2005 Guidelines for the Diagnosis and Management of Heart Failure in Adults: a report of the American College of Cardiology Foundation/American Heart Association Task Force on Practice Guidelines: developed in collaboration with the International Society for Heart and Lung Transplantation. Circulation 2009;119(14):e391–479.

11. Fonarow GC, Albert NM, Curtis AB, et al. Improving evidence-based care for heart failure in outpatient cardiology practices: primary results of the Registry to Improve the Use of Evidence-Based Heart Failure Therapies in the Outpatient Setting (IMPROVE HF). Circulation 2010;122(6):585–96.

12. Hlatky MA, Mark DB. The high cost of implantable defibrillators. Eur Heart J 2007;28(4):388–91.

13. Hlatky MA, Sanders GD, Owens DK. Cost-effectiveness of the implantable cardioverter defibrillator. Card Electrophysiol Rev 2003;7(4):479–82.

14. Moss AJ, Hall WJ, Cannom DS, et al. Cardiac-resynchronization therapy for the prevention of heart-failure events. N Engl J Med 2009;361(14):1329–38.

15. Linde C, Abraham WT, Gold MR, et al. Randomized trial of cardiac resynchronization in mildly symptomatic heart failure patients and in asymptomatic patients with left ventricular dysfunction and previous heart failure symptoms. J Am Coll Cardiol 2008;52(23):1834–43.

16. Yu CM, Chan JY, Zhang Q, et al. Biventricular pacing in patients with bradycardia and normal ejection fraction. N Engl J Med 2009;361(22):2123–34.

17. Cazeau S, Leclercq C, Lavergne T, et al. Effects of multisite biventricular pacing in patients with heart failure and intraventricular conduction delay. N Engl J Med 2001;344(12):873–80.

18. Abraham WT, Fisher WG, Smith AL, et al. Cardiac resynchronization in chronic heart failure. N Engl J Med 2002;346(24):1845–53.

19. Kramer DB, Josephson ME. Three questions for evidence-based cardiac electrophysiology. Circ Cardiovasc Qual Outcomes 2010;3(6):704–9.

20. Tang AS, Wells GA, Talajic M, et al. Cardiac-resynchronization therapy for mild-to-moderate heart failure. N Engl J Med 2010;363(25):2385–95.

21. Lubitz SA, Leong-Sit P, Fine N, et al. Effectiveness of cardiac resynchronization therapy in mild congestive heart failure: systematic review and meta-analysis of randomized trials. Eur J Heart Fail 2010;12(4):360–6.

22. Al-Majed NS, McAlister FA, Bakal JA, et al. Meta-analysis: cardiac resynchronization therapy for patients with less symptomatic heart failure. Ann Intern Med 2011;154(6):401–12.

23. Kaul S, Diamond GA. Trial and error. How to avoid commonly encountered limitations of published clinical trials. J Am Coll Cardiol 2010;55(5):415–27.

24. Tung R, Zimetbaum P, Josephson ME. A critical appraisal of implantable cardioverter-defibrillator therapy for the prevention of sudden cardiac death. J Am Coll Cardiol 2008;52(14):1111–21.

25. Myerburg RJ, Reddy V, Castellanos A. Indications for implantable cardioverter-defibrillators based on evidence and judgment. J Am Coll Cardiol 2009;54(9):747–63.

26. Jessup M. MADIT-CRT—breathtaking or time to catch our breath? N Engl J Med 2009;361(14):1394–6.

27. Bax JJ, Gorcsan J 3rd. Echocardiography and noninvasive imaging in cardiac resynchronization therapy: results of the PROSPECT (Predictors of Response to Cardiac Resynchronization Therapy) study in perspective. J Am Coll Cardiol 2009;53(21):1933–43.

28. Chung ES, Leon AR, Tavazzi L, et al. Results of the Predictors of Response to CRT (PROSPECT) trial. Circulation 2008;117(20):2608–16.

29. Achilli A, Peraldo C, Sassara M, et al. Prediction of response to cardiac resynchronization therapy: the selection of candidates for CRT (SCART) study. Pacing Clin Electrophysiol 2006;29(Suppl 2):S11–9.

30. Da Costa A, Thevenin J, Roche F, et al. Prospective validation of stress echocardiography as an identifier of cardiac resynchronization therapy responders. Heart Rhythm 2006;3(4):406–13.

31. Tedrow UB, Kramer DB, Stevenson LW, et al. Relation of right ventricular peak systolic pressure to major adverse events in patients undergoing cardiac resynchronization therapy. Am J Cardiol 2006;97(12):1737–40.

32. Singh JP, Klein HU, Huang DT, et al. Left ventricular lead position and clinical outcome in the multicenter automatic defibrillator implantation trial-cardiac

resynchronization therapy (MADIT-CRT) trial. Circulation 2011;123(11):1159–66.

33. Singh JP. QRS configuration and cardiac resynchronization therapy: do we need a patient-specific approach? Heart Rhythm 2009;6(10):1448–9.

34. Ellenbogen KA, Gold MR, Meyer TE, et al. Primary results from the SmartDelay determined AV optimization: a comparison to other AV delay methods used in cardiac resynchronization therapy (SMART-AV) trial: a randomized trial comparing empirical, echocardiography-guided, and algorithmic atrioventricular delay programming in cardiac resynchronization therapy. Circulation 2010;122(25):2660–8.

35. Kerlan JE, Sawhney NS, Waggoner AD, et al. Prospective comparison of echocardiographic atrioventricular delay optimization methods for cardiac resynchronization therapy. Heart Rhythm 2006;3(2):148–54.

36. Pfeffer MA, Jarcho JA. The charisma of subgroups and the subgroups of CHARISMA. N Engl J Med 2006;354(16):1744–6.

37. Rothwell PM. Treating individuals 2. Subgroup analysis in randomised controlled trials: importance, indications, and interpretation. Lancet 2005;365(9454):176–86.

38. Rothwell PM, Mehta Z, Howard SC, et al. Treating individuals 3: from subgroups to individuals: general principles and the example of carotid endarterectomy. Lancet 2005;365(9455):256–65.

39. Zareba W, Klein H, Cygankiewicz I, et al. Effectiveness of cardiac resynchronization therapy by QRS Morphology in the Multicenter Automatic Defibrillator Implantation Trial-Cardiac Resynchronization Therapy (MADIT-CRT). Circulation 2011;123(10):1061–72.

40. Epstein AE, DiMarco JP, Ellenbogen KA, et al. ACC/AHA/HRS 2008 Guidelines for Device-Based Therapy of Cardiac Rhythm Abnormalities: a report of the American College of Cardiology/American Heart Association Task Force on Practice Guidelines (Writing Committee to Revise the ACC/AHA/NASPE 2002 Guideline Update for Implantation of Cardiac Pacemakers and Antiarrhythmia Devices): developed in collaboration with the American Association for Thoracic Surgery and Society of Thoracic Surgeons. Circulation 2008;117(21):e350–408.

41. Beshai JF, Grimm RA, Nagueh SF, et al. Cardiac-resynchronization therapy in heart failure with narrow QRS complexes. N Engl J Med 2007;357(24):2461–71.

42. Stevenson LW. Challenges for the basis of practice in heart failure. Circ Heart Fail 2008;1(1):81–3.

43. Tricoci P, Allen JM, Kramer JM, et al. Scientific evidence underlying the ACC/AHA clinical practice guidelines. JAMA 2009;301(8):831–41.

44. Al-Khatib SM, Hellkamp A, Curtis J, et al. Non-evidence-based ICD implantations in the United States. JAMA 2011;305(1):43–9.

45. Kadish A, Goldberger J. Selecting patients for ICD implantation: are clinicians choosing appropriately? JAMA 2011;305(1):91–2.

46. Goldenberg I, Moss AJ. Implantable cardioverter defibrillator efficacy and chronic kidney disease: competing risks of arrhythmic and nonarrhythmic mortality. J Cardiovasc Electrophysiol 2008;19(12):1281–3.

47. Hager CS, Jain S, Blackwell J, et al. Effect of renal function on survival after implantable cardioverter defibrillator placement. Am J Cardiol 2010;106(9):1297–300.

48. Cuculich PS, Sanchez JM, Kerzner R, et al. Poor prognosis for patients with chronic kidney disease despite ICD therapy for the primary prevention of sudden death. Pacing Clin Electrophysiol 2007;30(2):207–13.

49. Van Bommel RJ, Mollema SA, Borleffs CJ, et al. Impaired renal function is associated with echocardiographic nonresponse and poor prognosis after cardiac resynchronization therapy. J Am Coll Cardiol 2011;57(5):549–55.

50. Lin G, Gersh BJ, Greene EL, et al. Renal function and mortality following cardiac resynchronization therapy. Eur Heart J 2011;32(2):184–90.

51. Reynolds CR, Jessup M. Translating the benefits of cardiac resynchronization therapy widely and wisely: challenges remain. Ann Intern Med 2011;154(6):436–8.

52. Hlatky MA, Sanders GD, Owens DK. Evidence-based medicine and policy: the case of the implantable cardioverter defibrillator. Health Aff (Millwood) 2005;24(1):42–51.

53. Desai AS, Fang JC, Maisel WH, et al. Implantable defibrillators for the prevention of mortality in patients with nonischemic cardiomyopathy: a meta-analysis of randomized controlled trials. JAMA 2004;292(23):2874–9.

54. Kadish A, Dyer A, Daubert JP, et al. Prophylactic defibrillator implantation in patients with nonischemic dilated cardiomyopathy. N Engl J Med 2004;350(21):2151–8.

55. Wikstrom G, Blomstrom-Lundqvist C, Andren B, et al. The effects of aetiology on outcome in patients treated with cardiac resynchronization therapy in the CARE-HF trial. Eur Heart J 2009;30(7):782–8.

56. Barsheshet A, Goldenberg I, Moss AJ, et al. Response to preventive cardiac resynchronization therapy in patients with ischaemic and nonischaemic cardiomyopathy in MADIT-CRT. Eur Heart J 2010;32(13):1622–30.

57. Bardy GH, Lee KL, Mark DB, et al. Amiodarone or an implantable cardioverter-defibrillator for congestive heart failure. N Engl J Med 2005;352(3):225–37.

58. Coceani M. Guideline challenge: has CRT earned a class I recommendation? Circ Heart Fail 2010;3(3):460–1.

59. Fein AS, Wang Y, Curtis JP, et al. Prevalence and predictors of off-label use of cardiac resynchronization therapy in patients enrolled in the National Cardiovascular Data Registry Implantable Cardiac-Defibrillator Registry. J Am Coll Cardiol 2010;56(10):766–73.

60. Bilchick KC, Kamath S, DiMarco JP, et al. Bundle-branch block morphology and other predictors of outcome after cardiac resynchronization therapy in Medicare patients. Circulation 2010;122(20):2022–30.

61. Cheng JW, Nayar M. A review of heart failure management in the elderly population. Am J Geriatr Pharmacother 2009;7(5):233–49.

62. Epstein AE, Kay GN, Plumb VJ, et al. Implantable cardioverter-defibrillator prescription in the elderly. Heart Rhythm 2009;6(8):1136–43.

63. Richardson DM, Bain KT, Diamond JJ, et al. Effectiveness of guideline-recommended cardiac drugs for reducing mortality in the elderly Medicare heart failure population: a retrospective, survey-weighted, cohort analysis. Drugs Aging 2010; 27(10):845–54.

64. Santangeli P, Di Biase L, Dello Russo A, et al. Meta-analysis: age and effectiveness of prophylactic implantable cardioverter-defibrillators. Ann Intern Med 2010;153(9):592–9.

65. Healey JS, Hallstrom AP, Kuck KH, et al. Role of the implantable defibrillator among elderly patients with a history of life-threatening ventricular arrhythmias. Eur Heart J 2007;28(14): 1746–9.

# Scar Mapping for Risk Stratification of Sudden Cardiac Death: Where Are We Now?

Antonio Dello Russo, MD, PhD*, Michela Casella, MD, PhD, Corrado Carbucicchio, MD, Claudio Tondo, MD, PhD

**KEYWORDS**
- Sudden cardiac death
- Implantable cardioverter-defibrillator • Scar mapping
- Risk stratification

Sudden cardiac death (SCD) accounts for 450,000 deaths yearly in the United States.[1] Overall, event rates in Europe are similar to those in the United States. In the past years, multiple clinical trials documented the effectiveness of the implantable cardioverter-defibrillator (ICD) to reduce SCD in high-risk patients. In particular, guideline-concluding trials have focused on left ventricular ejection fraction (EF) because of its demonstrated association with mortality risk in patients with recent myocardial infarction,[2] and current guidelines give prophylactic ICD indication based on EF only.[3,4] However, the absolute number of SCDs prevented applying current guidelines in the clinical practice is unacceptably low when compared with the total number of SCDs that occur yearly.[5,6] In particular, it is worrisome that most SCDs occur in the general population as the first and last manifestation of a subclinical cardiac disease.[6,7]

Moreover, a substantial proportion of patients who receive an ICD for primary prevention according to current recommendations will never experience arrhythmic events, thus, negating the potential benefit of ICDs while unnecessarily exposing to a risky and costly procedure.[8]

In the past years, multiple risk markers have been tested to improve current risk stratification. However, despite the initial enthusiasm, all the suggested risk markers have not been consistently demonstrated of incremental predictive value when compared with EF. On the other hand, recent evidence has suggested a striking association between anatomic substrate abnormalities and major arrhythmic events and mortality in patients with dilated cardiomyopathy (DCM). The novelty of these new risk markers mainly consists in their high positive and negative predictive value, although they have been mainly tested in a small population of patients and in retrospective analyses.

## CARDIAC MAGNETIC RESONANCE TO ASSESS ANATOMIC SUBSTRATE ABNORMALITIES

Cardiac magnetic resonance imaging (MRI) has been established as an accurate and reliable tool to distinguish between viable and fibrotic myocardial areas. In particular, gadolinium contrast-enhanced imaging protocols have demonstrated a close correlation with histologic data, especially in ischemic cardiomyopathy.[9–13] In the seminal study by Kim and colleagues,[12] 8 dogs were subjected to transient coronary occlusion (to produce transient myocardial ischemia), whereas 18 dogs underwent permanent coronary ligation (to produce irreversible myocardial injury). In vivo cine-MRI and delayed enhancement (DE) MRI were performed at various time points (1 day, 3 days, 8 weeks) following coronary manipulation. Animals were then sacrificed, and ex vivo DE-MRI was performed before histopathology analysis using triphenyl tetrazolium chloride (TTC) staining for the determination of infarct size. In animals subjected to coronary ligation, there was a near exact correlation between DE-MRI

Cardiac Arrhythmia Research Center, Centro Cardiologico Monzino, IRCCS, Via Parea 4, 20138 Milan, Italy
* Corresponding author.
*E-mail address:* antonio.dellorusso@ccfm.it

Card Electrophysiol Clin 3 (2011) 539–547
doi:10.1016/j.ccep.2011.08.001
1877-9182/11/$ – see front matter © 2011 Elsevier Inc. All rights reserved.

and histopathology-evidenced infarct size in the acute (r = .99, P<.001) and chronic (r = .97, P<.001) infarct settings. DE-MRI also provided accurate assessment of infarct morphology, closely replicating histopathology-evidenced infarct shape and contours. Conversely, in animals subjected to transient coronary occlusion, the affected coronary territories did not demonstrate hyperenhancement or histopathology-evidenced infarct despite transient impairment in myocardial contractility.

The reliability of MRI in myocardial tissue characterization has been consistently confirmed in further studies.[11,14–16] Since these demonstrations, the use of DE-MRI has dramatically expanded to better characterize the pathologic substrate underlying both ischemic and nonischemic cardiomyopathy. Highly specific patterns of fibrosis and scarring have been identified in many of cardiomyopathies.[17] Ischemic cardiomyopathy is characterized by subendocardial-based areas of late enhancement that correlate with myocardial fibrosis on histopathology, a pattern consistent with the wave front phenomenon as initially described by Reimer and colleagues.[18] Patients who have nonischemic DCM may also have DE evidence of scarring in up to 28% of cases; however, this is typically in a noncoronary distribution and is frequently seen in midwall or epicardial myocardium layers.[19]

Interestingly, the presence and distribution of myocardial scar tissue, as assessed by MRI, has been also found to carry important prognostic information. Nazarian and colleagues[20] reported that the volume and surface area of myocardial scars measured with MRI was well correlated with inducible ventricular arrhythmias on programmed stimulation in patients with ischemic and nonischemic cardiomyopathy. Recently, Yan and colleagues[21] showed that a larger scar border zone on MRI, which may indicate tissue heterogeneity and arrhythmogenic substrate, is actually predictive of all-cause and cardiovascular mortality independent of age and systolic function. It bears emphasis that this intriguing link between myocardial scar area and morphology, as assessed by MRI, and adverse cardiovascular outcome is being increasingly recognized in different myocardial diseases, including chronic myocarditis[22] and hypertrophic cardiomyopathy.[23,24]

## ELECTROANATOMIC MAPPING TO ASSESS ANATOMIC SUBSTRATE ABNORMALITIES AND SCARS IN ISCHEMIC CARDIOMYOPATHY

The role of electroanatomic mapping (EAM) in the risk stratification of patients undergoing prophylactic ICD implant has not been established. In recent years, high-density EAM has been used to characterize the electrical correlates of arrhythmogenic substrates in different clinical settings.[25,26] Regions with delayed and fragmented conduction bordering on scar tissue[27,28] and islets of surviving myocytes within otherwise dense scars[25–28] have all been demonstrated to be essential components of reentrant circuits that underlie ventricular tachycardia (VT).

However, several previous reports have suggested that EAM may represent a helpful tool to identify patients at risk of developing malignant ventricular arrhythmias, especially in patients with previous myocardial infarction. The earlier study by Cassidy and colleagues[29] was conducted on 132 patients with coronary artery disease and 26 patients with nonischemic DCM with different clinical presentation, ranging from no arrhythmias to cardiac arrest. They used a nondeflectable catheter with 1-cm bipolar spacing to sample from a mean of 11 left ventricular endocardial sites and found that patients presenting with sustained monomorphic VT had more abnormal endocardial electrograms and more evidence of slow endocardial conduction.

In the ablation era, high-density EAM has been used to characterize the electrophysiological substrate underlying malignant ventricular arrhythmias. Scar border zone regions as well as isolated and very late potentials within otherwise apparently dense scars have been consistently reported as critical components of the reentrant circuit and have all been successfully targeted for ablation (**Fig. 1**).[26–28] Recently, Haqqani and colleagues[30] reported a detailed left ventricular EAM case-control study, conducted on 17 patients with ischemic DCM and sustained monomorphic VT as compared with 17 patients with ischemic DCM and no history of arrhythmias. Patients with a history of VT showed wider low-voltage areas (55% of surface area vs 30%, P<.001) and more fractionated, isolated, and very late potentials. No other clinical or laboratory parameter, including EF, differed between the two groups.

## SUBSTRATE ABNORMALITIES AND SCAR MAPPING IN NONISCHEMIC CARDIOMYOPATHY

A major challenge in cardiology concerns the individuation of mechanisms underlying different clinical severity among patients with the same disease. Arrhythmogenic right ventricular cardiomyopathy (ARVC) is characterized by a progressive fibrofatty substitution of the ventricular myocardium, which leads to islets of residual myocytes

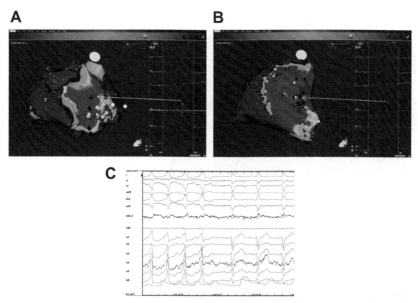

**Fig. 1.** A 64-year-old patient with ischemic dilated cardiomyopathy presenting with electrical storm. Endocardial (*A*) and epicardial (*B*) bipolar voltage maps of the left ventricle, obtained in sequence, showing a low-voltage area in the posterior perimitral region, including late and fragmented potentials (*white arrows*). Red dots mark ablation lesions, which were initially performed from the epicardial side targeting late potentials and subsequently performed on the endocardial side. (*C*) Clinical VT being interrupted during endocardial ablation.

interspersed among adipocytes and fibrous tissue.[31–33] Such pathologic substrates provide an ideal milieu for reentrant life-threatening ventricular arrhythmias.[33] However, it is unknown why only a subset of patients with ARVC develops clinical sustained VT despite the presence of myocardial fibrofatty tissue in all of these patients.

Although all patients with ARVC share the same substrate consisting of myocardial fibrofatty replacement, the clinical phenotypes are highly heterogeneous and span from no symptoms to congestive heart failure or arrhythmic sudden cardiac death.[31,34,35] In particular, arrhythmic events are the most important manifestation of ARVC and account for the greater part of ARVC-related mortality.[34,35] The correct identification of patients with ARVC at risk of arrhythmic events constitutes the major challenge of risk stratification because it would allow tailoring adequate and effective therapies to specific patients, such as ICD or substrate modification by catheter ablation.[36–38] Unfortunately, thus far, the identification of markers of increased arrhythmic risk has been elusive, and the most widespread practice is to implant an ICD in all patients with a definite diagnosis of ARVC, reserving substrate-based catheter ablation for patients with a clinical history of sustained ventricular arrhythmias.[36,37] The limitations of such an approach have been highlighted.[36] Data from large ICD registries of ARVC

support the concept that the risk of arrhythmic events in these patients is highly variable, and among clinical and instrumental findings, including programmed ventricular stimulation, only the history of syncope seems to independently predict the risk of subsequent arrhythmic events.[36] On the other hand, risk stratification based only on a history of syncope is still suboptimal because up to 20% of patients without such a history will develop major arrhythmic events.[36] Previous studies have demonstrated that EAM may represent a helpful strategy to identify substrate abnormalities in patients with ARVC.[38] Avella and colleagues[39] showed for the first time that endomyocardial biopsy (EMB) guided by right ventricular EAM could increase the sensitivity of the conventional biopsy technique in the diagnosis of ARVC.

Several studies demonstrated that fibrofatty tissue is predominant in the epicardial layers suggesting that the abnormal process of the disease begins in the epicardium and spreads toward the endocardium (**Fig. 2**).[40–43] Garcia and colleagues[44] recently demonstrated that a combined endocardial-epicardial ablation approach was useful in the control of life-threatening arrhythmias in patients with ARVC with VT and previous failed endocardial ablation. The same group recently described a new technique for identifying the presence and the anatomic extent of epicardial substrate

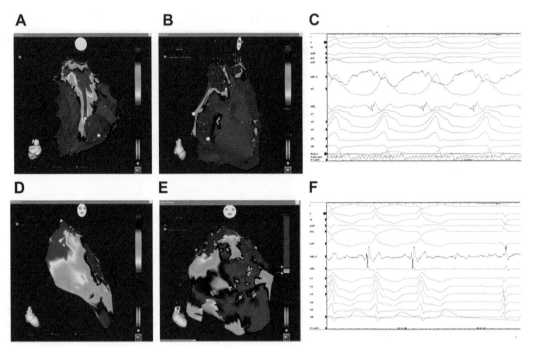

**Fig. 2.** A 66-year-old patient with ARVC who had previously undergone a failed endocardial catheter ablation and presented with electrical storm. (*A*) Endocardial bipolar voltage map of the right ventricle showing a low-voltage area in the posterior region of the outflow tract, extending to the tricuspid ring. (*B*) Extensive endocardial ablation lesions in the low-voltage area described previously. (*C*) Clinical VT persisting despite endocardial ablation and satisfactory early activation on the distal ablation catheter. (*D*) Epicardial bipolar voltage map of the right ventricle showing a corresponding low-voltage area in the posterior wall. (*E*) Extensive epicardial ablation lesions in the low-voltage area just described. (*F*) Clinical VT being interrupted during epicardial ablation.

abnormalities consistent with scar tissue in patients with ARVC.[45] The investigators demonstrated that endocardial unipolar mapping with a cutoff of 5.5 mV identifies more extensive areas of epicardial bipolar signal abnormalities in patients with arrhythmogenic right ventricular dysplasia/cardiomyopathy (ARVD/C) in comparison with the endocardial substrate EAM.[45]

*Myocarditis* is simply defined as an inflammatory condition mainly located in the heart muscle,[46–49] although considerable uncertainties still persist as to its etiological, pathologic, and clinical subclassifications. The clinical course is also variable[50,51]; a spontaneous recovery may occur after the acute phase in up to 50% of patients, but chronic inflammatory cardiomyopathy and DCM sustained by viral persistence or autoimmune self-perpetration represent a common evolution of the disease.

Myocarditis may cause arrhythmias both in its acute phase, caused by inflammatory infiltration and myocyte necrosis, and in its chronic phase, caused by immune reaction, fibrosis, and resulting electrical remodeling.[52–56] Previous studies have reported that EAM may be a helpful approach for the arrhythmic risk stratification in drug-refractory

patients with myocarditis VT.[38] Moreover, a recent study has demonstrated that EAM-guided EMB may be a safe and effective approach in the differential diagnosis of patients with myocarditis mimicking ARVC.[57]

## LESS-FREQUENT CARDIOMYOPATHIES

Sarcoidosis, amyloidosis, and hemochromatosis are systemic infiltrative disorders with a potential for diffuse organ involvement that also commonly affect the heart.

*Sarcoidosis* is an infiltrative disorder marked by granulomatous involvement of multiple organs and accounts for about 5 to 10 of nonischemic VTs. A cardiac involvement occurs in 20% to 40% of overall patients with sarcoidosis, and sudden cardiac death accounts for 30% to 70% of all deaths; even if severe conduction disturbances are frequent, tachyarrhythmias are supposed to be the most relevant cause for death,[58,59] and the degree of cardiac infiltration seems to be correlated with the risk of arrhythmic death.[60] According to etiopathology, granulomas or scars caused by deep subendocardial fibrous replacement represent the bases for reentry in both the right and the left ventricle; an epicardial or intramural origin of ventricular arrhythmias is likely in most patients. A prevalence of the peritricuspid and left basal regions is the rule, but multiple morphologies of VT (**Fig. 3**) frequently occur, even in cases of well-preserved ventricular function.

The clinical manifestations of cardiac sarcoidosis are largely nonspecific. As a result, diagnostic tests, such as EBM, or imaging may be required, particularly in patients without other manifestations of the disease.[61–63]

Transvenous EMB is an established diagnostic technique for evaluating cardiac involvement by sarcoidosis but carries a low sensitive value because of the inhomogeneous myocardial involvement (with a prevalence of the basal regions).[64]

Experience with MRI to diagnose or monitor myocardial sarcoidosis is somehow limited. A variety of findings have been noted, including a localized cardiac scar and localized high-intensity areas on T1- or T2-weighted images.[65]

However, gadolinium–diethylenetriamine penta-acetic acid enhancement permits earlier detection of cardiac involvement/scarring and the assessment of the efficacy of steroid therapy,[65–68] with a high sensitivity and specificity of late gadolinium enhancement. A previous case report study[69] suggests the usefulness of EAM to identify the cardiac substrate abnormalities in patients with sarcoidosis (see **Fig. 3**).

*Myotonic dystrophy type 1* (MD1), or Steinert disease, is the most common inherited muscular dystrophy in adults.[70,71] It is a genetic disorder with autosomal-dominant transmission. Sudden cardiac death represents 2% to 30% of fatalities.[72,73] Sudden cardiac death was previously ascribed to conduction blocks, but ventricular arrhythmias have recently been demonstrated to play a role, thus, suggesting alterations involving not only the conduction system, as initially proposed, but also the myocardium.[74,75]

A previous electroanatomic study[76] showed the presence of low voltage in both the right atrium

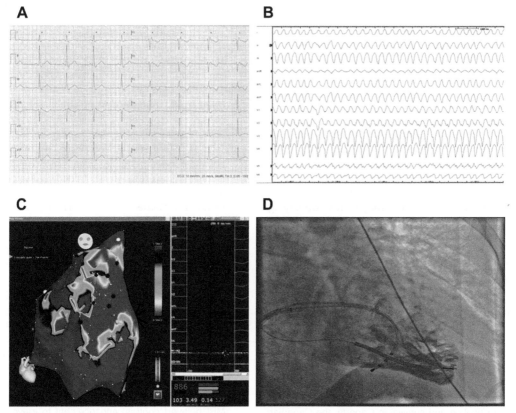

**Fig. 3.** A 38-year-old patient with suspected ARVC who presented with sustained VT. (*A*) A 12-lead electrocardiogram showing complete right bundle branch block and negative T waves in leads V$_1$ to V$_4$. (*B*) Clinical VT with left bundle branch morphology and superior axis. (*C*) Endocardial bipolar voltage map of the right ventricle showing a wide low-voltage area in the anterior-lateral wall. Blue dots mark the sites of late potentials that were then targeted for ablation. (*D*) Right ventricular angiography with abnormal gross trabeculations.

and ventricle confirming that not only the specialized conduction tissue but also the myocardium is affected in this disease. The EAM may be a useful tool to estimate the extent of cardiac involvement and the arrhythmic risk of patients with MD1.

In primary *amyloidosis*, the cardiac involvement and the correspondent clinical manifestations are common in about one-third of patients but are rarely isolated (4%); hemodynamic disturbances related to the restrictive pattern of cardiomyopathy are prevalent with progressive biventricular heart failure. Malignant ventricular arrhythmias present in the late stage of the disease and sudden cardiac death occurs in up to 30% of patients.

A less common cause for sudden cardiac death among infiltrative cardiomyopathies is represented by *hemochromatosis* in which the accumulation of iron in myocardial tissues leads to an arrhythmogenic substrate and an increased risk for VTs, especially in the juvenile-onset phenotype.

## SUMMARY

Sudden cardiac death still represents the most challenging and controversial issue in cardiology. Even though implementation of ICD in high-risk patients has been proved to be effective in reducing SCD, the occurrence of life-threatening arrhythmias in the general population is disproportionately high as the expression of latent cardiac disease. Substrate myocardial analysis seems to be of pivotal importance to detect anatomic abnormalities underlying clinical conditions predisposing major arrhythmic events. High-density EAM may be considered an effective technique to define substrate abnormalities in different clinical settings and its electrical correlates. Preliminary data have shown that EAM may help in identifying myocardial substrate abnormalities in patients with ventricular arrhythmic disorders. Therefore, this should prompt a widespread use of the technique in the attempt to improve the identification of markers of increased arrhythmic risk.

## REFERENCES

1. Zheng ZJ, Croft JB, Giles WH, et al. Sudden cardiac death in the United States, 1989 to 1998. Circulation 2001;104:2158–63.
2. Rouleau JL, Talajic M, Sussex B, et al. Myocardial infarction patients in the 1990s–their risk factors, stratification and survival in Canada: the Canadian Assessment of Myocardial Infarction (CAMI) study. J Am Coll Cardiol 1996;27:1119–27.
3. Zipes DP, Camm AJ, Borggrefe M, et al. ACC/AHA/ ESC 2006 guidelines for management of patients with ventricular arrhythmias and the prevention of sudden cardiac death: a report of the American College of Cardiology/American Heart Association Task Force and the European Society of Cardiology Committee for Practice Guidelines (writing committee to develop guidelines for management of patients with ventricular arrhythmias and the prevention of sudden cardiac death): developed in collaboration with the European Heart Rhythm Association and the Heart Rhythm Society. Circulation 2006;114: e385–484.
4. Epstein AE, DiMarco JP, Ellenbogen KA, et al. ACC/ AHA/HRS 2008 guidelines for device-based therapy of cardiac rhythm abnormalities: a report of the American College of Cardiology/American Heart Association Task Force on Practice Guidelines (writing committee to revise the ACC/AHA/NASPE 2002 guideline update for implantation of cardiac pacemakers and antiarrhythmia devices): developed in collaboration with the American Association for Thoracic Surgery and Society of Thoracic Surgeons. Circulation 2008;117:e350–408.
5. de Vreede-Swagemakers JJ, Gorgels AP, Dubois-Arbouw WI, et al. Out-of-hospital cardiac arrest in the 1990's: a population-based study in the Maastricht area on incidence, characteristics and survival. J Am Coll Cardiol 1997;30:1500–5.
6. Myerburg RJ, Kessler KM, Castellanos A. Sudden cardiac death: epidemiology, transient risk, and intervention assessment. Ann Intern Med 1993;119: 1187–97.
7. Myerburg RJ. Sudden cardiac death: exploring the limits of our knowledge. J Cardiovasc Electrophysiol 2001;12:369–81.
8. Tung R, Zimetbaum P, Josephson ME. A critical appraisal of implantable cardioverter-defibrillator therapy for the prevention of sudden cardiac death. J Am Coll Cardiol 2008;52:1111–21.
9. Amado LC, Gerber BL, Gupta SN, et al. Accurate and objective infarct sizing by contrast-enhanced magnetic resonance imaging in a canine myocardial infarction model. J Am Coll Cardiol 2004;44:2383–9.
10. Barkhausen J, Ebert W, Debatin JF, et al. Imaging of myocardial infarction: comparison of Magnevist and gadophrin-3 in rabbits. J Am Coll Cardiol 2002;39: 1392–8.
11. Fieno DS, Kim RJ, Chen EL, et al. Contrast-enhanced magnetic resonance imaging of myocardium at risk: distinction between reversible and irreversible injury throughout infarct healing. J Am Coll Cardiol 2000;36:1985–91.
12. Kim RJ, Fieno DS, Parrish TB, et al. Relationship of MRI delayed contrast enhancement to irreversible injury, infarct age, and contractile function. Circulation 1999;100:1992–2002.
13. Wagner A, Mahrholdt H, Holly TA, et al. Contrast-enhanced MRI and routine single photon emission

computed tomography (SPECT) perfusion imaging for detection of subendocardial myocardial infarcts: an imaging study. Lancet 2003;361:374–9.

14. Mahrholdt H, Wagner A, Holly TA, et al. Reproducibility of chronic infarct size measurement by contrast-enhanced magnetic resonance imaging. Circulation 2002;106:2322–7.

15. Wagner A, Mahrholdt H, Thomson L, et al. Effects of time, dose, and inversion time for acute myocardial infarct size measurements based on magnetic resonance imaging-delayed contrast enhancement. J Am Coll Cardiol 2006;47:2027–33.

16. Wu E, Judd RM, Vargas JD, et al. Visualisation of presence, location, and transmural extent of healed Q-wave and non-Q-wave myocardial infarction. Lancet 2001;357:21–8.

17. Mahrholdt H, Wagner A, Judd RM, et al. Delayed enhancement cardiovascular magnetic resonance assessment of non-ischaemic cardiomyopathies. Eur Heart J 2005;26:1461–74.

18. Reimer KA, Lowe JE, Rasmussen MM, et al. The wavefront phenomenon of ischemic cell death. 1. Myocardial infarct size vs duration of coronary occlusion in dogs. Circulation 1977;56:786–94.

19. Soriano CJ, Ridocci F, Estornell J, et al. Noninvasive diagnosis of coronary artery disease in patients with heart failure and systolic dysfunction of uncertain etiology, using late gadolinium-enhanced cardiovascular magnetic resonance. J Am Coll Cardiol 2005; 45:743–8.

20. Nazarian S, Bluemke DA, Lardo AC, et al. Magnetic resonance assessment of the substrate for inducible ventricular tachycardia in nonischemic cardiomyopathy. Circulation 2005;112:2821–5.

21. Yan AT, Shayne AJ, Brown KA, et al. Characterization of the peri-infarct zone by contrast-enhanced cardiac magnetic resonance imaging is a powerful predictor of post-myocardial infarction mortality. Circulation 2006;114:32–9.

22. De Cobelli F, Pieroni M, Esposito A, et al. Delayed gadolinium-enhanced cardiac magnetic resonance in patients with chronic myocarditis presenting with heart failure or recurrent arrhythmias. J Am Coll Cardiol 2006;47:1649–54.

23. Leonardi S, Raineri C, De Ferrari GM, et al. Usefulness of cardiac magnetic resonance in assessing the risk of ventricular arrhythmias and sudden death in patients with hypertrophic cardiomyopathy. Eur Heart J 2009;30:2003–10.

24. Satoh H, Matoh F, Shiraki K, et al. Delayed enhancement on cardiac magnetic resonance and clinical, morphological, and electrocardiographical features in hypertrophic cardiomyopathy. J Card Fail 2009; 15:419–27.

25. Callans DJ, Ren JF, Michele J, et al. Electroanatomic left ventricular mapping in the porcine model of healed anterior myocardial infarction. Correlation with intracardiac echocardiography and pathological analysis. Circulation 1999;100:1744–50.

26. Arenal A, Glez-Torrecilla E, Ortiz M, et al. Ablation of electrograms with an isolated, delayed component as treatment of unmappable monomorphic ventricular tachycardias in patients with structural heart disease. J Am Coll Cardiol 2003;41:81–92.

27. Marchlinski FE, Callans DJ, Gottlieb CD, et al. Linear ablation lesions for control of unmappable ventricular tachycardia in patients with ischemic and nonischemic cardiomyopathy. Circulation 2000;101: 1288–96.

28. Soejima K, Suzuki M, Maisel WH, et al. Catheter ablation in patients with multiple and unstable ventricular tachycardias after myocardial infarction: short ablation lines guided by reentry circuit isthmuses and sinus rhythm mapping. Circulation 2001;104:664–9.

29. Cassidy DM, Vassallo JA, Miller JM, et al. Endocardial catheter mapping in patients in sinus rhythm: relationship to underlying heart disease and ventricular arrhythmias. Circulation 1986;73:645–52.

30. Haqqani HM, Kalman JM, Roberts-Thomson KC, et al. Fundamental differences in electrophysiologic and electroanatomic substrate between ischemic cardiomyopathy patients with and without clinical ventricular tachycardia. J Am Coll Cardiol 2009;54:166–73.

31. Marcus FI, Fontaine GH, Guiraudon G, et al. Right ventricular dysplasia: a report of 24 adult cases. Circulation 1982;65:384–98.

32. Thiene G, Basso C. Arrhythmogenic right ventricular cardiomyopathy: an update. Cardiovasc Pathol 2001;10:109–17.

33. Corrado D, Basso C, Thiene G, et al. Spectrum of clinicopathologic manifestations of arrhythmogenic right ventricular cardiomyopathy/dysplasia: a multicenter study. J Am Coll Cardiol 1997;30:1512–20.

34. Dalal D, Nasir K, Bomma C, et al. Arrhythmogenic right ventricular dysplasia: a United States experience. Circulation 2005;112:3823–32.

35. Hamid MS, Norman M, Quraishi A, et al. Prospective evaluation of relatives for familial arrhythmogenic right ventricular cardiomyopathy/dysplasia reveals a need to broaden diagnostic criteria. J Am Coll Cardiol 2002;40:1445–50.

36. Corrado D, Calkins H, Link MS, et al. Prophylactic implantable defibrillator in patients with arrhythmogenic right ventricular cardiomyopathy/dysplasia and no prior ventricular fibrillation or sustained ventricular tachycardia. Circulation 2010;122:1144–52.

37. Verma A, Kilicaslan F, Schweikert RA, et al. Short- and long-term success of substrate-based mapping and ablation of ventricular tachycardia in arrhythmogenic right ventricular dysplasia. Circulation 2005; 111:3209–16.

38. Corrado D, Basso C, Leoni L, et al. Three-dimensional electroanatomic voltage mapping increases

accuracy of diagnosing arrhythmogenic right ventricular cardiomyopathy/dysplasia. Circulation 2005;111:3042–50.

39. Avella A, d'Amati G, Pappalardo A, et al. Diagnostic value of endomyocardial biopsy guided by electroanatomic voltage mapping in arrhythmogenic right ventricular cardiomyopathy/dysplasia. J Cardiovasc Electrophysiol 2008;19:1127–34.

40. Burke AP, Farb A, Tashko G, et al. Arrhythmogenic right ventricular cardiomyopathy and fatty replacement of the right ventricular myocardium: are they different diseases? Circulation 1998;97:1571–80.

41. Kies P, Bootsma M, Bax J, et al. Arrhythmogenic right ventricular dysplasia/cardiomyopathy: screening, diagnosis, and treatment. Heart Rhythm 2006;3:225–34.

42. Arruda M, Armaganijan L, Fahmy T, et al. Catheter ablation of ventricular tachycardia in arrhythmogenic right ventricular dysplasia. J Interv Card Electrophysiol 2009;25:129–33.

43. Fontaine G, Fontaliran F, Hebert JL, et al. Arrhythmogenic right ventricular dysplasia. Annu Rev Med 1999;50:17–35.

44. Garcia FC, Bazan V, Zado ES, et al. Epicardial substrate and outcome with epicardial ablation of ventricular tachycardia in arrhythmogenic right ventricular cardiomyopathy/dysplasia. Circulation 2009;120:366–75.

45. Polin GM, Haqqani H, Tzou W, et al. Endocardial unipolar voltage mapping to identify epicardial substrate in arrhythmogenic right ventricular cardiomyopathy/dysplasia. Heart Rhythm 2011;8:76–83.

46. Hufnagel G, Pankuweit S, Richter A, et al. The European Study of Epidemiology and Treatment of Cardiac Inflammatory Diseases (ESETCID). First epidemiological results. Herz 2000;25:279–85.

47. Howlett JG, McKelvie RS, Arnold JM, et al. Canadian Cardiovascular Society Consensus Conference guidelines on heart failure, update 2009: diagnosis and management of right-sided heart failure, myocarditis, device therapy and recent important clinical trials. Can J Cardiol 2009;25:85–105.

48. JCS Joint Working Group. Guidelines for diagnosis and treatment of myocarditis (JCS 2009). Circ J 2011;75:734–43.

49. Maisch B, Portig I, Ristic A, et al. Definition of inflammatory cardiomyopathy (myocarditis): on the way to consensus. A status report. Herz 2000;25:200–9.

50. Richardson P, McKenna W, Bristow M, et al. Report of the 1995 World Health Organization/International Society and Federation of Cardiology Task Force on the definition and classification of cardiomyopathies. Circulation 1996;93:841–2.

51. Magnani JW, Dec GW. Myocarditis: current trends in diagnosis and treatment. Circulation 2006;113:876–90.

52. Blauwet LA, Cooper LT. Myocarditis. Prog Cardiovasc Dis 2010;52:274–88.

53. Cooper LT Jr. Myocarditis. N Engl J Med 2009;360:1526–38.

54. Schultz JC, Hilliard AA, Cooper LT Jr, et al. Diagnosis and treatment of viral myocarditis. Mayo Clin Proc 2009;84:1001–9.

55. Kindermann I, Kindermann M, Kandolf R, et al. Predictors of outcome in patients with suspected myocarditis. Circulation 2008;118:639–48.

56. Magnani JW, Danik HJ, Dec GW Jr, et al. Survival in biopsy-proven myocarditis: a long-term retrospective analysis of the histopathologic, clinical, and hemodynamic predictors. Am Heart J 2006;151:463–70.

57. Pieroni M, Dello Russo A, Marzo F, et al. High prevalence of myocarditis mimicking arrhythmogenic right ventricular cardiomyopathy differential diagnosis by electroanatomic mapping-guided endomyocardial biopsy. J Am Coll Cardiol 2009;53(8):681–9.

58. Roberts WC, McAllister HA Jr, Ferrans VJ. Sarcoidosis of the heart. A clinicopathologic study of 35 necropsy patients (group 1) and review of 78 previously described necropsy patients (group 11). Am J Med 1977;63:86–108.

59. Smedema JP, Snoep G, van Kroonenburgh MP, et al. Cardiac involvement in patients with pulmonary sarcoidosis assessed at two university medical centers in the Netherlands. Chest 2005;128:30.

60. Padilla M. Cardiac sarcoidosis. In: Baughman R, editor. Lung biology in health and disease. Sarcoidosis, vol. 210. New YorK: Taylor & Francis Group; 2006. p. 515.

61. Chapelon-Abric C, de Zuttere D, Duhaut P, et al. Cardiac sarcoidosis: a retrospective study of 41 cases. Medicine (Baltimore) 2004;83:315.

62. Yoshida Y, Morimoto S, Hiramitsu S, et al. Incidence of cardiac sarcoidosis in Japanese patients with high-degree atrioventricular block. Am Heart J 1997;134:382.

63. Sekiguchi M, Yazaki Y, Isobe M, et al. Cardiac sarcoidosis: diagnostic, prognostic, and therapeutic considerations. Cardiovasc Drugs Ther 1996;10:495.

64. Uemura A, Morimoto S, Hiramitsu S, et al. Histologic diagnostic rate of cardiac sarcoidosis: evaluation of endomyocardial biopsies. Am Heart J 1999;138:299.

65. Smedema JP, Snoep G, van Kroonenburgh MP, et al. Evaluation of the accuracy of gadolinium-enhanced cardiovascular magnetic resonance in the diagnosis of cardiac sarcoidosis. J Am Coll Cardiol 2005;45:1683.

66. Shimada T, Shimada K, Sakane T, et al. Diagnosis of cardiac sarcoidosis and evaluation of the effects of steroid therapy by gadolinium-DTPA-enhanced magnetic resonance imaging. Am J Med 2001;110:520.

67. Tadamura E, Yamamuro M, Kubo S, et al. Effectiveness of delayed enhanced MRI for identification of

cardiac sarcoidosis: comparison with radionuclide imaging. AJR Am J Roentgenol 2005;185:110.

68. Smedema JP, Snoep G, van Kroonenburgh MP, et al. The additional value of gadolinium-enhanced MRI to standard assessment for cardiac involvement in patients with pulmonary sarcoidosis. Chest 2005; 128:1629.

69. Santucci PA, Morton JB, Picken MM, et al. Electroanatomic mapping of the right ventricle in a patient with a giant epsilon wave, ventricular tachycardia, and cardiac sarcoidosis. J Cardiovasc Electrophysiol 2004;15(9):1091–4.

70. Steinert H. Myopathologische Beitrage 1. Uber das klinische und anatomische Bild des Muskelschwunds der Myotoniker. Dtsch Z Nervenheikld 1909; 37:58–104 [in German].

71. Ashizawa T, Epstein HF. Ethnic distribution of myotonic dystrophy gene. Lancet 1991;338:642–3.

72. Mathieu J, Allard P, Potvin L, et al. A 10 year study of mortality in a cohort of patients with myotonic dystrophy. Neurology 1999;52:1658–62.

73. Die-Smulders CM, Howeler CJ, Thijs C, et al. Age and causes of death in adult-onset myotonic dystrophy. Brain 1998;121:1557–63.

74. Prystowsky EN, Pritchett EL, Roses AD, et al. The natural history of conduction system disease in myotonic muscular dystrophy as determined by serial electrophysiologic studies. Circulation 1979; 60:1360–4.

75. Pelargonio G, Dello Russo A, Sanna T, et al. Myotonic dystrophy and the heart. Heart 2002;88: 665–70.

76. Dello Russo A, Pelargonio G, Parisi Q, et al. Widespread electroanatomic alterations of right cardiac chambers in patients with myotonic dystrophy type 1. J Cardiovasc Electrophysiol 2006;17(1):34–40.

# ICD Efficacy Should Be Evaluated at Implantation

Steven M. Markowitz, MD

## KEYWORDS

- Implantable cardioverter defibrillator
- Defibrillation threshold • Clinical outcome • Testing protocol

Since the inception of implantable cardioverter defibrillator (ICD) implantation, intraoperative defibrillation testing has been considered integral to the procedure. The rationale for device testing was based on the assumption that demonstrating effective defibrillation below the maximum output of the device provides the confidence that the system would terminate spontaneous life-threatening arrhythmias. However, in the contemporary era of ICD implantation, advances in ICD technology and recent outcomes data have exposed this assumption to critical reevaluation, and the role of routine peri-implant defibrillation testing has increasingly been questioned.[1–3] This article reviews counterarguments that support the value of defibrillation testing at the time of implantation.

## THE CONCEPTS OF DEFIBRILLATION THRESHOLD AND SAFETY MARGIN

In experimental and clinical testing scenarios, defibrillation exhibits probabilistic behavior. Defibrillation success curves can be determined by repeating defibrillation multiple times at different energy levels. The resulting probabilities can be fitted to a logistic regression curve demonstrating a sigmoidal dose-response curve (**Fig. 1**). An exponential curve might better describe the relationship, because it identifies energies below which the probability of defibrillation is zero. It has also been suggested that the apparent probabilistic behavior of defibrillation is related to changes in current defibrillation requirements with increasing number of episodes tested.[4]

The defibrillation threshold (DFT) has been variously defined, but one rigorous scientific definition is an energy or voltage for a particular electrode configuration and pulse contour at which defibrillation is successful 50% of the time.[5,6] In clinical situations, it is impractical and possibly unsafe to perform a large number of defibrillation trials, and several protocols have been devised to approximate various points on the dose-response curve. These protocols essentially measure the lowest energy of defibrillation (LED) and include step-down, step-up, and binary search protocols.[7]

The concept of a safety margin is also subject to different interpretations and definitions. One way to conceptualize the safety margin is the difference between the DFT and the maximal output of the ICD (the measured safety margin). The importance of a 10-J safety margin emerged in a study of 33 patients in the era of epicardial defibrillation systems and monophasic shocks, in which patients with implant safety margins of less than 10 J were more likely to fail defibrillation during postoperative device testing.[8] Subsequent studies supported the observation that patients with low safety margins in epicardial systems had high rates of sudden or arrhythmic death.[9–11] Based on this relatively limited dataset, the 10-J safety margin has become a widely used implant criterion.

Methods for measuring the safety margin vary widely, depending on how many inductions are performed and what energies are tested. The number of tests chosen for any protocol is a compromise between the accuracy of estimating a particular point on the defibrillation success curve and the

Division of Cardiology, Department of Medicine, Cornell University Medical Center, Starr 4, 525 East 68th Street, New York, NY 10065, USA
E-mail address: smarkow@med.cornell.edu

Card Electrophysiol Clin 3 (2011) 549–558
doi:10.1016/j.ccep.2011.08.002
1877-9182/11/$ – see front matter © 2011 Elsevier Inc. All rights reserved.

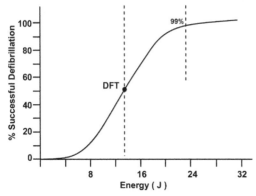

**Fig. 1.** The defibrillation dose-response curve describes the probability of successful defibrillation at different energy levels. The probability data can be modeled as a sigmoidal logistic regression curve. The defibrillation threshold (DFT) is defined here as the energy that produces a 50% probability of defibrillation success. Clinical testing protocols may estimate the DFT at other segments of the curve, depending on the characteristics of the protocol. The measured safety margin is the difference between the measured DFT and the maximum output of the device. An acceptable implant provides a sufficient safety margin to predict 99% defibrillation success at the device output. (*Adapted from* Singer I, Lang D. Defibrillation threshold: clinical utility and therapeutic implications. Pace 1992;15:932; with permission.)

safety of performing multiple ventricular fibrillation (VF) inductions. An implant criterion that has gained wide popularity is the demonstration of 2 sequential successful defibrillations at least 10 J below the maximum energy of the device. This technique predicts a high probability that the first shock at maximum energy will be successful. In a statistical analysis of ICD implant criteria, 2 sequential successful defibrillations with 24 J (using monophasic waveforms) predicted that the probability of a first shock success at 34 J is approximately 90%, and the annual sudden death rate expected in patients implanted with this criterion is less than 1% (considering that multiple shocks may be effective if the first shock fails).[12] This analysis supported an implant criterion of 2 sequential successful shocks at 24 J or less. Also, a requirement of a requirement of 3 out of 4 successes at 24 J or less predicted similar favorable outcomes at maximum energy. Other criteria that require successful defibrillation with one shock at even lower energy similarly predict high success rates at maximum output.[13]

Lower safety margins of 4 to 6 J were shown to be acceptable if the DFT was determined as the lowest energy that terminates VF on 3 trials, defined as the DFT++ in the Low Energy Safety Study (LESS).[14] This study, which excluded patients with DFT++

exceeding 21 J, showed that this criterion resulted in equivalent conversion rates for induced or spontaneous arrhythmias compared with much higher safety margins. An implication of this study is that, with more rigorous testing involving more inductions of VF, smaller minimum safety margins can be used.

## ARGUMENTS AGAINST ROUTINE DEFIBRILLATION TESTING

The arguments against routine implant defibrillation testing fall into the following categories:

1. Modern ICD systems, which use biphasic shocks, active pectoral cans, and high stored energies, are highly effective in terminating VF, and defibrillation failures are less common than with first-generation ICDs. The mean DFTs with biphasic shocks and active pectoral cans are in the range of 6 to 11 J[15–17] and inadequate safety margins are uncommon.[18,19]

2. Because defibrillation is a probabilistic phenomenon, it is inherently difficult to define whether any particular defibrillator/lead configuration is superior to another. If 1 or 2 shocks fail to defibrillate, a successful shock after a system modification could be related to chance rather than superior defibrillation efficacy.[12] Patients who fail shocks during testing may later have successful defibrillation of clinical VF because the failed shocks are false-negatives.[6]

3. There is a paucity of clinical evidence indicating that defibrillation testing alters clinical outcomes. Specifically, contemporary evidence does not show that implant DFTs or safety margins predict long-term mortality or first shock efficacy for spontaneous episodes of VF. Several single-center studies have failed to show differences in clinical outcomes among patients with high or low defibrillation margins,[20–23] an observation supported by an analysis of the Sudden Cardiac Death in Heart Failure Trial (SCD-HeFT).[18] A recent decision analysis model of defibrillation testing showed no significant survival advantage of a strategy of routine testing over not testing, with nearly identical 5-year survival rates.[1] These findings were robust for a wide range of assumptions. A small advantage to testing was found if high DFTs were common, defibrillation efficacy of clinical VF was 0% in high DFT patients, and the annual risk of lethal arrhythmias was high.

4. Safety concerns have been raised regarding defibrillation testing. In addition, system modifications that might be required to achieve

a higher safety margin also carry risks that might not be justified if defibrillation testing has little predictive value.

Based on these arguments, is there sufficient justification to abandon routine implant testing? This review focuses on the limitations of these arguments and concludes that the data do not necessarily negate the value of defibrillation testing.

## INCREASED DEFIBRILLATION THRESHOLDS WITH MODERN ICD SYSTEMS

Although DFTs are lower with active pectoral cans and biphasic waveforms, a substantial minority of patients with contemporary systems still have relatively low safety margins for defibrillation (**Table 1**). Using various definitions of high DFTs, the incidence of increased DFTs ranges from 3% to 12%.[17,19,22] For example, in a cohort of 1139 patients receiving transvenous ICDs for a variety of indications, including cardiac resynchronization therapy (CRT) implants, Russo and colleagues[21] found that more than 6% of recipients had inadequate safety margins (<10 J) and, therefore, required system revisions. With these modifications, adequate safety margins could be achieved in most patients. Even with the use of high-energy devices ($\geq$35 J), 3% of implanted patients had inadequate safety margins. In another study of 313 first-time ICD implants (26% of whom received CRT devices), a safety margin of less than 10 J was found in 5% of recipients despite various reprogramming and lead positioning attempts; these patients had subcutaneous arrays that effectively lowered the DFTs.[24] In a study of implants between 1996 and 2004, 10% of 632 patients who underwent DFT testing with either a step-down protocol or limited safety margin testing (with 1 or 2 shocks) had margins of less than 10 J.[25] Candidates for CRT have more advanced diseases and are more likely to have increased DFTs, as reported in 8% to 12% of CRT recipients.[26–28] Many of these high DFTs in CRT patients can also be lowered with system modifications.

Several factors have been identified as predictors of high DFTs with contemporary lead and defibrillator technology.[17,21,22,29–31] A consistent predictor to emerge from these various studies is left ventricular dilatation. Other predictors include increased left ventricular mass, amiodarone use, lower ejection fraction, worse heart failure class, increased body size, younger age, and ICD replacement/revision.

Although modern ICDs are highly effective in terminating ventricular tachycardia (VT) and VF, defibrillation failure of spontaneous arrhythmias remains a clinical problem.[32–34] Although most deaths in ICD patients are not sudden, deaths due to VT/VF do occur. In one study of 317 deaths in patients with transvenous ICDs, 17 of the deaths (5%) were caused by VT/VF uncorrected by ICD shocks; 20 had postshock pulseless electrical activity; and others had incessant VT/VF.[35] In another review of 4787 patients enrolled in clinical investigations (using both biphasic and monophasic devices, with and without tiered therapy), 74 cases of sudden death were identified, of which 49 were deemed tachyarrhythmic, 12 were nontachyarrhythmic, and 13 were indeterminate (overall rate of arrhythmic sudden death was at least 1%).[34]

It is not known if these victims of arrhythmic death could be identified earlier with implant or follow-up testing, because various dynamic clinical factors must contribute to defibrillation response. Ischemia, progressive heart failure, sympathetic activation, metabolic abnormalities, and antiarrhythmic drugs may all affect the DFT.[35] This may explain why first shock efficacy of spontaneous clinical arrhythmias is usually in the 80% to 90% range, lower than the success predicted with maximal output during device testing.[18,25] Thus, DFT testing in the laboratory is a best case scenario. Hypothetically, higher safety margins during implant might salvage patients prone to dynamic fluctuations in DFT.

Various methods are available to the implanting physician to lower DFTs.[36] These include lead repositioning, reprogramming the shock vector and polarity, removing or adding a superior vena cava coil, reprogramming the shock pulse width, and implanting subcutaneous or azygous vein leads (**Figs. 2** and **3**). No study has quantified the risks of these incremental interventions beyond the routine ICD implant.

## DEFIBRILLATION TESTING AND CLINICAL OUTCOMES

Several studies have compared the clinical outcomes of patients with high and low DFTs, as well as those implanted without testing, with regard to first shock success, survival, and sudden cardiac death. Contemporary studies are fairly consistent in demonstrating no difference in outcomes between those with high and low DFTs.[21–23,25,27] However, it cannot be concluded from these studies that DFTs are irrelevant to clinical outcome. One limitation of these studies is their retrospective design, and there is no randomized study of the testing versus no testing strategies. Furthermore, patients with high DFTs undergo system revisions to achieve more acceptable safety margins.[21] These revisions could mitigate the risk of high DFTs and mask the

**Table 1**
Representative studies reporting the incidence and outcomes in patients with low implant safety margins

| Study | Year | N[a] | Devices | Testing Protocol | Safety Margin <10 J (%) | Predictors of Inadequate Safety Margin | Complications[b] | Clinical Outcomes |
|---|---|---|---|---|---|---|---|---|
| Russo et al[21] | 2005 | 1085 | ICD/CRT | 2 terminations ≥10 J below max energy | 7 | Amiodarone Nonischemic heart disease Younger age Generator upgrade/revision | N/A | Mortality no different in low safety margin group |
| Theuns et al[23] | 2005 | 127 | ICD/CRT | Step down | 14 | None | N/A | Mortality no different in low safety margin group |
| Mainigi et al[26] | 2006 | 121 | CRT | 2 terminations ≥10 J below max energy | 12 | Prolonged QRS | 0% | Mortality no different in low safety margin group |
| Pires et al[25] | 2006 | 632 | ICD/CRT | Step down 1 or 2 shocks at 10–15 J | 10 | N/A | N/A | N/A |
| Schuger et al[28] (Ventak CHF/ Contak CD) | 2006 | 501 | CRT | (1) 2 terminations ≥10 J below max energy or (2) step down | 6 | Left ventricular dilatation Prolonged procedure time | 1.2% (6 hypotension and 1 death due to post shock pulseless electrical activity) | N/A |
| Blatt et al[18] (SCD-HeFT) | 2008 | 717 | ICD | Limited step up/step down with 2 inductions | 2 | N/A | N/A | Mortality and first shock efficacy no different in low safety margin group |
| Day et al[19] (Intrinsic RV) | 2008 | 1530 | ICD | 2 terminations ≥10 J below max energy | 4 | New York Heart Association class IV No prior myocardial infarction | 0% | N/A |
| Verma et al[25] | 2010 | 313 | ICD/CRT | 1 or more terminations ≥10 J below max energy | 5 | Amiodarone Left ventricular dilatation | 0.3% (1 with prolonged hypotension) | N/A |
| Michowitz et al[27] | 2011 | 204 | CRT | Defibrillation safety margin and vulnerability safety margin | 8 | N/A | 2% (4 cases of heart failure exacerbation, 1 leading to death) | N/A |

a N refers to the number of patients in the study who underwent defibrillation testing and excludes patients not subjected to testing.
b Complications attributable to defibrillation testing.

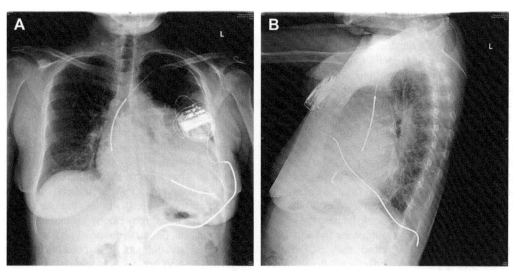

**Fig. 2.** (*A*) Subcutaneous lead implantation to lower DFT in a patient with severe left ventricular dilatation. The patient had nonischemic cardiomyopathy and an ICD implant for primary prevention. The left ventricular ejection fraction was 30% and the right ventricle was severely dilated. During a generator change, she was found to have high defibrillation requirements (>30 J). (*B*) After implantation of a subcutaneous lead, defibrillation was successful twice with 25 J. The posteroanterior (PA) and lateral (Lat) chest radiographs show the coil traversing from the flank to a position lateral to the spine. The resulting shock vector results in higher current density over the left ventricle.

differences between patients with adequate and inadequate safety margins detected with initial testing. Most of these studies do not address the outcomes of patients with high DFTs if no mitigation is provided to lower the DFT.

A subanalysis of SCD-HeFT examined the predictive value of DFT testing in the multicenter randomized trial, in which patients received transvenous ICDs, regardless of implant safety margin.[18] Using a stratifier of 10 J to assign patients to high

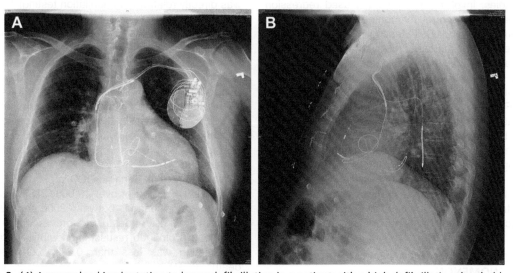

**Fig. 3.** (*A*) Azygous lead implantation to lower defibrillation in a patient with a high defibrillation threshold and severe left ventricular dilatation. The patient had severe aortic regurgitation with a left ventricular ejection fraction of 24% and diastolic dimension of 7.8 cm. He underwent implantation of a biventricular ICD following cardiac arrest after aortic valve replacement. During device testing at implant, maximal energy shocks of 41 J failed to achieve defibrillation in 2 successive tests. The defibrillation lead was placed in a nonapical location to avoid long-term apical pacing in this pacing-dependent patient. (*B*) After addition of the azygous vein lead, 2 successive tests with 31 J were successful. The posteroanterior (PA) and lateral (Lat) chest radiographs show a coil in the azygous vein, which is posterior to the left ventricle.

and low DFT groups, this analysis showed no difference in first shock efficacy (which was 83% overall) or survival in patients with low or high DFTs. A close examination of the SCD-HeFT experience reveals that all 717 patients implanted with ICDs who underwent implant testing had successful defibrillation with 30 J or less, which was the maximum output of devices in this study, and 98% had successful defibrillation with 20 J or less. Because all patients tested at implant had successful defibrillation with 30 J or less, it is not possible to predict outcomes of patients with DFTs exceeding the maximum output of the device. Only 16 patients in this study had a DFT between 21 and 30 J, 3 of whom had an appropriate shock, limiting the ability of the study to examine outcomes in high DFT patients. It should be noted that SCD-HeFT enrolled stable patients with class II to III heart failure who were treated with optimal medical therapy. It is likely that sicker patients are now implanted with ICDs and it is unrealistic to expect uniform defibrillation success with 30 J or less.

In several studies, patients who did not undergo defibrillation testing typically demonstrated high long-term mortality.[21,25,37] In these retrospective studies, the reasons for not testing included hemodynamic instability, severe occlusive coronary disease or other structural heart disease (such as aortic stenosis), intracavitary thrombus or atrial fibrillation without therapeutic anticoagulation, or a recent cerebrovascular event. One of these studies, involving 112 patients, used regression analysis to control for confounding factors and found that no DFT testing was a significant predictor of mortality.[37] Nevertheless, it is likely that the poor long-term outcomes were related to severe underlying disease, and the data are not conclusive in showing that a strategy of no DFT testing results in higher mortality. One investigation that does address this issue is a study from Italy that compared outcomes of patients implanted in Italian centers that routinely test at implant with those from centers that do not test at implant.[38] While no difference was found in outcomes between these groups, the study was retrospective and of a relatively small size and included only 291 patients overall.

## DEFIBRILLATION AS A PROBABILISTIC PHENOMENON

Defibrillation testing needs to be interpreted in light of the dose-response probability curve. It has been shown that 2 out of 2 successful defibrillations predict a high likelihood of shock success with an energy 10 J higher. Conversely, 2 out of 2 unsuccessful shocks predict a lower likelihood of success at a 10-J higher energy. Failure of multiple shocks during testing should predict unsuccessful defibrillation in clinical situations. A logical hypothesis is that reproducible shock failures may identify patients likely to benefit from a system revision. Because a shock failure usually results in a system modification, the prognostic significance of multiple failed shocks has not been addressed in clinical studies. Defibrillation requirements may increase with increasing number of VF episodes tested.[4] Therefore, it is not uncommon for a second test to fail after a single successful defibrillation.

One implication of this discussion is that limited testing protocols at 10 J below the device output (with 1 or 2 tests) may poorly predict subsequent defibrillations, because the point on the DFT curve is imprecisely defined. It is possible that more rigorous testing protocols would better define the safety margin, and it is unknown if such protocols would have better predictive value.[6]

## COMPLICATIONS OF DEFIBRILLATION TESTING

Complications attributed to defibrillation testing during implantation are uncommon but include intractable VT/VF, pulseless electrical activity, heart failure exacerbation, and cerebral/systemic embolism. A single-center study of 440 implants reported 2 strokes and one perioperative death caused by heart failure (but it is unclear if this was directly related to defibrillation testing).[39] Another study of 501 patients reported one death due to pulseless electrical activity.[28] The complication rate of defibrillation testing in another series was 1/313 due to prolonged hypotension after testing.[24] A study of 256 CRT implantations reported a higher complication rate of 2% due to 4 heart failure exacerbations, one of which resulted in death.[27] The most significant predictor of hemodynamic compromise with defibrillation testing seems to be severe left ventricular systolic dysfunction.[40]

In a survey of all Canadian ICD implant centers, comprising a cohort of over 19,000 ICD implants and generator changes between 2000 and 2006, the combined risk of death, cerebrovascular accident, and prolonged resuscitation with defibrillation testing was less than 0.2%.[41] Of the 3 deaths (0.016%), 2 occurred in patients who underwent lead revision and developed pulseless electrical activity after a second VF induction, and 1 was due to an embolic stroke that occurred after defibrillation also converted atrial fibrillation. All 5 cerebrovascular events in this cohort (0.026%) occurred in patients with atrial fibrillation who were bridged or treated with intravenous heparin, which was temporarily interrupted for the implantation.

Defibrillation shocks have been shown to acutely worsen left ventricular contractility and cause release of cardiac enzymes.[42] Myocardial dysfunction can occur as a result of VF, high-energy shock, or both. There are reasons to believe that the shocks independently contribute to left ventricular dysfunction and hemodynamic compromise. Limited data demonstrate that shocks without VF can cause transient left ventricular dysfunction.[43,44]

In response to these rare but potentially serious outcomes, alternative protocols relying on single shock success rates might be considered in patients at higher risk.[13] Alternatively, a protocol to measure the upper limit of vulnerability could be used to eliminate or reduce the number of shocks delivered.[45,46] For prevention of defibrillation-related stroke, options are: to defer implant testing until an adequate course of anticoagulation is delivered; to perform testing on therapeutic anticoagulation (at least 3 weeks of warfarin or clearance of a left atrial thrombus with transesophageal echocardiography); or reinduction of atrial fibrillation immediately following conversion to sinus rhythm.

## OTHER ADVANTAGES TO DEFIBRILLATION TESTING

1. *Sensing Verification*: Implant testing verifies appropriate sensing and detection of VF. It has been suggested that sinus rhythm R-waves greater than 5 mV predict a high likelihood of appropriate sensing of VF.[46] Yet, modern lead systems have demonstrated unpredictable reductions in R-wave amplitudes following implantation.[47] Undersensing of VF may occur after ineffective shocks.[48] Also, postshock undersensing or oversensing after return to sinus rhythm may be detected during implant testing and should be corrected to prevent delivery of secondary inappropriate shocks.

2. *Device Integrity*: Implant testing allows verification of device function in delivering a high-voltage shock, with assessment of charge time and integrity of the high-voltage and pacing/sensing components. Although rare, device malfunction might be detected only through high-voltage testing (**Fig. 4**). This consideration may be even more important in patients having generator changes or revisions, in whom lead abnormalities are more likely.[49]

3. *Programming Considerations*: A theoretic argument in favor of defining the DFT with better precision is the ability to program lower first shock energies for VF.[14,50,51] The benefit of lower energies rests on the recognition that higher shock energies have more profound effects on hemodynamics.[52] It is possible that lower energy shocks would be less likely to result in pulseless electrical activity, a cause of sudden death in ICD recipients.[33] Lower energies also result in shorter charge times, which may reduce the likelihood of syncope. These considerations have not been addressed

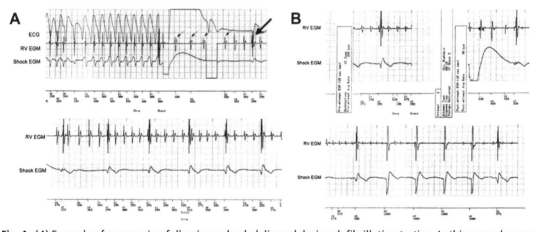

**Fig. 4.** (*A*) Example of oversensing following a shock delivered during defibrillation testing. In this example, oversensing of large-amplitude nonphysiologic signals followed delivery of a high-voltage shock to terminate induced VT. Oversensing of these signals resulted in inappropriate redetection of VT and delivery of a second shock. (*B*) In this case, oversensing was due to seal-plug damage, which resulted in heated air escaping through the damaged seal plug after the shock. Oversensing occurred only with the electrical stress of a high-voltage shock and would not be detected in the absence of shock delivery. (*Reproduced from* Cheung JW, Iwai S, Lerman BB, et al. Shock-induced ventricular oversensing due to seal plug damage: a potential mechanism of inappropriate device therapies in implantable cardioverter-defibrillators. Heart Rhythm 2005;2:1373; with permission.)

by the various retrospective studies that examined outcomes following defibrillation testing.

4. *Single Versus Dual-Coil ICD Leads*: It has been demonstrated that dual-coil ICD leads have, on average, lower DFTs than unipolar ICD leads;[53] yet, there is increasing interest in implanting single-coil leads in most patients because of easier extractability. Most of the studies cited in this review article used dual-coil leads. If a single-coil lead is implanted, defibrillation testing might be important, particularly in those patients who have risk factors for high DFTs.

5. *Unconventional Lead Locations*: Most of the data on the incidence of high safety margins and clinical outcomes involved ICD leads implanted in the right ventricular apex. In some centers, a location in the septum or right ventricular outflow tract is advocated. Preliminary evidence suggests that DFTs in these locations are acceptable,[54] but large-scale and long-term outcome studies are not available.

## SUMMARY

The clinical studies which seem to weigh against routine defibrillation testing have limitations that prevent using these to change clinical practice. A more nuanced approach is called for rather than complete elimination of defibrillation testing. One reasonable approach is to test patients most likely to have increased DFTs, such as those with significant left ventricular dilatation or those on amiodarone. At the same time, testing would be deferred in patients at highest risk for complications, such as those with hemodynamic instability or at risk for thromboembolism. Also, appreciation of defibrillation probabilities allows the implanter to make more informed decisions regarding implant criteria and system modifications. At the same time, prospective investigations are needed into different implant testing protocols that can define safety margins with better precision and better predict clinical outcomes.

## REFERENCES

1. Gula LJ, Massel D, Krahn AD, et al. Is defibrillation testing still necessary? A decision analysis and Markov model. J Cardiovasc Electrophysiol 2008; 19:400.

2. Strickberger SA, Klein GJ. Is defibrillation testing required for defibrillator implantation? J Am Coll Cardiol 2004;44:88.

3. Viskin S, Rosso R. The top 10 reasons to avoid defibrillation threshold testing during ICD implantation. Heart Rhythm 2008;5:391.

4. Deale OC, Wesley RC Jr, Morgan D, et al. Nature of defibrillation: determinism versus probabilism. Am J Physiol 1990;259:H1544.

5. Singer I, Lang D. Defibrillation threshold: clinical utility and therapeutic implications. Pacing Clin Electrophysiol 1992;15:932.

6. Swerdlow CD, Russo AM, Degroot PJ. The dilemma of ICD implant testing. Pacing Clin Electrophysiol 2007;30:675.

7. Shorofsky SR, Peters RW, Rashba EJ, et al. Comparison of step-down and binary search algorithms for determination of defibrillation threshold in humans. Pacing Clin Electrophysiol 2004;27:218.

8. Marchlinski FE, Flores B, Miller JM, et al. Relation of the intraoperative defibrillation threshold to successful postoperative defibrillation with an automatic implantable cardioverter defibrillator. Am J Cardiol 1988;62:393.

9. Epstein AE, Ellenbogen KA, Kirk KA, et al. Clinical characteristics and outcome of patients with high defibrillation thresholds. A multicenter study. Circulation 1992;86:1206.

10. Lehmann MH, Thomas A, Nabih M, et al. Sudden death in recipients of first-generation implantable cardioverter defibrillators: analysis of terminal events. Participating investigators. J Interv Cardiol 1994;7:487.

11. Pinski SL, Vanerio G, Castle LW, et al. Patients with a high defibrillation threshold: clinical characteristics, management, and outcome. Am Heart J 1991; 122:89.

12. Degroot PJ, Church TR, Mehra R, et al. Derivation of a defibrillator implant criterion based on probability of successful defibrillation. Pacing Clin Electrophysiol 1924;20:1997.

13. Higgins S, Mann D, Calkins H, et al. One conversion of ventricular fibrillation is adequate for implantable cardioverter-defibrillator implant: an analysis from the Low Energy Safety Study (LESS). Heart Rhythm 2005;2:117.

14. Gold MR, Higgins S, Klein R, et al. Efficacy and temporal stability of reduced safety margins for ventricular defibrillation: primary results from the Low Energy Safety Study (LESS). Circulation 2002; 105:2043.

15. Bardy GH, Ivey TD, Allen MD, et al. A prospective randomized evaluation of biphasic versus monophasic waveform pulses on defibrillation efficacy in humans. J Am Coll Cardiol 1989;14:728.

16. Block M, Hammel D, Bocker D, et al. A prospective randomized cross-over comparison of mono- and biphasic defibrillation using nonthoracotomy lead configurations in humans. J Cardiovasc Electrophysiol 1994;5:581.

17. Hodgson DM, Olsovsky MR, Shorofsky SR, et al. Clinical predictors of defibrillation thresholds with an active pectoral pulse generator lead system. Pacing Clin Electrophysiol 2002;25:408.

18. Blatt JA, Poole JE, Johnson GW, et al. No benefit from defibrillation threshold testing in the SCD-HeFT (Sudden Cardiac Death in Heart Failure Trial). J Am Coll Cardiol 2008;52:551.

19. Day JD, Olshansky B, Moore S, et al. High defibrillation energy requirements are encountered rarely with modern dual-chamber implantable cardioverter-defibrillator systems. Europace 2008;10:347.

20. Anvari A, Gottsauner-Wolf M, Turel Z, et al. Predictors of outcome in patients with implantable cardioverter defibrillators. Cardiology 1998;90:180.

21. Russo AM, Sauer W, Gerstenfeld EP, et al. Defibrillation threshold testing: is it really necessary at the time of implantable cardioverter-defibrillator insertion? Heart Rhythm 2005;2:456.

22. Shukla HH, Flaker GC, Jayam V, et al. High defibrillation thresholds in transvenous biphasic implantable defibrillators: clinical predictors and prognostic implications. Pacing Clin Electrophysiol 2003;26:44.

23. Theuns DA, Szili-Torok T, Jordaens LJ. Defibrillation efficacy testing: long-term follow-up and mortality. Europace 2005;7:509.

24. Verma A, Kaplan AJ, Sarak B, et al. Incidence of very high defibrillation thresholds (DFT) and efficacy of subcutaneous (SQ) array insertion during implantable cardioverter defibrillator (ICD) implantation. J Interv Card Electrophysiol 2010;29:127.

25. Pires LA, Johnson KM. Intraoperative testing of the implantable cardioverter-defibrillator: how much is enough? J Cardiovasc Electrophysiol 2006;17:140.

26. Mainigi SK, Cooper JM, Russo AM, et al. Elevated defibrillation thresholds in patients undergoing biventricular defibrillator implantation: incidence and predictors. Heart Rhythm 2006;3:1010.

27. Michowitz Y, Lellouche N, Contractor T, et al. Defibrillation threshold testing fails to show clinical benefit during long-term follow-up of patients undergoing cardiac resynchronization therapy defibrillator implantation. Europace 2011;13(5):683–8.

28. Schuger C, Ellenbogen KA, Faddis M, et al. Defibrillation energy requirements in an ICD population receiving cardiac resynchronization therapy. J Cardiovasc Electrophysiol 2006;17:247.

29. Khalighi K, Daly B, Leino EV, et al. Clinical predictors of transvenous defibrillation energy requirements. Am J Cardiol 1997;79:150.

30. Raitt MH, Johnson G, Dolack GL, et al. Clinical predictors of the defibrillation threshold with the unipolar implantable defibrillation system. J Am Coll Cardiol 1995;25:1576.

31. Schwartzman D, Concato J, Ren JF, et al. Factors associated with successful implantation of nonthoracotomy defibrillation lead systems. Am Heart J 1996;131:1127.

32. Anderson KP. Sudden cardiac death unresponsive to implantable defibrillator therapy: an urgent target for clinicians, industry and government. J Interv Card Electrophysiol 2005;14:71.

33. Mitchell LB, Pineda EA, Titus JL, et al. Sudden death in patients with implantable cardioverter defibrillators: the importance of post-shock electromechanical dissociation. J Am Coll Cardiol 2002;39:1323.

34. Pires LA, Hull ML, Nino CL, et al. Sudden death in recipients of transvenous implantable cardioverter defibrillator systems: terminal events, predictors, and potential mechanisms. J Cardiovasc Electrophysiol 1999;10:1049.

35. Lerman BB, Engelstein ED. Metabolic determinants of defibrillation. Role of adenosine. Circulation 1995;91:838.

36. Mainigi SK, Callans DJ. How to manage the patient with a high defibrillation threshold. Heart Rhythm 2006;3:492.

37. Hall B, Jeevanantham V, Levine E, et al. Comparison of outcomes in patients undergoing defibrillation threshold testing at the time of implantable cardioverter-defibrillator implantation versus no defibrillation threshold testing. Cardiol J 2007;14:463.

38. Bianchi S, Ricci RP, Biscione F, et al. Primary prevention implantation of cardioverter defibrillator without defibrillation threshold testing: 2-year follow-up. Pacing Clin Electrophysiol 2009;32:573.

39. Alter P, Waldhans S, Plachta E, et al. Complications of implantable cardioverter defibrillator therapy in 440 consecutive patients. Pacing Clin Electrophysiol 2005;28:926.

40. Steinbeck G, Dorwarth U, Mattke S, et al. Hemodynamic deterioration during ICD implant: predictors of high-risk patients. Am Heart J 1994;127:1064.

41. Birnie D, Tung S, Simpson C, et al. Complications associated with defibrillation threshold testing: the Canadian experience. Heart Rhythm 2008;5:387.

42. Runsio M, Kallner A, Kallner G, et al. Myocardial injury after electrical therapy for cardiac arrhythmias assessed by troponin-T release. Am J Cardiol 1997; 79:1241.

43. Rollan MJ, San Roman JA, Bratos JL, et al. Acute pulmonary edema secondary to myocardial damage after electrical cardioversion. Pacing Clin Electrophysiol 2003;26:2330.

44. Stein KM, Devereux RB, Hahn RT, et al. Effect of transthoracic shocks on left ventricular function. Resuscitation 2005;66:309.

45. Day JD, Doshi RN, Belott P, et al. Inductionless or limited shock testing is possible in most patients with implantable cardioverter- defibrillators/cardiac resynchronization therapy defibrillators: results of the multicenter ASSURE Study (Arrhythmia Single Shock Defibrillation Threshold Testing Versus Upper Limit of Vulnerability: Risk Reduction Evaluation with Implantable Cardioverter-Defibrillator Implantations). Circulation 2007;115:2382.

46. Swerdlow CD. Implantation of cardioverter defibrillators without induction of ventricular fibrillation. Circulation 2001;103:2159.

47. Kenigsberg DN, Mirchandani S, Dover AN, et al. Sensing failure associated with the Medtronic Sprint Fidelis defibrillator lead. J Cardiovasc Electrophysiol 2008;19:270.

48. Natale A, Sra J, Axtell K, et al. Undetected ventricular fibrillation in transvenous implantable cardioverter-defibrillators. Prospective comparison of different lead system-device combinations. Circulation 1996; 93:91.

49. Kron J, Herre J, Renfroe EG, et al. Lead- and device-related complications in the antiarrhythmics versus implantable defibrillators trial. Am Heart J 2001;141:92.

50. Neuzner J. Safety margins: lessons from the Low Energy Endotak Trial (LEET). Am J Cardiol 1996; 78:26.

51. Strickberger SA, Daoud EG, Davidson T, et al. Probability of successful defibrillation at multiples of the defibrillation energy requirement in patients with an implantable defibrillator. Circulation 1997; 96:1217.

52. Tokano T, Bach D, Chang J, et al. Effect of ventricular shock strength on cardiac hemodynamics. J Cardiovasc Electrophysiol 1998;9:791.

53. Gold MR, Olsovsky MR, Pelini MA, et al. Comparison of single- and dual-coil active pectoral defibrillation lead systems. J Am Coll Cardiol 1998;31:1391.

54. Reynolds CR, Nikolski V, Sturdivant JL, et al. Randomized comparison of defibrillation thresholds from the right ventricular apex and outflow tract. Heart Rhythm 2010;7:1561.

# Evaluation of Defibrillation Efficacy at Implantation is Unnecessary

Ganesh Venkataraman, MD*, S. Adam Strickberger, MD

**KEYWORDS**

- Implantable defibrillator • Defibrillation threshold testing
- Defibrillation efficacy • Sudden cardiac death

Implantable defibrillator (ICD) therapy improves mortality in several subsets of patients at risk for sudden cardiac death.[1–3] Defibrillation efficacy (DE) testing is routinely performed at initial ICD implantation, although it is associated with a small but finite risk of complications, including worsening heart failure, stroke, pulseless electrical activity, and death. Over the past 2 decades, several major advances have been made in ICD technology, including adjustable biphasic waveforms, active can technology, and higher output devices, which have greatly enhanced DE. Moreover, there is no data to suggest that DE testing at the time of ICD implantation predicts first-shock success for termination of ventricular tachycardia (VT) or ventricular fibrillation (VF), or improves survival. The purpose of this article is to demonstrate that the evaluation of DE at the time of initial ICD implantation is unnecessary.

## HISTORY OF DEFIBRILLATION EFFICACY TESTING

DE testing has been integral to ICD implantation since the inception of ICD therapy. DE testing was first performed with epicardial ICD systems, which were implanted via a thoracotomy or subxiphoid approach. Two or more defibrillation patches were arranged in various configurations on the epicardium or pericardium. Generally, implantation of an ICD generator mandated successful defibrillation. These systems from the 1980s and early 1990s frequently required that the shock polarity, location, or number of electrodes be altered to achieve reliable defibrillation. With the introduction of transvenous endocardial leads in combination with monophasic waveforms, DE testing remained an important aspect of implantation; approximately 30% of patients were found to have elevated defibrillation requirements and required system revision with additional defibrillation electrodes or a change in shock polarity.[4,5] Active can technology, adjustable biphasic waveforms, and higher output devices have greatly enhanced DE in the newer generation of implantable defibrillators.[6,7]

DE testing has been performed at implantation in randomized trials that have shown the survival benefit of ICD therapy.[1–3] Both primary and secondary prevention trials of ICD therapy required DE testing as a critical component of ICD implantation.[1–3] Therefore, DE testing remains a standard part of the ICD implant procedure.

### Evaluation of Defibrillation Efficacy

Defibrillation efficacy is probabilistic in nature, and is represented by a sigmoidal dose–response curve (**Fig. 1**A). That is, a specific defibrillation energy is associated with a probability of successful defibrillation.[8] $DE_{50}$ is the energy associated with a 50% probability of successful defibrillation.

This work was not supported by external funding.

Washington Electrophysiology, and Cardiovascular Research Institute, Washington Hospital Center, 106 Irving Street, NW, South #204, Washington, DC 20010-2975, USA

\* Corresponding author.

*E-mail address:* Ganesh.S.Venkataraman@medstar.net

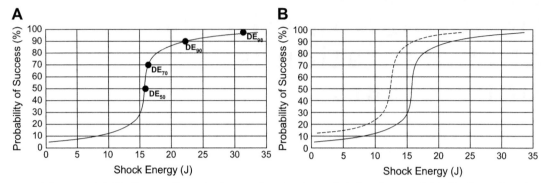

**Fig. 1.** (*A*) A typical defibrillation efficacy (DE) curve showing the probability of successful defibrillation based on the shock energy. Various methods of DE testing (see text for details) are associated with different probabilities of successful defibrillation ($DE_{50}$ to $DE_{98}$). (*B*) Two different DE curves. The curve to the left (*dashed line*) is associated with improved DE compared with the curve on the right (*solid black line*). Note that factors that improve DE, such as adjustable biphasic waveforms, shift the curve to the left, whereas factors that negatively impact DE shift the curve to the right.

The probability of defibrillation can vary from day to day because of physiologic changes. In addition, factors such as the shock waveform or pulse duration, and the number and position of defibrillation electrodes, can move the curve left or right and alter the defibrillation curve (see **Fig. 1**B). The probability of successful defibrillation may also vary based on conduction properties of myocardial cells, random changes in the volume of the myocardial mass that is depolarized, or other factors.

Safety margin testing is the most common method of DE testing. Most, if not all, of the randomized trials that have shown improved survival with an ICD have mandated safety margin testing.[1–3] Successful safety margin testing requires two consecutive successful defibrillation shocks at an energy requirement 10 to 15 J less than the maximum output of the ICD. This approach is associated with an approximately 90% probability of successful defibrillation (see **Fig. 1**A). The 10-J safety margin was first validated by Marchlinski and colleagues[9] who showed that a 10-J difference between the intraoperative defibrillation energy requirement and the maximum energy output of the ICD generator predicted successful defibrillation postoperatively.

The step-down protocol to assess DE involves the serial reduction in shock energy until defibrillation failure occurs. The lowest successful shock defines the defibrillation threshold. This approach identifies the energy associated with approximately a 70% rate of successful defibrillation.[10] Given the shape of the DE curve and the probabilistic nature of successful defibrillation, a shock energy equal to twice the $DE_{70}$ is associated with a 98% probability of successful defibrillation[10] (see **Fig. 1**A). As with safety margin testing, two successive successful defibrillation shocks with

a step-down protocol increase the likelihood that these shock energies are located on the upper portion of the DE curve.

The step-down, step-up protocol is primarily used for research purposes. A step-down protocol is performed until defibrillation failure occurs. The shock energy is then increased until successful defibrillation is again achieved. This approach has the advantage of giving a more accurate estimate of the $DE_{50}$, but it requires numerous shocks (see **Fig. 1**A). In the Low Energy Safety Study (LESS), a rigorous step-down/step-up protocol that began with a single successful defibrillation of VF at 14 J provided a similar positive predictive accuracy as two successive successful defibrillations at 17 or 21 J.[11]

An alternative approach to the evaluation of DE is identification of the upper limit of vulnerability (ULV). According to the ULV theory of defibrillation, there is a period near the peak of the T wave, known as the *vulnerable period*, at which a shock of a certain magnitude will induce VF. As one raises the shock energy, there is a limit above which VF will no longer be induced. This so-called ULV to VF has been shown to correlate well with the defibrillation threshold.[12,13] The attractiveness of the ULV approach is that it provides the possibility of determining DE without VF induction. The T wave must be scanned with shocks delivered at varying intervals, such as 0, 20, and 40 ms, before and after the peak of the T wave. Although the number of shocks to be delivered for reliable determination of DE is greater with the ULV approach, the number of VF inductions is minimized. A study of 426 patients undergoing ICD implantation found that the ULV achieved similar first-shock efficacy as in patients who underwent safety margin testing.[14]

## EVALUATION OF DEFIBRILLATION EFFICACY: WHAT ARE THE DATA?

Despite the fact that every major randomized trial which demonstrated a mortality benefit of ICD therapy has required the evaluation of DE at the time of initial device implantation, there is no evidence that the evaluation of DE adds any prognostic value or benefit to the patient. Inadequate safety margins are seen in only approximately 5% of patients undergoing ICD implantation.[15,16] Conflicting data exist between the association of an inadequate safety margin and clinical outcomes. Moreover, in some locales, the evaluation of DE is performed in approximately 65% of initial ICD implants and 25% of ICD generator replacements.[17]

Several single-center, nonrandomized, retrospective registries question the need for intraoperative evaluation of DE.[18–21] The largest series evaluated 835 patients undergoing ICD implantation. Routine DE testing was performed with either a standard step-down protocol or with limited safety margin testing, or not performed entirely in a nonrandomized manner. These investigators found no difference in first-shock efficacy and sudden death–free survival rates among the three groups. Total mortality was higher in the group that did not undergo DE testing, most likely because of comorbidities that precluded the evaluation of DE.[18] In a series of patients undergoing ICD implantation with cardiac resynchronization therapy, the evaluation of DE was associated with no difference in successful device therapy or overall survival.[19] Smaller series have similarly found no difference in first-shock efficacy[20] or total mortality[21] with DE testing. A decision analysis that evaluated the impact of the evaluation of DE at ICD implantation using a Markov model showed similar 1- and 5-year survival rates in both groups, regardless of the strategy chosen.[22]

Perhaps the best available data evaluating the clinical impact of an elevated defibrillation energy requirement during evaluation of DE are from a prespecified analysis of the Sudden Cardiac Death in Heart Failure Trial (SCD-HeFT).[23] In this trial, 711 patients underwent single-chamber ICD implantation for primary prevention of sudden cardiac death and were prospectively followed based on their baseline DE data. All patients received an ICD with a 30-J maximum output. DE was evaluated in all patients using a modified step-up/step-down protocol that started at 20 J and ended at either 10 or 30 J, based on first-shock successful defibrillation. A high-energy DE group, defined as greater than 10 J, was found in 24% of patients. At a mean follow-up of 45 months, no significant difference were seen in all-cause mortality between patients with a defibrillation energy requirement of 10 J or less or greater than 10 J. In addition, first-shock efficacy for VT/VF was independent of the baseline DE. In three patients, 30 J was required for successful defibrillation at implantation. Each of these patients had an episode of VT or VF, which was successfully treated with the first shock. These data suggest that evaluation of DE, and its results, do not correlate with first-shock efficacy or overall survival.

## WHAT IS THE ARGUMENT FOR EVALUATION OF DE?

The major argument for the evaluation of DE is that all randomized trials that have shown a mortality benefit with ICD therapy have required this evaluation during device implantation. Until a randomized trial demonstrates that omitting DE testing does not adversely affect mortality, abandoning the practice of DE testing will be difficult. However, some patients will require a system modification to achieve an adequate defibrillation safety margin. The evaluation of DE may allow for better programming of the device, with faster and lower energy shocks, potentially decreasing the risk of hemodynamic instability or syncope. Finally, a patient undergoing ICD implantation without the evaluation of DE presents a potential medicolegal concern. Many physicians believe that the evaluation of DE represents the standard of care. In general, these arguments for the evaluation of DE are historical, with few data to support them.

## WHAT IS THE ARGUMENT AGAINST THE EVALUATION OF DE?

The major argument against the evaluation of DE is that, as an additional part of the ICD implant procedure, it presents a risk for complications and has never been proven to independently improve mortality. Shocks, even in sinus rhythm, adversely affect hemodynamics.[24] In a Canadian registry of more than 19,000 ICD implants with DE testing, three deaths, five strokes, and 29 episodes of prolonged resuscitation occurred, some of which resulted in significant clinical consequences.[25]

Second, major advances in ICD technology have significantly decreased the frequency of inadequate DE at ICD implantation. Higher output devices, adjustable biphasic waveforms, and active can technology have all contributed to achieving an adequate safety margin during evaluation of DE with "out of the box" programming. The data on the clinical significance of an inadequate safety margin are unclear and do not support DE testing.

Third, most patients receiving ICD therapy are unlikely to experience a sustained ventricular arrhythmia. Most ventricular arrhythmias in patients with an ICD are VT, not VF. Most VT episodes are terminated by antitachycardia pacing, and the shock energy required to successfully terminate VT is significantly less than that required to terminate VF. Finally, the evaluation of DE is probabilistic in nature and can change. Therefore, a "subthreshold" shock may be effective after two, three, or four attempts. Moreover, an inadequate safety margin at implant does not preclude a patient from having successful defibrillation in the future. Likewise, a small percentage of patients with adequate safety margins at ICD implantation die of unsuccessful defibrillation of VF or electromechanical dissociation after successful defibrillation. Based on the available data, evaluation of DE at ICD implantation does not seem to improve first-shock efficacy or survival.

## FUTURE DATA NEEDED

A randomized trial seems critical to answer the question of whether evaluation of DE is necessary. Healey and colleagues[26] describe a trial that randomizes patients undergoing ICD implantation to either DE testing or no testing, although the details of this study have not been reported. The number of patients needed to enroll may limit the feasibility of this type of trial.

To calculate the number of patients needed to conduct this type of trial, a few assumptions are necessary. First, approximately 5% of patients undergoing ICD implantation will have inadequate DE. Assuming that 20% of patients with an ICD have an episode of VF, only 1% who are at risk for VF have inadequate DE. Assuming an annual mortality rate of 10% for patients undergoing ICD implantation, and an additional 1% mortality rate for patients undergoing ICD implantation without evaluation of DE, 29,000 patients must be randomized to achieve a statistical power of 80%. Of course, a noninferiority study may require a smaller sample size by an order of magnitude.

## SUMMARY

ICD therapy improves survival of patients at risk for sudden cardiac death. The evaluation of DE at implantation has long been the standard of care. Advances in ICD technology have led to a dramatic reduction in the percentage of patients with inadequate DE. The evaluation of DE has small but finite

risks. Available data suggest that the evaluation of DE during ICD implantation does not improve first-shock efficacy or survival and may not be necessary. Prospective randomized trials and long-term follow-up are warranted to clarify whether the evaluation of DE at ICD implantation can be safely abandoned.

## REFERENCES

1. The Antiarrhythmics versus Implantable Defibrillators (AVID) Investigators. A comparison of antiarrhythmic-drug therapy with implantable defibrillators in patients resuscitated from near-fatal ventricular arrhythmias. N Engl J Med 1997;337:1576–83.
2. Moss AJ, Zareba W, Hall WJ, et al. Prophylactic implantation of a defibrillator in patients with myocardial infarction and reduced ejection fraction. N Engl J Med 2002;346:877–83.
3. Bardy GH, Lee KL, Mark DB, et al. Amiodarone or an implantable cardioverter-defibrillator for congestive heart failure. N Engl J Med 2005;352:225–37.
4. Strickberger SA, Hummel JD, Daoud E, et al. Implantation by electrophysiologists of 100 consecutive cardioverter defibrillators with nonthoracotomy lead systems. Circulation 1994;90:868–72.
5. Strickberger SA, Hummel JD, Horwood LE, et al. Effect of shock polarity on ventricular defibrillation threshold using a transvenous lead system. J Am Coll Cardiol 1994;24:1069–72.
6. Gold MR, Foster AH, Shorofsky SR. Effects of an active pectoral-pulse generator shell on defibrillation efficacy with a transvenous lead system. Am J Cardiol 1996;78:540–3.
7. Olsovsky MR, Hodgson DM, Shorofsky SR, et al. Effect of biphasic waveforms on transvenous defibrillation thresholds in patients with coronary artery disease. Am J Cardiol 1997;80:1098–100.
8. Rattes MF, Jones DL, Sharma AD, et al. Defibrillation threshold: a simple and quantitative estimate of the ability to defibrillate. Pacing Clin Electrophysiol 1987;10:70–7.
9. Marchlinski FE, Flores B, Miller JM, et al. Relation of the intraoperative defibrillation threshold to successful postoperative defibrillation with an automatic implantable cardioverter defibrillator. Am J Cardiol 1988;62:393–8.
10. Strickberger SA, Daoud EG, Davidson T, et al. Probability of successful defibrillation at multiples of the defibrillation energy requirement in patients with an implantable defibrillator. Circulation 1997;96:1217–23.
11. Higgins S, Mann D, Calkins H, et al. One conversion of ventricular fibrillation is adequate for implantable cardioverter-defibrillator implant: an analysis from

the Low Energy Safety Study (LESS). Heart Rhythm 2005;2:117–22.

12. Chen PS, Feld GK, Kriett JM, et al. Relation between upper limit of vulnerability and defibrillation threshold in humans. Circulation 1993;88:186–92.

13. Hwang C, Swerdlow CD, Kass RM, et al. Upper limit of vulnerability reliably predicts the defibrillation threshold in humans. Circulation 1994;90:2308–14.

14. Day JD, Doshi RN, Belott P, et al. Inductionless or limited shock testing is possible in most patients with implantable cardioverter- defibrillators/cardiac resynchronization therapy defibrillators: results of the multicenter ASSURE Study (Arrhythmia Single Shock Defibrillation Threshold Testing Versus Upper Limit of Vulnerability: risk reduction evaluation with implantable cardioverter-defibrillator implantations). Circulation 2007;115:2382–9.

15. Epstein AE, Ellenbogen KA, Kirk KA, et al. Clinical characteristics and outcome of patients with high defibrillation thresholds. A multicenter study. Circulation 1992;86:1206–16.

16. Russo AM, Sauer W, Gerstenfeld EP, et al. Defibrillation threshold testing: is it really necessary at the time of implantable cardioverter-defibrillator insertion? Heart Rhythm 2005;2:456–61.

17. Healey JS, Birnie DH, Lee DS, et al, Ontario ICD Database Investigators. Defibrillation testing at the time of ICD Insertion: an analysis from the Ontario ICD registry. J Cardiovasc Electrophysiol 2010;21:1344–8.

18. Pires LA, Johnson KM. Intraoperative testing of the implantable cardioverter-defibrillator: how much is enough? J Cardiovasc Electrophysiol 2006;17:140–5.

19. Michowitz Y, Lellouche N, Contractor T, et al. Defibrillation threshold testing fails to show clinical benefit during long-term follow-up of patients undergoing cardiac resynchronization therapy defibrillator implantation. Europace 2011;13:683–8.

20. Calvi V, Dugo D, Capodanno D, et al. Intraoperative defibrillation threshold testing during implantable cardioverter-defibrillator insertion: do we really need it? Am Heart J 2010;159:98–102.

21. Bianchi S, Ricci RP, Biscione F, et al. Primary prevention implantation of cardioverter defibrillator without defibrillation threshold testing: 2-year follow-up. Pacing Clin Electrophysiol 2009;32: 573–8.

22. Gula LJ, Massel D, Krahn AD, et al. Is defibrillation testing still necessary? a decision analysis and Markov model. J Cardiovasc Electrophysiol 2008; 19:400–5.

23. Blatt JA, Poole JE, Johnson GW, et al. No benefit from defibrillation threshold testing in the SCD-HeFT (Sudden Cardiac Death in Heart Failure Trial). J Am Coll Cardiol 2008;52:551–6.

24. Tokano T, Bach D, Chang J, et al. Effect of ventricular shock strength on cardiac hemodynamics. J Cardiovasc Electrophysiol 1998;9:791–7.

25. Birnie D, Tung S, Simpson C, et al. Complications associated with defibrillation threshold testing: the Canadian experience. Heart Rhythm 2008;5:387–90.

26. Healey JS, Hohnloser SH, Glikson M, et al. A novel design for a randomized trial to test if ICD implantation without any defibrillation testing is as effective as standard treatment. Heart Rhythm 2009;6:S374.

# Should You Use DFT or ULV to Assess Defibrillation Efficacy?

Charles D. Swerdlow, MD[a],*,
Ulrika Birgersdotter-Green, MD[b]

## KEYWORDS

- Implantable cardioverter defibrillator
- Upper limit of vulnerability • Ventricular fibrillation
- Vulnerability testing

Two methods are used to assess defibrillation efficacy at implantable cardioverter defibrillator (ICD) implant.[1–3] The direct, defibrillation method requires one or more sequences of induced ventricular fibrillation (VF) followed by defibrillation shocks. The pattern of success and failure of these shocks is used to estimate either the defibrillation safety margin or the defibrillation threshold (DFT). The indirect, vulnerability method relies on the close correlation between the upper limit of vulnerability (ULV), determined by delivering shocks in regular rhythm and the minimum shock strength that defibrillates reliably. The vulnerability method is less intuitive than the defibrillation method, but, in most patients, it can determine defibrillation safety margin without inducing VF. Which method is better?

## PROBABILISTIC NATURE OF DEFIBRILLATION

Probability of defibrillation success is a continuous function of shock strength (**Fig. 1**).[4,5] There is a wide range of clinically relevant shocks strengths over which defibrillation may either succeed or fail but no true threshold above which shocks always succeed. The outcomes of a series of defibrillation test shocks at the same shock strength gives an estimate of the probability of success at that shock strength. For example, if 5 of 10 defibrillation shocks (50%) are successful at 1 the shock strength, approximates the $DFT_{50}$. Multiple series of test shocks at different shock strengths provide an estimate of the entire defibrillation probability-of-success curve.[5–7]

Determination of a complete defibrillation probability of success curve requires more fibrillation-defibrillation episodes than is practical or safe in humans. Furthermore, only the upper portion of the probability of success curve is of clinical interest. To address the needs of clinical practice and research, more limited patient-specific and safety margin testing strategies have been developed. These two strategies are summarized in **Fig. 2**.

## PATIENT-SPECIFIC VERSUS SAFETY MARGIN TESTING STRATEGIES

In clinical research, the principal goal is to determine a patient-specific estimate of defibrillation efficacy so that defibrillation can be compared under different experimental conditions. The objective of patient-specific strategies is an accurate estimate of the minimum shock strength that achieves a specific, high probability of success (eg, $DFT_{90}$). Defibrillation efficacy must be assessed at several shock strengths chosen in

[a] Cedars Sinai Heart Center, Cedars-Sinai Medical Center, 414 North Camden Dr Beverly Hills, Los Angeles, CA 90210, USA
[b] University of California San Diego, 5512 Chelsea Avenue, La Jolla, San Diego, CA 92037, USA
* Corresponding author.
E-mail address: swerdlow@ucla.edu

Card Electrophysiol Clin 3 (2011) 565–576
doi:10.1016/j.ccep.2011.08.011
1877-9182/11/$ – see front matter © 2011 Published by Elsevier Inc.

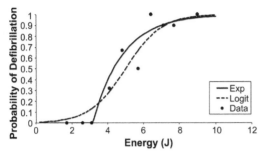

**Fig. 1.** Defibrillation probability of success curve for one dog. The abscissa plots shock strength in joules, and the ordinate plots the fraction of shocks that defibrillated at each shock strength. Each data point was computed from the results of 7 to 10 shocks. Best-fit curves are shown for exponential (Exp) and logit (sigmoid-shaped) models. The exponential curve fits the data better, primarily because of the absence of successful defibrillation at shock strengths less than or equal to 3 J. (*Adapted from* Gliner BE, Murakawa Y, Thakor NV. The defibrillation success rate versus energy relationship: part I—curve fitting and the most efficient defibrillation energy. Pacing Clin Electrophysiol 1990;13:326–38.)

relation to an estimate of the probability of success curve.

In clinical practice, the principal goal of assessing defibrillation efficacy is to identify those patients who do not have an adequate safety margin between the maximum output of the ICD and the shock strength that defibrillates reliably. Safety margin strategies limit testing to the minimum necessary to determine if there is a sufficient safety margin. Defibrillation efficacy is assessed one or more times, but usually at only 1

shock strength chosen in relation to the maximum shock strength of the ICD being tested. The outcome of each assessment is classified as successful or unsuccessful, and the cumulative result is compared with an implant criterion, which is the level of defibrillation success that is predicted to result in clinically adequate defibrillation of spontaneous VF. Performance that does not meet the implant criterion requires revising the ICD system.

## FIBRILLATION-DEFIBRILLATION TESTING

In the more commonly used defibrillation testing, VF is induced one or more times by rapid pacing, direct current, or T-wave shocks, and defibrillation test shocks of varying strengths are delivered. If the test shock is unsuccessful, a stronger rescue shock is delivered.

### The Defibrillation Threshold in Relation to the Probability-of-Success Curve

In physiology, a threshold stimulus is the minimum stimulus strength required to evoke a response. Weaker stimuli never evoke a response; stronger stimuli always evoke a response. The threshold concept does not apply to defibrillation. The probabilistic nature of defibrillation ensures that, over the clinically relevant range of shock strengths, the same shock strength may either succeed or fail on successive attempts. The term, DFT, is deeply established, so it is important to understand what it means. The DFT is calculated from pattern of successes/failures of a few shocks at different strengths along the probability of success

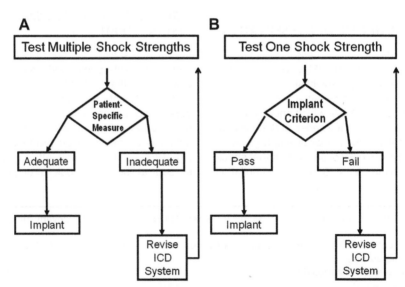

**Fig. 2.** Patient-specific (*A*) versus safety margin (*B*) strategies for implant testing. See text for details.

curve. Thus, the DFT is based on a limited, discrete sampling of a continuous statistical distribution. The probability of success and range of error at the DFT depends on the details of how this sampling is performed: the shock protocol, initial shock strength, and shock step size.[1]

### Methods for Measuring the DFT

In general, the pattern of outcomes (success or failure) of the sequence of defibrillation (and rescue) shocks is used to estimate a specific point on the probability-of-success curve. A multiple reversal protocol with equal steps estimates the $DFT_{50}$ accurately by averaging the values of successful and unsuccessful shocks but is usually considered too rigorous for clinical testing (**Fig. 3**).[8] The most commonly used clinical DFT methods include binary search, step down, and step up (**Fig. 4A–C**). In contrast to the method for estimating the $DFT_{50}$, clinically used methods define the DFT as the weakest shock strength that defibrillates. The number of fibrillation-defibrillation episodes is fixed in the binary search method but variable in the step up and step down methods. The step up method permits assessing more shock strengths with fewer VF episodes, but it results in longer VF episodes if a strong shock is required for defibrillation. For this reason, some investigators question its safety. Other protocols require 2 or 3 consecutive defibrillation successes to define enhanced thresholds, referred to as the DFT+ and DFT++, respectively.[9] The DFT++ corresponds to a higher point on the probability-of-success curve, probably near the $DFT_{90}$.

What are the probabilities of successful defibrillation and confidence intervals at the DFT as measured clinically? Different methods of measuring the DFT approximate different points on the probability-of-success curve. Within the range of starting shock strengths and step sizes used clinically, these methods approximate the $DFT_{60}$ to $DFT_{80}$.[10,11] Clinical measurement of DFT has only fair reproducibility. In a study of 25 patients, the correlation coefficient between two successful determinations of the DFT was 0.64.[12] Two patients (8%) had differences between first and second determinations of greater than or equal to 10 J.

### Safety Margin Testing, DFT Testing, and the Implant Criterion

Safety margin (see **Fig. 4** D) testing is more reproducible than DFT testing.[1] Whether safety margin or DFT testing is used, there is an inverse relationship between specificity of failing high-DFT patients and sensitivity for passing low-DFT patients, depending on the implant criterion used. Smits and Virag[1] compared the ability of different implant criteria to identify patients with a 90% probability of a successful first shock at the maximum output of a 35-J ICD.[11] The specificity of classifying high-DFT patients correctly varied from 11% for a binary search protocol requiring DFT less than or equal to 24 J to 74% for a step-down protocol requiring DFT less than or equal to 18 J. **Table 1** shows sensitivity and specificity of various implant criteria.

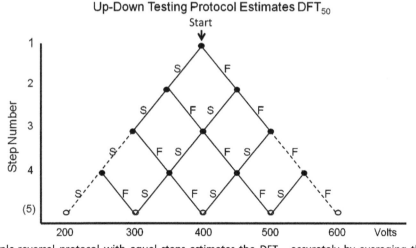

**Fig. 3.** Multiple-reversal protocol with equal steps estimates the $DFT_{50}$ accurately by averaging the values of successful and unsuccessful shocks. The starting shock strength should be near the population mean $DFT_{50}$. The $DFT_{50}$ is calculated as the average of the strengths of the 4 delivered shocks and fifth shock, which is calculated but not delivered. (*Data from* McDaniel W, Schuder J. An up-down algorithm for estimation of the cardiac ventricular defibrillation threshold. Med Instrum 1988;22:286–92.)

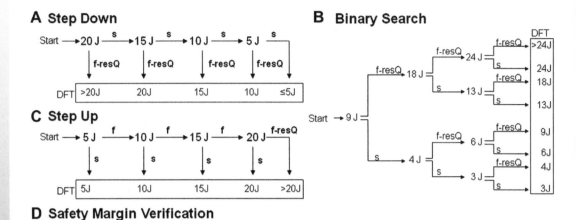

**Fig. 4.** Commonly used methods for assessing defibrillation efficacy at implant of an ICD with a maximum shock strength of 30 J. Panels A–C illustrate protocols to determine the patient-specific DFT. Panel D illustrates a method to verify a defibrillation safety margin between the maximum shock strength of the ICD and the shock strength required for consistent defibrillation. In each panel, "s" indicates defibrillation success, and "f-resQ" indicate defibrillation failure followed by a strong rescue shock. The rescue shock may be delivered internally from the ICD or externally from a transthoracic defibrillator. Panel A illustrates the Step Down method. Panel B illustrates the Binary Search method. In both Panel A and Panel B, each failed defibrillation shock is followed by a rescue shock Thus each fibrillation-defibrillation episode provides data regarding the efficacy of one shock strength. Panel C illustrates the Step Up method. Panel D illustrates the Safety Margin method. This method limits testing to the minimum necessary to determine if there is a sufficient safety margin between the maximum shock strength of the ICD and the shock strength required for consistent defibrillation. LED indicates lowest tested energy that defibrillates.

### Regression to the Mean: Implications for High DFTs and Retesting

Any defibrillation failure may be a low probability event due to chance alone rather than evidence of substandard defibrillation performance. For example, a defibrillation system with an acceptable 95% success rate is expected to fail in 5% of attempts. If a shock at the $DFT_{95}$ fails to defibrillate, defibrillation of a second episode of VF at the same shock strength is likely to succeed, because it has the same 95% probability of success. To

generalize, when a single measurement is an outlier in a statistical distribution, a repeat measurement likely is closer to the mean. This behavior, called regression to the mean, applies to repeated measurements in the same subject of a variable that follows a statistical distribution[13]: outlier values (high or low) are likely to be followed by less extreme ones nearer a subject's true mean.

The first clinical implication, illustrated in the preceding paragraph, is that a single defibrillation failure may be a low probability event. Thus, an ICD system should not be revised after a single

**Table 1**
**Predicted performance of different implant criteria**

| Protocol | Criterion | Passing (%) | Sensitivity (%) | Specificity (%) |
|---|---|---|---|---|
| 2 Inductions | 2/2 Successes at 24 J | 93 | 96 | 53 |
| 1 Induction | 1/1 Success at 15 J | 91 | 94 | 52 |
| 1 Induction | 1/1 Success at 12 J | 87 | 90 | 61 |
| Step down | DFT $\leq$24 J | 96 | 98 | 32 |
| Step down | DFT $\leq$18 J | 87 | 91 | 74 |
| Binary search | DFT $\leq$24 J | 99 | 100 | 11 |
| Binary search | DFT $\leq$12 J | 87 | 90 | 61 |

defibrillation failure without other evidence that the tested shock strength is insufficient. The second clinical implication relates to retesting. If selective retesting is performed only on high-DFT patients, the likely result is lower DFTs on retesting, even if no change is made to the system. If a system is revised and retesting results in a lower DFT, the anticipated regression to the mean must be accounted for before concluding that the lower, post-revision DFT represents a treatment effect. Usually, the optimal method for discriminating regression to the mean from treatment effect is not known for an individual patient and testing protocol.

## VULNERABILITY TESTING

In vulnerability testing, shocks are delivered at the most vulnerable interval in the cardiac cycle. The ULV is the weakest shock strength at or above which VF is not induced when the shock is delivered at this interval. A shock is considered strong enough to defibrillate if VF is not induced and insufficient if VF is induced.

### The Vulnerable Zone

The vulnerable period is that portion of the cardiac cycle during which shocks induce VF. Shocks in the vulnerable period induce VF only if their strength is in an intermediate range, at or above the VF threshold and less than the ULV. The combination of shock coupling intervals (relative to the R wave or pacing stimulus) and shock strengths that induce VF in a regular rhythm define the vulnerable zone. It is displayed as a bounded, homogeneous, spatiotemporal region in a 2-D display defined by time (coupling interval) on the abscissa and shock strength on the ordinate (**Fig. 5**).[3,14–16]

### The ULV Hypothesis of Defibrillation

Successful defibrillation must necessarily fulfill two sequential requirements: the shock must interrupt all VF wavefronts and, then, it must not reinitiate VF. Although the precise mechanism of defibrillation is not known with certainty, any successful theory must explain how these two requirements are fulfilled. The ULV hypothesis[17] postulates a mechanistic relationship between the ULV—measured during regular rhythm—and the minimum shock strength that defibrillates reliably. It rests on three assumptions: first, local vulnerable periods exist during VF; second, the ULV in VF approximates the ULV in normal rhythm; and third, the ULV during VF exceeds the shock strength required to stop all VF wavefronts.

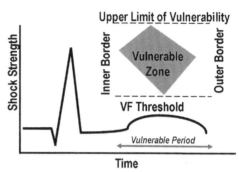

**Fig. 5.** The vulnerable zone displayed as a bounded, homogeneous region in a 2-D space defined by time (coupling interval) on the abscissa and shock strength on the ordinate. The ULV is the weakest shock strength at or above which VF is not induced when the shock is delivered at any time during the vulnerable period. The upper border (ULV) and the lower borders (VF threshold) are defined by shock strength. The inner (*left*) and outer (*right*) borders are defined by time (coupling interval).

According to the ULV hypothesis, a shock always defibrillates if it terminates all VF wavefronts and prevents reinitiation of VF. The latter requirement implicitly includes both spatial and temporal components: the shock must not reinitiate VF even if the spatial region of weakest field strength (lowest voltage gradient) is temporally coincident with the local vulnerable period. The minimum required shock strength is the ULV. Thus, there is a close correlation between the ULV and the weakest shock strength that defibrillates reliably.[17] Two corollaries of this hypothesis have clinical relevance: (1) the ULV provides a patient-specific measure of defibrillation efficacy, usually with a single fibrillation-defibrillation episode and (2) the safety margin for ICD shocks can be assessed without inducing VF. Multiple lines of evidence support this hypothesis.[3,18–20]

The response to a shock that stops all wavefronts but is weaker than the ULV varies depending on the unpredictable fibrillatory pattern of pre-shock activation and repolarization in the region of weakest field strength. If the shock times in the local vulnerable period, then it reinitiates VF and is unsuccessful. Otherwise it terminates VF and is successful. Thus the ULV hypothesis predicts that defibrillation will be probabilistic on a macroscopic level.[21]

### Establishing the ULV as a Clinical Tool

For an estimate of the ULV in regular rhythm to provide a useful measure of defibrillation efficacy, 3 conditions must be met: (1) the most vulnerable part of the human cardiac cycle corresponding to the ULV must be identified; (2) the ULV in regular rhythm must identify a specific point on the defibrillation probability of success curve; and (3) the method for estimating the ULV must be reproducible.

### Timing of the Peak of the Human Vulnerable Zone

The most vulnerable part of the human vulnerable zone is narrow and no fiducial timing marker identifies it in all patients.[3,22–24] Thus a scan of 3 or 4 shocks separated by 20-ms intervals is used to ensure that at least one is delivered at on the most vulnerable interval (**Fig. 6**).

### Measurements from the surface ECG

An easily measured fiducial marker of repolarization is the maximum absolute value of the latest peaking monophasic T wave opposite in polarity from the R wave during right-ventricular apical pacing.[22,23] For a single-coil shock vector, a 4-shock scan should be delivered at −40 ms, −20 ms, 0 ms, and +20 ms relative to the peak of the T wave.[22] For a dual-coil shock vector, a 4-shock scan should be delivered at −20, 0, +20, and +40 ms relative to the peak (see **Fig. 6**).[3,22–24]

### Measurements from the endocardial electrograms

Vulnerability testing would be more efficient if ICDs selected timing intervals for T-wave shocks

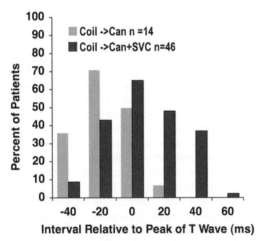

**Fig. 6.** Histograms show timing of most vulnerable intervals (peak of vulnerable zone) relative to peak of T wave during ventricular paced rhythm at cycle length 500 ms. Separate histograms show data for 14 patients with single-coil leads and 46 patients with dual-coil leads. Percentages add to greater than 100% because the peak of the vulnerable zone contains a median of 2 coupling intervals. The distribution for single-coil leads is shifted to shorter intervals relative to the distribution for dual-coil leads.

automatically. Because ICD electrograms typically have biphasic T waves, their peaks are difficult to measure. The recovery time, however, which is the maximum of the first derivative (dV/dt) of the T wave, is a reliable measure of local repolarization. The recovery time of the far-field (shock) electrogram has been used as a fiducial marker of global repolarization to time T-wave shocks accurately.[23] This permits automated selection of the fiducial interval used for timing T-wave shocks.[24,25] The global recovery time occurs approximately 15 to 30 ms after the peak of the T wave.[23–25] Accounting for delays in processing times, a 4-shock T-wave scan should be delivered at −50, −30, −10, and +10 ms relative to the recovery time (**Fig. 7**).

### ULV: Probability of Successful Defibrillation and Reproducibility

As measured clinically, the ULV correlates closely with the shock strength that defibrillates with 90% probability (DFT$_{90}$).[26] The acute success rate at ICD implantation for shocks with strength of 3 J to 5 J above the ULV approximates 100%.[12,26]

Because the ULV depends on predictable patterns of activation and repolarization during normal rhythm, it is highly reproducible.[12] Thus the probability of success curve for not inducing VF is steep, and the range of appropriately timed shocks, which can either induce or not induce VF, is narrow (**Fig. 8**).

### Inductionless Implantation of ICDs Using only Vulnerability Safety Margin Testing

Instead of determining a patient-specific shock strength based on the ULV, a vulnerability safety margin safety can be determined relative to maximum output of the ICD, analogous to a defibrillation safety margin. By definition, this shock strength equals or exceeds the ULV. The advantage of this approach is that it does not require induction of VF to determine a safety margin for shocks that defibrillate reliably. It has been validated prospectively in single-center[27,28] studies and in multicenter studies.[25,29]

Day and colleagues[29] assessed acute vulnerability safety margin using a 3-shock T-wave scan at 14 J in 421 patients. The 77% of patients who passed vulnerability safety margin testing without induction of VF at 14 J underwent fibrillation-defibrillation testing with defibrillation shock strength of 21 J. The success rate for defibrillation of induced VF was 98.5%.

Based on population estimates of the distribution of individual patient probability of success curves, approximately 90% of ICD recipients will

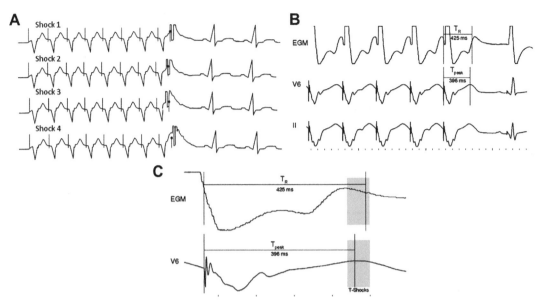

**Fig. 7.** Schematic representation of automated vulnerability testing based on the intracardiac electrogram (EGM) after pacing trains at 500 ms. (*A*) Surface ECG recordings during T-wave shocks delivered at four coupling intervals in relation to a fiducial point selected using the ICD's far-field EGM. (*B*) Far-field electrogram and representative surface ECG leads during right ventricular pacing at cycle length 500 ms in an individual patient during vulnerability testing for a dual-coil lead. The last 5 beats of the pacing train and the subsequent sinus beat are shown. The fiducial point measured from the ECG ($T_{peak}$) occurs at 396 ms in V6. The fiducial point measured from the electrogram (recovery time, $T_R$) occurs at 425 ms. (*C*) High resolution image of the repolarization phase of the last paced beat. The gray rectangles represent the 60 ms window scanned by four T-wave shocks, −20 to +40 ms relative to $T_{peak}$ and −50 to +10 ms relative to $T_R$. These windows align because of the offset between $T_{peak}$ and $T_R$.

pass vulnerability safety margin testing at 20 J, allowing an adequate safety margin for ICDs with shock strength greater than or equal to 30 J.[30] In a recent multicenter study, 54 patients underwent automated vulnerability safety margin testing at

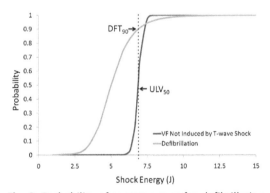

**Fig. 8.** Probability of success curves for defibrillation and not inducing VF by T-wave shocks in regular rhythm. The vulnerability curve for T-wave shocks is steeper than the defibrillation curve, and the range of shocks over which defibrillation may succeed or fail is wider than that over which VF may or may not be induced. The DFT$_{90}$ is near the midrange of the vulnerability curve.

18 J based on the intracardiac electrogram.[25] Modeling predicted that VF will be induced in 12% of patients; VF was induced in 10 patients (19%). All 44 patients who passed testing (81%) without induction of VF had successful defibrillations at 25 J (10-J safety margin). Of the 10 patients in whom VF was induced, 3 had unsuccessful defibrillation at 22 J and 2 had unsuccessful defibrillation at 25 J ($P = .04$).[25]

## Sensing During VF in Relation to Vulnerability Testing

In addition to testing defibrillation efficacy, VF is induced to ensure reliable sensing. ULV testing, which requires induction of 1 episode of VF, permits assessment of sensing during VF but vulnerability safety margin testing does not. Studies of vulnerability safety margin testing have required adequate R waves ($\geq$5–7 mV) in native rhythm because there is an approximate correlation between R-wave amplitude in native rhythm and the amplitude of VF electrograms.[31] Using this approach, VF was not undersensed at implant[24,27,29,32] or follow-up.[27] In modern ICDs, clinically significant undersensing of VF is rare, even if R waves are small,[33,34] and cannot be predicted or reproduced at ICD implant.[2,35] Ruetz and colleagues[34] reported no correlation between baseline R-wave amplitude and sensing of induced VF (n = 1177) or spontaneous device-detected VF (n = 1235).

### How to Use Vulnerability Testing to Assess Defibrillation Safety Margin Without Inducing VF

Box 1 summarizes the steps of vulnerability testing for left pectoral ICDs in which the housing (the can)

---

**Box 1**

**How to do vulnerability testing**

1. Record all 12 surface ECG leads at speed $\geq$100 mm/s.

2. Deliver pacing train from right ventricular apex at cycle length 500 ms.

3. Determine $S_1$–$T_{peak}$ of latest peaking monophasic T wave.

4. Select the strength of the test shock (see text).

5. Give scan of 4 T shocks

   a. Single-coil leads: 0, −20, −40, and +20 ms relative to $T_{peak}$

   b. Dual-coil leads: 0, −20, +20, and +40 ms relative to $T_{peak}$

6. Wait at least 60 seconds between shocks.

7. If the 4-shock scan does not induce VF,

   a. Testing is completed if the goal is to determine a safety margin.

7a. Remeasure the $S_1$–$T_{peak}$ interval, decrease the test shock strength and repeat the 4-shock scan if the goal is to determine the ULV. Repeat this process until VF is induced.

8. If VF is induced

   a. At the initial test shock strength, the shock strength is below the ULV.

   b. Otherwise the previous tested shock strength is the ULV

9. Wait 4 to 5 minutes. Then remeasure the $S_1$–$T_{peak}$ interval.

10. Rescan the vulnerable zone using stronger shocks at the same and adjacent coupling intervals relative to the T wave if any of these intervals were not tested.

11. Program the first ICD shock to at least 5 J greater than or equal to the ULV or the shock strength in step 8a.

---

serves as defibrillation electrodes (see previous review for details[3]):

1. Record all 12 surface ECG leads at a minimum speed of 100 mm/s if testing is based on the surface ECG.

2. Deliver an R-wave synchronized 8-beat pacing train from the right ventricular apex at cycle length 500 ms. Unpublished data indicate that the method applies equally well to apical septal pacing and is insensitive to pacing cycle lengths greater than the range of 400 to 600 ms. (Charles Swerdlow, MD, unpublished data, 2001). In some patients with rapidly conducted atrial fibrillation, pacing must be performed at cycle length 400 ms to achieve a stable rhythm for vulnerability testing.

3. Review the pacing train to ensure capture of all 8 beats. Using the last complex of the pacing train, determine the interval from the pacing stimulus to the peak of the latest peaking monophasic T wave ($S_1$–$T_{peak}$) that has opposite polarity to the QRS complex. The last complex is easiest to measure because it is usually followed by a pause, which prevents superimposition of the terminal portion of a T wave with the next pacing stimulus. Measurements based on only a few leads may underestimate the $S_1$–$T_{peak}$ interval.

4. Select an initial test-shock strength for scanning the vulnerable zone. The optimal shock depends on the trade-off between the value of avoiding VF and that of programming the lowest effective shock strength. If maximal priority is assigned to not inducing VF, the shock strength should be 5 J to 10 J below the maximum output of the ICD. If the goal is to determine the ULV—not just a safety margin—then the shock strength should be a few joules higher than the population's mean DFT, usually in the 10-J to 12-J range. Because VF may be induced, vulnerability testing requires the same preparation for external rescue defibrillation as defibrillation testing.

5. Deliver up to 4 T-wave shocks in the sequence indicated. Coupling intervals are ordered based on their probability of inducing VF.

6. Wait at least 60 seconds for recovery of circulation between shocks that do not induce VF. The authors wait 90 to 120 seconds in the sickest of patients.

7. If the 4-shock scan does not induce VF, the shock strength is greater than or equal to the ULV. If the goal is to determine an ICD safety margin rather than the ULV, testing is complete. Program the first ICD shock greater than or

equal to the tested shock strength +5 J. If VF is not induced as in step 5 and the goal is to determine the ULV, remeasure the $S_1-T_{peak}$ interval, decrease the test shock strength, and repeat the 4-shock scan. If VF is induced, the previous tested shock strength is the ULV. If VF is not induced, iterate the process. The lowest shock strength that ensures near 100% defibrillation success is a 3 J to 5 J greater than the ULV.

8. If VF is induced as in step 5, the shock strength is below the ULV. Nonsustained polymorphic VT lasting longer than 3 seconds with cycle length less than 250 ms is considered equivalent to VF for the purpose of estimating the ULV. Rarely, sustained VT is induced. Initiation of either nonsustained VF or sustained VT usually indicates that the shock strength is near a border of the vulnerable zone. If the induced VT or VF requires defibrillation, wait 4 to 5 minutes. Then remeasure the $S_1-T_{peak}$ interval and rescan the vulnerable zone using stronger shocks, starting at the same coupling interval relative to the T wave. The $S_1-T_{peak}$ interval changes significantly in 10% to 20% of clinical ICD implants, depending on the number of shocks, number of VF episodes, and patient's autonomic tone.

Once an interval that induces VF is identified and a stronger shock at the same interval does not induce VF, the homogenous property of the vulnerable zone ensures that the scan at the higher shock strength need include only a 20-ms window on each side of the inducing interval, providing the $S_1-T_{peak}$ interval is constant. If VF is induced at this stronger shock strength, either repeat step 8 or revise the defibrillation system.

## COMPARISON OF DEFIBRILLATION AND VULNERABILITY TESTING
### Accuracy of Assessing Defibrillation Efficacy

Clinically, the ULV provides a superior measure of defibrillation efficacy than the DFT for two reasons. First, it is more reproducible than the DFT.[12] Second, it provides a direct estimate of a more clinically relevant point on the defibrillation probability of success curve. The ULV provides a good estimate of the $DFT_{90}$ with a mean of 1.2 episodes of VF. In contrast, defibrillation testing using the DFT++ method requires 5 to 6 episodes of VF for a comparably accurate assessment of the $DFT_{90}$. Typical DFT testing requiring approximately 3 episodes of VF results in less accurate assessment of the clinically less useful $DFT_{60-80}$. Furthermore, because therapeutic ICD shocks can be programmed to 5 J above the ULV (vs 10

J above the DFT), on average, programmed shock strengths are lower for ULV testing than DFT testing.[36]

There are fewer data comparing safety margin testing via the defibrillation and vulnerability methods. Available data indicate that vulnerability safety margin testing is as least as reliable as defibrillation safety margin testing.[27,29,32]

### Sensing During VF

Clinically significant undersensing is sufficiently rare and not reproducible that VF does not need to be induced to confirm sensing during VF. Sensing should be confirmed, however, if patients have separate electrical devices that may interfere with ICD sensing, such as neurostimulators or cardiac contractility modulation devices.

### Risks

The risks of defibrillation testing are related to VF, shocks alone, and anesthesia required for shocks (**Table 2**). The principal risk of shocks alone is arterial thromboembolism if intracardiac thrombus is present. Vulnerability testing does not reduce this risk.

The greatest risk of inducing VF is pulseless electrical activity (PEA) caused by electromechanical dissociation, which may occur in clinically stable patients. Fatal electromechanical dissociation has been reported only after defibrillation from VF[37–40] but not after shocks during paced or normal rhythm. This distinction applies during both implant testing and follow-up. Some patients with post-VF PEA had severe left-ventricular dysfunction or underwent many fibrillation-defibrillation episodes, but PEA has been reported in stable patients during

**Table 2**
**Risks of vulnerability testing (shocks alone) versus defibrillation testing (shocks and VF) at ICD implant testing**

| | Defibrillation Testing | Vulnerability Testing |
|---|---|---|
| Risks of VF | | |
| Prolonged resuscitation | + | ± |
| Postshock PEA | + | 0 |
| Risks of shocks alone | | |
| Thromboembolism if intracardiac thrombus | + | + |
| Anesthesia required | + | + |

Abbreviations: +, definite risk; ±, low risk; 0, no risk.

the first or second fibrillation-defibrillation episode. In one large study, 2 of 3 deaths attributable to defibrillation testing in a study of 19,067 patients were caused by PEA in clinically stable patients.[38] In addition, prolonged resuscitation from PEA or refractory VF occurred in 27 patients (0.14%). To the best of the authors' knowledge, PEA has not been reported as a result of T-wave shocks that did not induce VF.

Additional risks of inducing VF include central nervous system hypoperfusion, resulting in electroencephalographic changes,[41] myocardial ischemia, prolonged resuscitation, and myocardial depression. Although shocks alone may depress myocardial contractility,[42] significant hypotension is more common after a single fibrillation-defibrillation episode than after 3 T-wave shocks that do not induce VF (8% vs 2%, $P = .006$).[43] In another study, prolonged hypotension did not occur in any of 394 patients during vulnerability safety margin testing, whereas it occurred in 2% of a subgroup of patients after 1 episode of induced VF.[29]

Vulnerability testing reduces the risks associated with VF to the extent that it minimizes induction of VF. It permits safety margin testing without inducing VF in 80% to 90% of patients and determination of the minimum patient-specific shock strength that defibrillates with fewer episodes of VF (approximately 1 vs at least 3). But it does not reduce risks associated with shocks alone or anesthesia. Overall, it is probably safer than defibrillation testing.

## Convenience

Both vulnerability safety margin testing and defibrillation safety margin testing with 2 induced VF episodes take approximately 5 minutes to complete. Occasionally VF can be difficult to induce, despite the multiple options provided by ICD programmers.[25] In a prospective multicenter study, the mean time required by investigators with varying prior experience was 4.5 minutes for vulnerability safety margin testing versus 2.4 minutes for a single episode of VF.[29] Three-fourths of all vulnerability safety margin tests were performed within 5 minutes.

Until vulnerability testing is automated in ICDs, it requires accurate measurement of the interval between S1 and the peak of the T wave in multiple ECG leads. The vulnerability method is subject to operator error, and it is impractical if only 1 to 3 ECG leads are recorded or if measurements can be made only at 25 to 50 mm/s. In contrast, commercially available ICD programmers all incorporate technology designed to induce VF for defibrillation testing.

## SUMMARY

The pacing threshold is assessed at pacemaker implantation to ensure a safety margin for cardiac stimulation. By analogy, the DFT has been assessed at ICD implantation to ensure a safety margin for defibrillation. Because of the statistical nature of defibrillation, however, there is no threshold for defibrillation. The ULV, a measurement made in regular rhythm, provides a more reproducible estimate of the minimum shock strength required for defibrillation than the DFT, and it measures a clinically more relevant point on the defibrillation probability of success curve than the DFT ($DFT_{90}$ vs $DFT_{60-80}$). The apparent paradox of the ULV's superiority to the DFT is explained by the fact that the critical event in reliable defibrillation is preventing shocks from reinitiating fibrillation, not terminating all VF wavefronts. Of greatest clinical importance, vulnerability safety margin testing can confirm an adequate defibrillation safety margin without inducing VF in 80% to 90% of ICD recipients. Even without automated vulnerability testing, operator-performed testing can be completed rapidly and accurately with limited training. The authors consider it to be the preferred method for assessing defibrillation efficacy at ICD implants.

## REFERENCES

1. Smits K, Virag N. Impact of Defibrillation Test Protocol and Test Repetition on the Probability of Meeting Implant Criteria. Pacing Clin Electrophysiol 2011. [Epub ahead of print].
2. Swerdlow CD, Russo AM, DeGroot PJ. The dilemma of icd implant testing. Pacing Clin Electrophysiol 2007;30:675–700.
3. Swerdlow CD, Shehata M, Chen PS. Using the upper limit of vulnerability to assess defibrillation efficacy at implantation of icds. Pacing Clin Electrophysiol 2007;30:258–70.
4. McDaniel WC, Schuder JC. The cardiac ventricular defibrillation threshold: inherent limitations in its application and interpretation. Med Instrum 1987;21:170–6.
5. Davy JM, Fain ES, Dorian P, et al. The relationship between successful defibrillation and delivered energy in open-chest dogs: reappraisal of the "defibrillation threshold" concept. Am Heart J 1987;113:77–84.
6. Gliner BE, Murakawa Y, Thakor NV. The defibrillation success rate versus energy relationship: part I–curve fitting and the most efficient defibrillation energy. Pacing Clin Electrophysiol 1990;13:326–38.
7. Malkin RA, Souza JJ, Ideker RE. The ventricular defibrillation and upper limit of vulnerability dose-response curves. J Cardiovasc Electrophysiol 1997; 8:895–903.

8. McDaniel W, Schuder J. An up-down algorithm for estimation of the cardiac ventricular defibrillation threshold. Med Instrum 1988;22:286–92.

9. Gold MR, Higgins S, Klein R, et al. Efficacy and temporal stability of reduced safety margins for ventricular defibrillation: primary results from the low energy safety study (less). Circulation 2002;105:2043–8.

10. DeGroot PJ, Church TR, Mehra R, et al. Derivation of a defibrillator implant criterion based on probability of successful defibrillation. Pacing Clin Electrophysiol 1997;20:1924–35.

11. Smits K, DeGroot P. A bayesian approach to reduced implant testing of a ventricular defibrillator: a computer simulation [abstract]. Europace 2004;6:S97.

12. Swerdlow CD, Davie S, Ahern T, et al. Comparative reproducibility of defibrillation threshold and upper limit of vulnerability. Pacing Clin Electrophysiol 1996;19:2103–11.

13. Barnett AG, van der Pols JC, Dobson AJ. Regression to the mean: what it is and how to deal with it. Int J Epidemiol 2005;34:215–20.

14. Winfree AT. Sudden cardia death: a problem in topology. Sci Am 1983;248:144–9.

15. Yamanouchi Y, Cheng Y, Tchou PJ, et al. The mechanisms of the vulnerable window: the role of virtual electrodes and shock polarity. Can J Physiol Pharmacol 2001;79:25–33.

16. Efimov IR, Gray RA, Roth BJ. Virtual electrodes and deexcitation: new insights into fibrillation induction and defibrillation. J Cardiovasc Electrophysiol 2000; 11:339–53.

17. Chen PS, Shibata N, Dixon E, et al. Comparison of the defibrillation threshold and the upper limit of ventricular vulnerability. Circulation 1986;73:1022–8.

18. Chen PS, Wolf PD, Ideker RE. The mechanism of cardiac defibrillation: a different point of view. Circulation 1991;84:913–9.

19. Efimov IR, Cheng Y, Yamanouchi Y, et al. Direct evidence of the role of virtual electrode-induced phase singularity in success and failure of defibrillation. J Cardiovasc Electrophysiol 2000;11:861–8.

20. Evans FG, Ideker RE, Gray RA. Effect of shock-induced changes in transmembrane potential on reentrant waves and outcome during cardioversion of isolated rabbit hearts. J Cardiovasc Electrophysiol 2002;13:1118–27.

21. Yashima M, Kim YH, Armin S, et al. On the mechanism of the probabilistic nature of ventricular defibrillation threshold. Am J Physiol Heart Circ Physiol 2003;284:H249–55.

22. Swerdlow C, Martin D, Kass R, et al. The zone of vulnerability to t-wave shocks in humans. J Cardiovasc Electrophysiol 1997;8:145–54.

23. Swerdlow C, Shivkumar K, Zhang J. Determination of the upper limit of vulnerability using implantable cardioverter-defibrillator electrograms. Circulation 2003;107:3028–33.

24. Shehata M, Belk P, Kremers M, et al. Automatic determination of timing intervals for upper limit of vulnerability using icd electrograms. Pacing Clin Electrophysiol 2008;31:691–700.

25. Birgersdotter-Green U, Monir G, Ruetz L, et al. Automated vulnerability testing accurately identifies patients with inadequate defibrillation safety margin. Circulation 2010;122:A20654.

26. Swerdlow CD, Ahern T, Kass RM, et al. Upper limit of vulnerability is a good estimator of shock strength associated with 90% probability of successful defibrillation in humans with transvenous implantable cardioverter-defibrillators. J Am Coll Cardiol 1996; 27:1112–8.

27. Swerdlow CD. Implantation of cardioverter defibrillators without induction of ventricular fibrillation. Circulation 2001;103:2159–64.

28. Green UB, Garg A, Al-Kandari F, et al. Successful implantation of cardiac defibrillators without induction of ventricular fibrillation using upper limit of vulnerability testing. J Interv Card Electrophysiol 2003;8:71–5.

29. Day JD, Doshi RN, Belott P, et al. Inductionless or limited shock testing is possible in most patients with implantable cardioverter- defibrillators/cardiac resynchronization therapy defibrillators: results of the multicenter assure study (arrhythmia single shock defibrillation threshold testing versus upper limit of vulnerability: risk reduction evaluation with implantable cardioverter-defibrillator implantations). Circulation 2007;115:2382–9.

30. Ruetz L, Belk P, Stromberg K. A model of defibrillation efficacy for comapring upper limit of vulnerability to conventional implant testing. Heart Rhythm 2008;5:S240.

31. Ellenbogen KA, Wood MA, Stambler BS, et al. Measurement of ventricular electrogram amplitude during intraoperative induction of ventricular tachyarrhythmias. Am J Cardiol 1992;70:1017–22.

32. Birgersdotter-Green U, Garg A, Al-Kandari F, et al. Implantation of cardiac defibrillators without induction of ventricular fibrillation using upper limit of vulnerability testing. J Interv Card Electrophysiol 2003;8:71–5.

33. Kenigsberg DN, Mirchandani S, Dover AN, et al. Sensing failure associated with the medtronic sprint fidelis defibrillator lead. J Cardiovasc Electrophysiol 2008;19:270–4.

34. Ruetz L, Koehler J, Jackson T, et al. Sinus-rhythm r-wave amplitude does not predict undersensing of ventricular fibrillation by implantable cardioverter-defibrillators [abstract]. Circulation 2009;120:S650.

35. Dekker LR, Schrama TA, Steinmetz FH, et al. Undersensing of vf in a patient with optimal r wave sensing during sinus rhythm. Pacing Clin Electrophysiol 2004;27:833–4.

36. Swerdlow C, Peter C, Hwang C, et al. Programming of implantable defibrillators based on the upper limit

of vulnerability rather than the defibrillation threshold. Circulation 1997;95:1497–504.

37. Russo AM, Sauer W, Gerstenfeld EP, et al. Defibrillation threshold testing: is it really necessary at the time of implantable cardioverter-defibrillator insertion? Heart Rhythm 2005;2:456–61.

38. Birnie D, Tung S, Simpson C, et al. Complications associated with defibrillation threshold testing: the canadian experience. Heart Rhythm 2008;5: 387–90.

39. Schuger C, Ellenbogen KA, Faddis M, et al. Defibrillation energy requirements in an icd population receiving cardiac resynchronization therapy. J Cardiovasc Electrophysiol 2006;17:247–50.

40. Frame R, Brodman R, Furman S, et al. Clinical evaluation of the safety of repetitive intraoperative defibrillation threshold testing. Pacing Clin Electrophysiol 1992;15:870–7.

41. de Vries JW, Bakker PF, Visser GH, et al. Changes in cerebral oxygen uptake and cerebral electrical activity during defibrillation threshold testing. Anesth Analg 1998;87:16–20.

42. Tokano T, Bach D, Chang J, et al. Effect of ventricular shock strength on cardiac hemodynamics. J Cardiovasc Electrophysiol 1998;9:791–7.

43. Day J, Freedman R, Zubair I, et al. Most patients may safely undergo inductionless ICD implants [abstract]. Circulation 2003;108(suppl 4):324.

# Is a Dual-Chamber ICD Always Better in Patients Requiring an ICD?

Renee M. Sullivan, MD, Brian Olshansky, MD*

**KEYWORDS**
- Implantable cardioverter defibrillator • Dual chamber
- Pacemaker • Mortality • Heart failure

Implantable cardioverter defibrillators (ICDs) were developed to interrupt life-threatening ventricular tachycardia (VT) and ventricular fibrillation (VF). Based on large, well-controlled, randomized clinical trials with long-term follow-up, guidelines have been established for the use of ICDs in individuals at risk for sudden cardiac death suspected because of ventricular arrhythmias.[1] Data from these trials show improvement in multiple end points, including risk of death[2–4] for primary and secondary prevention.[5]

Since the inception of these devices, major technological advances have altered the construction of the ICD generator and leads to improve shock efficacy, reduce device size, and improve ease of implantation, without compromising the delivery of life-saving therapy. The single-chamber shock box has been transformed into a device that discriminates arrhythmia types and stores data regarding tachyarrhythmias at different programmable rates and durations.

These devices can deliver antitachycardia pacing (ATP) as a treatment option to reduce the need for ICD shocks. ICDs can now data log and report episodes and burden of atrial and ventricular arrhythmias, as well as determine the percentage of atrial and ventricular pacing. Algorithms have been developed to better determine whether a tachycardia is supraventricular or ventricular thereby, it is hoped, averting the need for inappropriate shocks. These devices can also deliver rate-responsive atrioventricular (AV) pacing as necessary.

For those ICD candidates who do not need cardiac resynchronization therapy (CRT), dual-chamber ICDs advantages that single-chamber devices do not offer. The question remains: is a dual-chamber ICD always better in patients requiring an ICD? The answer seems clear but, surprisingly, the role of the dual-chamber ICD is highly debated and, to many who voice an opinion, a dual-chamber device has no role whatsoever.

Although there is evidence that dual-chamber ICDs can be potentially harmful and may not offer benefits compared with a single-chamber ICD, most devices implanted in the United States, outside those for CRT, are dual-chamber ICDs. This is with good reason. Physicians prefer dual-chamber ICDs and have not been convinced by literature to the contrary. The reasons that physicians prefer dual-chamber ICDs are complex and cannot be understood simply by looking at controlled clinical trials and opinions voiced. In lieu of the literature, the consistency of the use of the dual-chamber ICD attests that there is no specific disadvantage of using this device over another. We agree with the majority opinion and provide our reasons in this article.

Department of Internal Medicine, University of Iowa Hospital and Clinics, 200 Hawkins Drive, Iowa City, IA 52242, USA
* Corresponding author.
E-mail address: brian-olshansky@uiowa.edu

Card Electrophysiol Clin 3 (2011) 577–592
doi:10.1016/j.ccep.2011.08.003
1877-9182/11/$ – see front matter © 2011 Elsevier Inc. All rights reserved.

cardiacEP.theclinics.com

## ARE THERE BENEFITS OF A DUAL-CHAMBER DEVICE?

Based on technological advancements, expectations have changed. A realistic goal, to discriminate and treat arrhythmias effectively for optimal outcomes, remains. Dual-chamber devices have several potential advantages over single-chamber devices: (1) they may provide atrial-based rate-responsive pacing to ameliorate sinus node dysfunction and chronotropic incompetence; (2) they may help discriminate atrial tachycardias automatically, thereby preventing unnecessary shocks; (3) they allow retrospective analysis of data so that appropriateness of shock and tachycardia characteristics may be determined to assist the physician with future programming; (4) they may reduce atrial fibrillation and heart failure and associated hospitalizations; and (5) they provide flexibility of programming over time to meet individual patient needs.

On the other hand, dual-chamber devices have potential disadvantages: (1) they require a second lead, with the risk of dislodgment and problems with implantation; (2) they may lead to unnecessary right ventricular pacing; and (3) they may increase cost.

## A DUAL-CHAMBER ICD: THE ICD CAN PACE

Patients may require pacing for sinus node dysfunction, chronotropic incompetence, transient or complete AV block, or sudden asystolic episodes. Having the capability of dual-chamber rate-responsive atrial-based pacing allows flexibility for proper rate appropriate AV synchrony under physiologic conditions. Backup ventricular pacing is a poor substitute.

Pacing is not necessarily required for all patients who receive ICDs but having this option can be useful. Over time, most ICD patients benefit from β-blocker therapy. It can be difficult to optimize the dose without compromising heart rate response. Medications, including digoxin, to control rate during atrial fibrillation and for heart failure, and amiodarone, prescribed for supraventricular and ventricular tachyarrhythmias, including atrial fibrillation, can compromise AV conduction and sinus node rate response to decrease baseline heart rate. In these patients, at any time, and unpredictably, it is possible for bradycardia or chronotropic incompetence to develop. Progressive sinus node dysfunction or AV block is possible for ICD candidates who have ischemic and nonischemic cardiomyopathy. In clinical practice, having an atrial lead can be helpful.

Although there may be an occasional patient in whom there is never a question about the need for pacing, such as an otherwise young and healthy patient with Brugada syndrome, most patients who receive ICDs do not fit into this category. Even young, otherwise healthy, patients with channelopathies, such as those with long QT interval syndrome, may benefit from atrial pacing because it can facilitate overdrive suppression of ventricular ectopy and prevent long-short episodes that may initiate ventricular tachyarrhythmias. Nevertheless, some suggest that in young patients, dual-chamber ICDs may not provide protection or benefit and cite a risk of lead fracture, especially in athletes.[6]

Methods to determine exactly who will and will not benefit from atrial-based, rate-responsive pacing with backup ventricular pacing remain uncertain when it comes to use of pacemakers for sinus node dysfunction and even AV block. For patients with complete heart block, there may be a survival benefit, but for most patients who have transient asystolic episodes or sinus node dysfunction, the indications are soft.

It is similarly difficult to know who will benefit from pacing a priori in an ICD cohort. ICD data in this regard are based on retrospective analyses and outcomes unrelated to functionality or quality of life.[7] Chronotropic incompetence was evaluated in 123 ICD patients with a single-chamber ICD in sinus rhythm, a dual-chamber ICD in sinus rhythm, and a single-chamber ICD in permanent atrial fibrillation. Of those evaluated, 38% were considered to have chronotropic incompetence. Significant predictors were coronary disease ($P = .036$), cardiac surgery ($P = .037$), β-blocker ($P = .032$), and amiodarone ($P = .025$) use alone, and the combined use of these drugs ($P = .01$).[8] Although only 30% of ICD patients may have a pacing indication, it is not always evident at implant which patients these are.[9]

It is also uncertain how to best program ICDs to improve outcomes. Physicians involved in day-to-day management of patients who have pacemakers or ICDs know that specific programming adjustments in rate response, baseline rate, upper rate, and AV relationships can have dramatic effects despite large randomized clinical trials that show little benefit from atrial-based rate-responsive pacing.[10]

## ADDED VALUE OF A DUAL-CHAMBER ICD: ARRHYTHMIA DISCRIMINATION

For many patients, a wide overlap in rates makes it difficult to distinguish a supraventricular tachycardia from VT. In the Inhibition of Unnecessary

RV Pacing with AVSH in ICDs (INTRINSIC RV) study,[11,12] monomorphic VT occurred in 42% of the population, with 59% of those episodes having rates between 200 and 250 beats per minute (bpm) with all remaining episodes less than 200 bpm.[13] Similarly, in the ALTITUDE study,[14] there was a wide overlap of rates of supraventricular tachycardia and VT episodes. Rate, by itself, therefore, may not be a good indicator of VT but this may be patient dependent. In younger patients, sinus rates can exceed 200 bpm with intense physical activity. Alternatively, in patients with heart failure or those with sustained VT, the risk of monomorphic VT occurring at rates similar to sinus tachycardia and atrial fibrillation may be high. A dual-chamber device has enhanced options to better discriminate the arrhythmia mechanism.

## Automatic Tachyarrhythmia Discrimination

Patients do not appreciate shocks, even when they are delivered for appropriate reasons. It is more difficult to accept an inappropriate shock, for example, for atrial fibrillation with a rapid ventricular response or for sinus tachycardia. Inappropriate shocks represent 8% to 40% of shocks and occur in 12% to 21% of ICD patients. Inappropriate shocks cause pain, fear, anxiety, syncope, proarrhythmia, and may be associated with increased mortality.[15,16] Aside from ablation of or medications to suppress a tachycardia, methods to reduce inappropriate shocks include ICD programming of tachycardia zones to higher rates, programming ATP, extending detection times, and use of algorithms to automatically discriminate supraventricular tachycardia from VT. With regard to discrimination algorithms, dual-chamber devices have the advantage.

Some algorithms exist in both single-chamber and dual-chamber ICDs. Morphology discrimination to detect changes in local electrogram morphology in VT versus baseline rhythm are not specific to dual-chamber ICDs. Morphology algorithms to evaluate local and far-field bipolar right ventricular electrogram characteristics may have some potential advantage to discriminate arrhythmias[17]; this may vary by electrogram vector[18] but, by no means, is discrimination 100% accurate. Gradations in electrogram characteristics and changes over time can make it difficult to rely solely on this criterion to determine when an ICD shock should be delivered. The lack of specificity of morphology discrimination can be improved by a V >A rate discriminator in a dual-chamber device.[19]

Sudden onset and heart rate irregularity may point toward the presence of VT (vs sinus tachycardia) or atrial fibrillation (vs VT), respectively. These algorithms work both for single-chamber and dual-chamber devices and therefore there is no specific advantage to having a dual-chamber device in this regard.

Relationships between atrial and ventricular activation are the sine quo non to distinguish supraventricular tachycardia from VT. Whereas VT can occur with AV association (in a 1:1 fashion or in a fixed multiple) or with AV dissociation, supraventricular tachycardias almost never occur with ventricular rates greater than the atrial rate. Therefore, AV relationship may help determine automatically whether a tachycardia is VT or not.

In one trial,[20] 400 ICD patients from 27 centers received a dual-chamber ICD programmed to minimize ventricular pacing but to have single-chamber or dual-chamber detection. The odds of inappropriate detection were decreased by almost half with dual-chamber detection enhancements (odds ratio [OR] = 0.53; 95% confidence interval [CI] 0.30–0.94; $P$ = .03). In this trial, dual-chamber ICDs, programmed to optimize detection enhancements and to minimize ventricular pacing, significantly decreased inappropriate detections. The rate of inappropriate detections for supraventricular tachycardia was 39.5% in the single-chamber arm compared with 30.9% in the dual-chamber arm.

More recently, AV relationships, considered in lieu of other discriminators such as lead noise discrimination, lead integrity, electrogram morphology, and T-wave discrimination, as is present in the Medtronic Protecta device (Medtronic, St Paul, MN, USA), may help reduce the incidence of inappropriate shocks (although not validated in a large clinical population).[21] Using the PR Logic dual-chamber detection algorithm, in a prospective, large, multicenter cohort, the relative sensitivity to detect VT or VF was 100%. The positive predictive value for supraventricular tachycardia was 100%.[22] Boston Scientific uses Rhythm ID in some dual-chamber devices. An electrogram vector timing and correlation algorithm integrated with ventricular and atrial rate comparison (V >A) and stability above an atrial fibrillation rate threshold is reported to have a sensitivity of 100% and specificity of 97%, suggesting that development of proper algorithms may effectively discriminate ventricular from supraventricular arrhythmias.[23] In another study, prospectively programmed enhanced-detection algorithms (stability 24 milliseconds, onset 9%, atrial fibrillation threshold 200 bpm, V >A, and sustained rate duration at least at 30 seconds) were associated on a per episode basis with the detection algorithm sensitivity of 99% and specificity of

89%. Discrimination of VT with 1:1 AV conduction remains an issue,[24] and the superiority to a single-chamber device remains arguable.

One additional problem with discrimination algorithms is that ICDs may deliver shocks even if discrimination algorithms point toward supraventricular tachycardia when tachycardia is prolonged, the so-called sustained rate duration. This is the case for many supraventricular tachycardias and therefore therapies may be delivered despite the discrimination algorithms mentioned earlier. Not well tested but possible would be to turn sustained rate duration to "off" if the algorithms were effective discriminators.

Automatic discrimination remains problematic; it is not clear that these algorithms are completely effective. The benefits are, at best, modest. In many instances, the algorithms may work for a selected time but sustained rate duration may lead to a shock anyway. While efforts continue, automatic algorithms in a dual-chamber device may be slightly better than single-chamber devices to discriminate supraventricular from ventricular arrhythmias.[25] Part of the problem is that discrimination of a rhythm disturbance with a stable AV relationship is difficult to classify,[26] although not all agree that this is a major issue.[27]

In a study of 2244 arrhythmia events in ICD patients, believed to be ventricular in origin, 431 (19.2%) were misclassified and resulted in inappropriate ICD shocks. Of these events, 42% were atrial arrhythmias. No significant difference was seen in the rate of inappropriate therapy because of a rapid supraventricular rhythm between patients with single-chamber versus dual-chamber ICDs.[28]

A meta-analysis of five prospective trials of dual-chamber ICD implants using standard arrhythmia classification algorithms in 802 patients (generally for secondary prevention) in 74 medical centers evaluated 9690 events over $302 \pm 113$ days of follow-up; 62 episodes were treated inappropriately by shocks in 40 patients, representing 5% of the population. Events were classified as oversensing (1.4%), sinus tachycardia (66%), supraventricular tachycardia (13%), slow (<150 bpm) VT (8.7%), and VT or VF (10.3%). The sensitivity of slow VT detection was 94%; for VT and VF, detection was 99.3%. The specificity of sinus rhythm, sinus tachycardia, and supraventricular tachycardia recognition was 94%, positive predictive value was 79.3%, and negative predictive value was 99.2%. The specificity of standard dual-chamber arrhythmia detection settings was 94%.[29]

In another meta-analysis of five prospective trials comparing single-chamber with dual-chamber ICDs, inappropriate shocks/patient were similar (OR 1.23; 95% CI, 0.83–1.81; $P = .31$) but there were fewer episodes with dual-chamber ICDs (OR 0.64; 95% CI, 0.52–0.78; $P<.001$). However, the mean reduction was only 1.1 episode/patient ($P<.001$).[25]

### Tachycardia Therapy Programming: Rate and Length of Episodes

The Primary Prevention Parameters Evaluation (PREPARE) study[30] evaluated long detection duration (with supraventricular discriminators for those with dual-chamber devices) in an attempt to reduce the inappropriate and unnecessary shock rate, yet allow for appropriate therapy as needed. PREPARE programming significantly reduced the morbidity index incidence density (0.26 events/patient-year for PREPARE study patients vs 0.69 events/patient-year from the Comparison of Empiric to Physician-Tailored Programming of Implantable Cardioverter-Defibrillators [EMPIRIC] and Multicenter InSync Randomized Clinical Evaluation Implantable Cardioverter Defibrillator [MIRACLE] trial comparator, $P = .003$). PREPARE patients were less likely to receive a shock in the first year versus control (9% vs 17%, $P<.01$). Although PREPARE did not show harm with long detection intervals, this programming is potentially risky and the control group was not adequate. PREPARE was a study performed by the group reporting outcomes from the Dual Chamber and VVI Implantable Defibrillator (DAVID)[31] trial, who argued in favor of using single-chamber devices. In PREPARE, of those patients not receiving biventricular devices, 110 of 452 received a single-chamber and 342 of 452 received a dual-chamber device.

The Multicenter Automatic Defibrillator Implantation Trial–Reduce Inappropriate Therapy (MADIT–RIT), an ongoing dual-chamber ICD study, is evaluating 3 programming modalities to determine which best reduces inappropriate therapies. In this study, standard modality programming (170 bpm and VT zone with ATP and shock, and 200 bpm VF zone with shock) is compared with a high rate cutoff arm and with an arm in which there is delayed detection (with discrimination algorithms), with no sustained rate duration but with slower rates programmed on. The recommended backup pacing is dual-chamber with AV Search Hysteresis. The investigators decided against studying a single-chamber programmed device.

### IMPORTANCE OF ATRIAL ELECTROGRAMS

Although automatic detection algorithms are far from foolproof and are in need of further refinement, when a patient receives an ICD shock, information derived from the ICD can be helpful to determine the next step. It is almost inconceivable that a clinical trial using an ICD can determine with any degree of certainty whether a monomorphic tachycardia is supraventricular or ventricular with only a ventricular lead present. The Sudden Cardiac Death in Heart Failure Trial (SCD-HeFT)[4,16] evaluated appropriate versus inappropriate activations and their prognostic significance. The MADIT II also evaluated inappropriate shocks, and many of the patients in this trial had a single-chamber device.[15] It can be difficult, even for the best-trained eye, to determine which patient with a single-chamber device has received an appropriate or inappropriate shock without an atrial electrogram. Whereas episodes of VF and polymorphic VT can be determined with a high degree of certainty, monomorphic tachycardias are more prevalent and are harder to distinguish.

In clinical practice, if a patient receives an ICD activation, the cause for the activation can be determined with better certainty if an atrial lead is present. Although it might not necessarily offset the first ICD activation or even the second (appropriate or inappropriate), having this information makes it easier to determine the cause of the tachycardia and how to manage the patient.

Several examples of how atrial electrograms can be used to make diagnoses are shown in **Fig. 1**. In one example, there is an abrupt onset of tachycardia that has a similar, if not identical, appearance to the slower rate in sinus rhythm (**Fig. 2**). The arrhythmia is not perfectly regular and electrogram appearance in the far-field is slightly different. From the atrial tracing, it is clear that this arrhythmia is supraventricular tachycardia. In another patient (**Fig. 3**), an irregular tachycardia occurs. The electrograms

appear similar to the slower rate. Nevertheless, by evaluating intracardiac electrograms, it is clear this is not a supraventricular tachycardia, but is VT. This condition is difficult to diagnose without an atrial lead. In another example (**Fig. 4**), a sustained tachycardia is present and the ventricular electrogram appears regular. There is no baseline for comparison. There are some slight changes between some beats but it is not clear what this is. By observing the atrial electrogram, it is clear that this is a VT. For another patient (**Fig. 5**), on the left side of this tracing, the electrogram morphology is regular, rapid, and appears different from the rhythm on the right side of the tracing. By having the atrial electrogram, it is clear that this is supraventricular tachycardia. The problem of discerning supraventricular from VT is compounded when there is ventricular pacing, which alters the local ventricular electrogram.

One key reason to implant an atrial lead is to help decipher one arrhythmia from another. In some instances, it can be difficult even with the atrial lead to know for sure if the rhythm is supraventricular or not, but the atrial lead provides incremental benefit.

Not only is recording atrial electrograms important for understanding ICD activations better but the atrial electrogram can also help determine the presence of atrial fibrillation. Atrial fibrillation may be associated with symptoms, congestive heart failure exacerbations, and risk of stroke. Atrial fibrillation burden may provide some evidence that there is need for anticoagulation to prevent thromboembolic events,[32,33] point to failure of previous therapies (drugs or ablation), and assist in determining if worsening symptoms or outcomes may be caused by atrial fibrillation. In addition, events such as stroke may be stood better by atrial recordings if these rercordings show newly detected episodes of atrial fibrillation.[34]

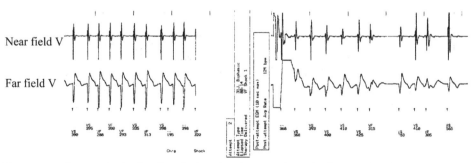

**Fig. 1.** Electrogram, from a single-chamber device, showing a tachycardia for which a shock was delivered. The cause of the tachycardia cannot be easily determined without an atrial lead.

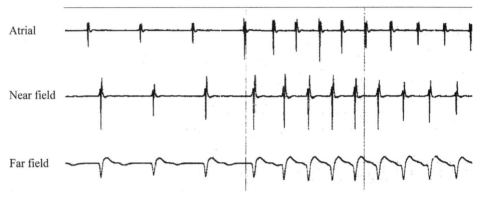

Atrial

Near field

Far field

**Fig. 2.** Intracardiac electrogram showing the abrupt onset of tachycardia with a morphology similar to that in sinus rhythm. The presence of an atrial lead helps make the diagnosis of supraventricular tachycardia in this case.

## IS POTENTIAL HARM ASSOCIATED WITH A DUAL-CHAMBER ICD?
### The DAVID Trial and Misconceptions About Harm for a Dual-Chamber ICD

Controlled clinical trials of ICDs that have shown improved survival have incorporated the use, in some cases, of single-chamber and dual-chamber (MADIT II[2]) or single-chamber devices only (SCD HeFT[4]). The DAVID trial[31] attempted to address whether dual-chamber devices were potentially harmful. However, the trial did not evaluate single-chamber versus dual-chamber ICDs. This 1-year follow-up study of 506 patients with an indication for an ICD randomized patients who underwent dual-chamber implant to VVI-40 (40 bpm pacing backup) or DDDR-70 (70 bpm lower rate pacing, no specific AV interval mentioned but commonly set at 180 milliseconds and with a range of 100–250 milliseconds). The combined end point of heart failure hospitalization and total mortality was greater in the group with DDDR pacing (**Fig. 6**).

Although the exact reason for the result is unclear, several issues are apparent: (1) the DDDR group had lower rate programming at 70

bpm, whereas the VVI programmed devices were set at 40 bpm; (2) the DDDR programmed group had a mean right ventricular pacing at one year of $58.9 \pm 36.0\%$, whereas the mean right ventricular pacing in the VVI arm was $3.5 \pm 14.9\%$; (3) the cumulative probability of heart failure hospitalization and total mortality was higher in the DDDR arm (relative hazard ratio [HR] 1.61, CI 1.06–2.44; $P \leq .03$), but for each end point separately, there was only an insignificant trend in heart failure or death between groups. Abnormal ventricular contraction, abnormal electrical activation, changes in the AV interval or changes in heart rate could be responsible for these findings. However, based on the programming characteristics, most conclude that a high percentage of pacing in the right ventricle was responsible for the differences.

A common misconception of the DAVID trial is that it showed single-chamber ICDs to be superior to dual-chamber ICDs; this was not the case because no patient had a single-chamber device. Another misconception is that the DAVID trial showed DDDR programming was inferior to VVI programming. The DAVID trial showed that DDDR programming, as was performed in this

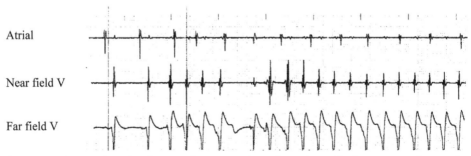

Atrial

Near field V

Far field V

**Fig. 3.** Electrogram from a dual-chamber ICD showing an irregular tachycardia that starts and stops. Analysis of both the atrial and ventricular leads shows this rhythm to be VT.

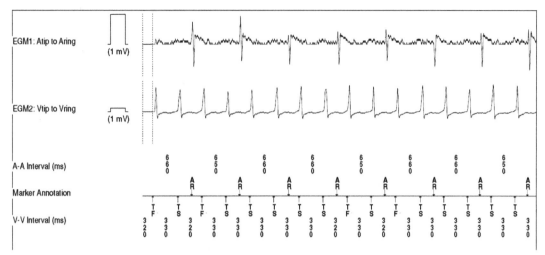

**Fig. 4.** Electrogram from a dual-chamber device showing sustained tachycardia with no baseline rhythm for comparison. After evaluating the atrial and ventricular tracings, the diagnosis of VT is made.

trial, was inferior to VVI programming based on the primary composite end point.

The DAVID trial did not prove that any degree of right ventricular pacing is harmful. It showed that right ventricular pacing at a rate greater than 50% at one year is associated with adverse outcomes. It did not show that lesser amounts of right ventricular pacing, or pacing from other sites in the right ventricle, affected outcomes. These data applied only to the DAVID population; these data might not apply to patients who have channelopathies or other medical conditions warranting ICD therapies, for example.

## RIGHT VENTRICULAR PACING: POTENTIALLY HARMFUL

Right ventricular pacing may influence outcomes deleteriously as shown in pacemaker and ICD trials. It increases the risk of atrial fibrillation, heart failure hospitalizations, ventricular arrhythmias, and mortality. Right ventricular pacing can lead to desynchronization that may cause acute changes in ventricular function and hemodynamics and may have long-standing effects on remodeling.

Data reporting the experience of patients who received extensive right ventricular pacing exist for pacemaker populations in which ventricular pacing was forced versus reduced or nearly eliminated by managed ventricular pacing (MVP). In the Search AV Extension and Managed Ventricular Pacing for Promoting Atrioventricular Conduction (SAVE Pace) trial,[35] those patients who had greater amounts of ventricular pacing had increased risk of atrial fibrillation. In this study, 1065 patients with sinus-node disease, intact AV conduction, and a normal QRS were randomized to MVP or to

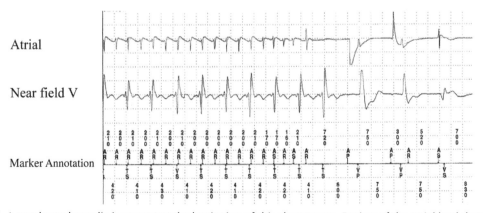

**Fig. 5.** A regular tachycardia is present at the beginning of this electrogram. Review of the atrial lead shows the rhythm to be supraventricular tachycardia.

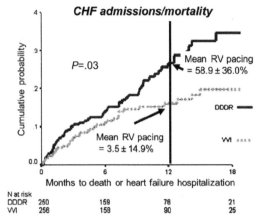

Fig. 6. Data from the DAVID trial showed patients receiving DDDR pacing compared with VVI pacing had more congestive heart failure admissions or mortality. (*Data from* Wilkoff BL, Cook JR, Epstein AE, et al. Dual-chamber pacing or ventricular backup pacing in patients with an implantable defibrillator: the Dual Chamber and VVI Implantable Defibrillator (DAVID) trial. JAMA 2002;288(24):3121–3.)

standard dual-chamber pacing with a forced ventricular pacing percentage of 99%. Persistent atrial fibrillation developed in 12.7% in the group assigned to conventional dual-chamber pacing and 7.9% in the group assigned to MVP, but the mortality was similar in both groups.

In a recent prospective trial of 177 patients with a biventricular pacemaker randomized to biventricular pacing or right ventricular apical pacing, ventricular function was reduced in those with nearly 100% right ventricular pacing compared with those who had biventricular pacing. At 12 months, the mean left ventricular ejection fraction was lower (54.8 ± 9.1% vs 62.2 ± 7.0%, P<.001) and the left ventricular end-systolic volume was higher in the right-ventricular-pacing group (35.7 ± 16.3 mL vs 27.6 ± 10.4 mL, P<.001).[36] The changes in ejection fraction and volumes were not associated with adverse outcomes and may not apply directly to an ICD population.

In the Mode Selection Trial (MOST),[37] high levels of right ventricular pacing, regardless of the programming (DDD or VVI), was associated with deleterious outcomes, more so than the mode of pacing in patients with sinus node dysfunction. In this study, patients with sinus-node dysfunction were randomized to dual-chamber pacing (1014 patients) or ventricular pacing (996 patients) and followed for a median of 33.1 months. In patients assigned to dual-chamber pacing, the risk of atrial fibrillation was lower (HR 0.79; 95% CI 0.66–0.94; P = .008), and heart failure scores were better (P<.001).[37] If RV pacing was more than 80% (VVIR) or more than 40% (DDDR), patients were at higher risk.[38]

A MADIT II retrospective subanalysis[39] showed that ventricular pacing at a rate greater than 50% increased the risk of heart failure hospitalization and death compared with those pacing 50% or less but most patients were pacing nearly 100% or not at all (**Fig. 7**). More recently, over an 8-year follow-up, mortality data were obtained from MADIT II ICD patients. The cumulative percentage of right ventricular pacing was categorized as low (≤ 50%, n = 369) or high (>50%, n = 198). Survival

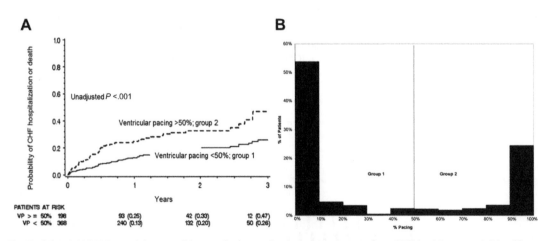

Fig. 7. (A) In MADIT II, participants with ventricular pacing at a rate greater than 50% had increased risk of heart failure hospitalization and death compared with participants with pacing less than 50%. (B) shows that despite the cutoff of less than 50% or greater than 50% right ventricular pacing, most participants in MADIT II were paced almost not at all or 100% of the time. (*From* Steinberg JS, Fischer A, Wang P, et al. The clinical implications of cumulative right ventricular pacing in the multicenter automatic defibrillator trial II. J Cardiovasc Electrophysiol 2005;16(4):361, 362; with permission.)

benefit was maintained among patients with a low percentage right ventricular pacing (HR = 0.60, $P<.001$) but not for those with high percentage right ventricular pacing (HR = 0.89, $P = .45$), suggesting long-term harm of right ventricular pacing.[40]

Right ventricular pacing was evaluated to see if it increased the risk of heart failure in an asymptomatic ICD population of 456 patients with mean left ventricular ejection fraction 40% ± 13% followed over 31 ± 22 months. With a right ventricular pacing cut point of 50%, heart failure occurred more often in the group paced greater than 50% (20% vs 9%; $P<.001$). Multivariate analysis identified right ventricular pacing greater than 50% (HR 1.85; 95% CI 1.08–3.15; $P = .03$) as a cause for more heart failure events in patients with ejection fraction 25% or less. Right ventricular pacing greater than 50% predicted appropriate shocks (HR 1.50; 95% CI 1.02–2.20; $P = .04$).[41]

In the ALTITUDE study,[14] 130,000 patients were enrolled, for whom 34,514 data sets were examined. In this study, patients were programmed DDD(R), VVI(R), and DDI(R) for a total of 15,426, 16,631, and 2097 patients. Many in the DDD(R) group were pacing at high rates in the right ventricle, whereas most of the VVI(R) patients were not. Those pacing between 1% and 4% did slightly worse than the group not pacing at all. Those doing the worst had progressively greater amounts of right ventricular pacing. Participants pacing between 35% and 100% had a poorer survival (HR 1.72, $P<.001$). The cut point of 40% showed a difference in outcomes with regard to survival as presented at Heart Rhythm by Hayes in 2009. Because high amounts of right ventricular pacing are a concern, some implanters attempt to minimize right ventricular pacing at all costs, assuming the optimal percentage of right ventricular pacing is zero. This is not necessarily the case.

## RIGHT VENTRICULAR PACING: A MARKER FOR COMORBIDITIES

Patients with ICDs who pace more in the right ventricle have greater risk of comorbidities. A recent analysis from MADIT II[40] evaluated long-term follow-up and cumulative amounts of right ventricular pacing (low [≤50%] or high [>50%]). The group with right ventricular pacing greater than 50% had high risk of mortality throughout the trial. However, there were differences between the groups; those pacing in the right ventricle greater than 50% were older (≥65 years, $P<.001$), had a wider baseline QRS (≥0.12, $P<.001$), had a longer PR interval (≥0.21, $P<.001$), had more renal insufficiency (blood urea nitrogen level >25 mg/dL, $P<.001$) and had worse

heart failure class (New York Heart Association functional class II–IV, $P = .003$). Furthermore, patients were right ventricular pacing either close to 0% or nearly 100% of the time. In the INTRINSIC RV trial, patients who were pacing more in the right ventricle were a sicker group.[42]

## DATA REFUTING HARM FROM A DUAL-CHAMBER ICD

There are many potential ways to program dual-chamber devices. Right ventricular pacing is not always required. The device could be programmed AAI(R), DDI, AAI(R) ↔ (ie, managed ventricular pacing [MVP]) DDD(R) with AV Search Hysteresis or some other modality that may reduce right ventricular pacing.

DDIR is a limited solution. It permits long AV delays. There is no upper rate tracking and there are limitations with long AV delays and lack of AV synchronization. Operationally, DDIR is VVIR during AV block if the sinus rate is greater than the lower rate limit. There is competitive atrial pacing during sensor modulation that may precipitate atrial fibrillation. There may be underdetection of VT.

Other trials have evaluated modalities in which dual-chamber devices can be implanted with low amounts of right ventricular pacing. These trials included the DAVID II trial,[43] which compared AAI-70 with VVI-40 programming, the INTRINSIC RV trial, which compared VVI programming with DDDR with AV Search Hysteresis,[11] the Dual Chamber and Atrial Tachyarrhythmias Adverse Events Study (DATAS),[44] which compared DDD versus VVI programming, and the Managed Ventricular Pacing (MVP) trial[45] which compared MVP with VVI back up.

The INTRINSIC RV trial[11] was designed to evaluate the importance of programming characteristics related to heart failure hospitalization and total mortality. Patients with standard primary or secondary indications for an ICD (none with long-standing atrial fibrillation or CRT indications) underwent dual-chamber ICD implantation. The device was programmed DDDR with AV Search Hysteresis for 1 week. Those randomized at 1-week follow-up to DDDR-60 to DDDR-130 or VVI-40 had no more than 20% right ventricular pacing (it was felt that >20% right ventricular pacing may be dangerous and these patients were followed in an observational arm). Proper adjustments to allow for greater than 80% recruitment and less than 20% pacing required an amendment,[46] testifying that specific programming characteristics are important and challenging. At 12 months, DDDR with AV Search Hysteresis was not inferior to VVI programming; there was even a trend toward superiority (relative risk reduction = 0.67, P = .07) in favor of dual-chamber programmed devices (**Fig. 8**). The 12-month mean percentage right ventricular pacing rate was 10%, substantially lower than in the DAVID trial.

An INTRINSIC RV subanalysis, considering right ventricular pacing as a continuous variable, showed an association with increased risk of heart failure hospitalization and total mortality in patients with a high percentage of right ventricular pacing (OR = 1.27, P = .003). When considering right ventricular pacing as a discrepancy variable (vs 0%–9% pacing), those pacing 30% had an OR of 3.09 (CI 1.21–7.87, P = .018) (**Fig. 9**).[42]

When considering only the DDDR with AV Search Hysteresis arm, heart failure hospitalization and total mortality were lowest in those who had right ventricular pacing 10% to 19% of the time, remarkably better than those pacing 50% or greater (**Fig. 10**). As right ventricular pacing increased, adverse outcomes increased but the group pacing 0% to 9% of the time had a higher rate of heart failure hospitalization and total mortality than the group pacing 10% to 19% of the time. These data suggest that some degree of right ventricular pacing may be beneficial by an unknown mechanism. More importantly, some degree of right ventricular pacing was not necessarily harmful. The outcome in this population was at least as good, if not better, than the VVI programmed group. One possible explanation for a small amount of ventricular pacing is that AV synchrony was maintained and that there may be a dynamic relationship between the extent of right ventricular pacing and AV dyssynchrony in this specific population.

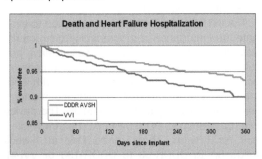

**Fig. 8.** Data from the INTRINSIC RV study showed DDDR with AV Search Hysteresis programming was not inferior to VVI programming with regard to heart failure hospitalizations or mortality. (*From* Olshansky B, Day JD, Moore S, et al. Is dual-chamber programming inferior to single-chamber programming in an implantable cardioverter-defibrillator? Results of the INTRINSIC RV (Inhibition of Unnecessary RV Pacing With AVSH in ICDs) study. Circulation 2007;115(1):13; with permission.)

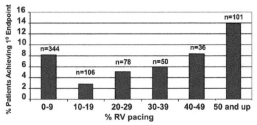

**Fig. 9.** A subanalysis of the INTRINSIC RV study showed the percentage of right ventricular pacing was associated with outcomes. Participants with 10% to 19% right ventricular pacing had fewer heart failure hospitalizations or death compared with participants with other degrees of right ventricular pacing. (*From* Olshansky B, Day JD, Lerew DR, et al. Eliminating right ventricular pacing may not be best for patients requiring implantable cardioverter-defibrillators. Heart Rhythm 2007;4(7):889; with permission.)

Many of the studies that have looked at the percentage of right ventricular pacing and outcomes have not carefully considered what degree of right ventricular pacing is important. For example, data from MADIT II[39] have considered a cutoff point at which there is risk from right ventricular pacing. Although that rate may be at 40%, most patients in this trial had either no ventricular pacing or nearly 100% pacing. Gradations were hardly present, similar to other trials. It is only the INTRINSIC RV trial[11,42] that had a gradation in the amount of pacing present.

There may be other potential benefits of AV Search Hysteresis that are not well understood. Data from the ALTITUDE study showed that DDDR with AV Search Hysteresis programmed "on" had an HR of 0.844 (P = .06) in favor of AV Search Hysteresis versus VVI programming for survival. With AV Search Hysteresis "off" and DDDR programming, the HR was in the other direction, 1.138 (P = .046) in favor of VVI programming. Although the ALTITUDE data were not prospective, DDD(R) programming with AV Search Hysteresis makes sense because it does not affect survival in a negative way and may have benefit, as presented by David Hayes at the 2009 HRS meeting.

In a subanalysis of the DAVID trial,[47] patients who were right ventricular pacing at a rate greater than 40% had a remarkably different outcome with respect to heart failure hospitalization and total mortality compared with those pacing 40% or less (**Fig. 11**). Those who had pacing less than 40% did as well, if not better, than the VVI arm. Those who were pacing greater than 40% did worse than the VVI arm. The difference between the outcome of heart failure hospitalization and total mortality in the DDDR arms with pacing

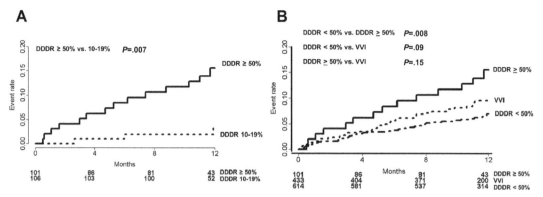

**Fig. 10.** (*A*) Data from the INTRINSIC RV study showed fewer heart failure hospitalizations and deaths in participants with DDDR with right ventricular pacing 10% to 19% compared with participants with DDDR programming and 50% or greater right ventricular pacing. (*B*) There were fewer heart failure hospitalizations and deaths amongst participants in the DDDR arm with less than 50% right ventricular pacing compared with those with 50% or greater right ventricular pacing in the DDDR arm. There was a trend for fewer events in participants with less than 50% right ventricular pacing in the DDDR arm versus the VVI arm.

greater than or less than 40% was significant (*P* = .03). It seems that a certain level of right ventricular pacing is not harmful and may help. These data corroborate the data in the INTRINSIC RV trial[42] (when looking at the pacing data with similar cut points), but the DAVID subanalysis was a small population.

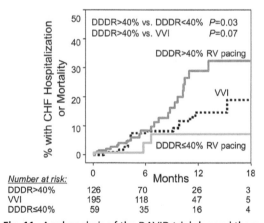

**Fig. 11.** A subanalysis of the DAVID trial showed there to be more heart failure hospitalizations or mortality in patients programmed DDDR with greater than 40% right ventricular pacing compared with DDDR with 40% or less right ventricular pacing. There was no difference in outcomes when comparing patients programmed DDDR with greater than 40% pacing and those programmed VVI. Although the population is small, these data suggest that some degree of right ventricular (RV) pacing (≤40%) is not inferior to VVI programming similar to the data from the INTRINSIC RV trial seen in **Fig. 10**B. (*From* Sharma AD, Rizo-Patron C, Hallstrom AP, et al. Percent right ventricular pacing predicts outcomes in the DAVID trial. Heart Rhythm 2005;2(8):832; with permission.)

The DATAS study[48] compared patients with dual-chamber programmed devices with those with single-chamber devices and with those with single simulated (ie, dual-chamber devices programmed single-chamber) devices in which an atrial lead was placed. There was no difference between outcomes in the group that had an atrial lead but was programmed as a single-chamber device compared with a single-chamber device, but dual-chamber devices had a better score when it came to clinically significant adverse events by 33% (*P* = .0028). The dual-chamber device showed a trend toward improved survival and fewer inappropriate shocks.

The MVP trial[45] compared dual-chamber devices that were programmed as dual-chamber, MVP, with VVI-40 backup programming to determine risk for heart failure hospitalization and total mortality. In the dual-chamber programmed "on" group, rate-responsive atrial-based pacing occurred but with MVP, ventricular pacing occurred only if there was a blocked P wave. The rate of ventricular pacing was low but long-short episodes could occur. In this study, there was no improvement in outcomes with MVP programming. Nevertheless, in a dual-chamber programmed device, with rate-responsive atrial-based programming (which is generally similar to atrial-based rate-responsive pacemaker), outcomes were no worse than VVI programming but potentially offered atrial detection and atrial pacing capabilities. One interesting subgroup analysis of the MVP trial looked at patients with long PR intervals. If the PR interval was 230 milliseconds or greater, the outcome with VVI was better than MVP (HR = 2.79, *P* = .019). It is possible that rate-responsive atrial-based pacing prolongs the PR interval, causing hemodynamic problems, or that a long-short interval led to proarrhythmia. Disadvantages of MVP programming, therefore, include AV decoupling[49] and proarrhythmia.[50] Although MVP programming may lead to proarrhythmia, even VVI backup programming can do the same thing.[51]

The DAVID II trial[43] evaluated AAI-70 to VVI-40 programming in a population of primary prevention patients. In this study, there was no potential advantage of atrial-based programming but no harm was created either. AAI pacing could serve as another safe modality for pacing using a dual-chamber ICD device.

## ICD COMPLICATIONS: IS A DUAL-CHAMBER DEVICE WORTH IT?

There is concern that implanting an atrial lead can create additional comorbidities and risks to the patient. Having a second lead can cause thrombosis of the subclavian vein. The atrial lead can also dislodge, requiring subsequent procedures, or cause ventricular ectopy if the lead falls into the ventricle. In addition, there is a risk of a second stick into the vein that may increase the risk of pneumothorax or bleeding. Nevertheless, when considering data from several large studies, the risk of ICD complications is not much greater with an atrial lead.

In the DATAS trial, the atrial lead dislodged in 4 of 223 patients (1.8%).[44] In the INTRINSIC RV trial, atrial lead issues occurred in 26 of 1530 patients (1.6%).[11] In the Centers for Medicare and Medicaid Services (CMS) National Cardiovascular Data Registry (NCDR) database, atrial lead dislodgement occurred in 1.3%. These data are in concert with previous pacemaker lead data that have been recorded from experienced implanters.[52–54]

Another evaluation of the NCDR database, which included 104,049 first-time device implants, showed that dual-chamber (n = 64,489) compared with single-chamber ICD implantation was more frequently associated with cardiac arrest (0.31% vs 0.23%, $P$ = .01), hematoma (0.92% vs 0.71%, $P<$.001), pneumothorax (0.53% vs 0.36%, $P<$.001), pericardial tamponade (0.09% vs 0.05%, $P$ = .01), lead dislodgement (0.88% vs 0.5%, $P<$.001), and any complication (3.2% vs 2.1%, $P<$.001).[55] Although these numbers are significant, the complication rates reported are low, acceptable, and hardly important clinically. Moreover, there are likely differences between the groups that explain the complications and adverse outcomes.

In another report from the NCDR database, implants were considered to fall within Combined Medicaid and Medicare recommended time guidelines or implants were placed earlier than recommended.[56] Those ICDs placed early were more likely to be dual-chamber implants (63.3% vs 58.4%, $P<$.001). Early implants were placed in an older and sicker population with a greater chance of having heart failure, diabetes, end-stage renal disease, atrial fibrillation and flutter, and chronic lung disease. Therefore, the dual chamber implant may not be the only explanation for adverse outcomes.

In a multivariable model, the prospective multicenter Canadian registry of patients undergoing first-time implantation of an ICD found an increased risk of major complications for patients receiving a dual-chamber device versus a single-chamber device (adjusted HR 1.82, 95% CI 1.19–2.79, $P$ = .006).[57] Direct and indirect implant-related complications were associated with increased death. These findings are not explained. For patients in the Canadian registry undergoing ICD replacement, there were no significant differences in complication rates between single-chamber and dual-chamber implants.[58]

## IS COST AN ISSUE?

Having a dual-chamber ICD system is potentially more costly but cost is a moving target. Prices of devices are negotiated heavily. Reimbursement rates may not be in line with costs. The cost difference may not translate to patient expense. Furthermore, there is similar longevity of single-chamber and dual-chamber devices and the replacement frequency is about the same.

Goldberger and colleagues[59] considered the cost advantage of dual-chamber versus single-chamber devices. Although the initial upfront costs of a single-chamber device may be less, other considerations come into play. In some cases, it is clear that an upgrade is required for pacing. When this situation occurs, the ICD pocket must be opened and a new lead placed. It is clear that opening an ICD pocket increases risk to the patient, including risk of infection and damage to the implanted system. Major complications occurred in about 5.8% of patients, whereas minor complications occurred in about 2.3%. Cost is also an issue. As Goldberger found, the dual-chamber ICD device remained the cheapest device, with upgrade rates in the range of 10%. A DDD ICD remains the cheapest device; the cost differential was $1568. From our own clinical experience, when a single-chamber ICD device is implanted, the options for patient care are limited year after year.

## WHAT DO THESE DATA MEAN?

The totality of the data indicate that (1) the implantation of a dual-chamber, rate-responsive ICD, by itself, adds little additional risk compared with a single-chamber ICD; (2) dual-chamber devices, by themselves, do not increase risk for adverse outcomes; (3) dual-chamber devices programmed to allow for high rates of right ventricular apical pacing may increase the risk of heart failure hospitalization and total mortality; (4) dual-chamber devices, by themselves, do not necessitate high rates of right ventricular pacing (this is based only on programming characteristics); (5) some right ventricular pacing is not necessarily harmful (low amounts may even be beneficial to patients).

## WHAT DO OUR COLLEAGUES DO?

The CMS NCDR database collects information from hospitals throughout the United States regarding ICD implants in the Medicare population. The data are consistent on one specific issue: more dual-chamber ICDs are implanted than single-chamber ICDs. This number has not changed. If anything, more dual-chamber devices are implanted now than single-chamber devices compared with several years ago. When it comes to non-CRT ICDs, approximately 62% are dual-chamber devices and 38% are single-chamber devices. Our colleagues, therefore, vote every day about which type of device they want to implant in their patients and they choose, for good reason, a dual-chamber device.

Data from other countries are in concert with data from the United States. In Australia and New Zealand, when a non-CRT ICD device is implanted, it tends to be a dual-chamber device.[60] In an analysis of the INTRINSIC RV trial, physicians continued to use dual-chamber programming even if patients were right ventricular pacing more than 20%.[61]

## NEXT STEPS

There may be other ways to program dual-chamber devices to make them even more effective to detect arrhythmias and to deliver dual-chamber pacing as necessary. New technologies are being developed such that a single lead could be used for atrial sensing and ventricular pacing but, nevertheless, atrial pacing is not available with these devices yet.[62]

## SUMMARY: SINGLE-CHAMBER VERSUS DUAL-CHAMBER ICDs

Single-chamber ICDs are not superior to dual-chamber ICDs. They limit the flexibility of programming and detection of arrhythmias that dual-chamber ICDs provide. Single-chamber ICDs lack the capability to provide AV synchronous rate-responsive bradycardia pacing when required. Many patients who are candidates for ICDs are treated with medications that can create chronotropic incompetence and bradycardia, which can lead to symptoms. Rate-responsive pacing is capable in a dual-chamber device but not a single-chamber device. Single-chamber devices can compromise arrhythmia management, whereas dual-chamber devices can help provide evidence that an arrhythmia is supraventricular or ventricular, either by automatic detection algorithms or by manual interpretation of data. In either case, a dual-chamber device can provide a better glimpse of the arrhythmias that may be causing problems for a patient and help guide proper therapy. They can also be useful to determine the need for anticoagulation should atrial fibrillation be present.

Single-chamber devices have no specific cost advantage. The advantage based on risk is small. There is really no advantage of a single-chamber device compared with a dual-chamber device. In most cases, single-chamber ICDs do not make sense.

## IS THERE EVER A REASON TO USE A SINGLE-CHAMBER ICD?

Patients who have long-standing atrial fibrillation, in whom sinus rhythm is never expected to be achieved, will not benefit in any way from a dual-chamber device and may experience only harm. With usefulness of ablation in patients with heart failure, some of the patients with long-standing atrial fibrillation may be allowed to maintain sinus rhythm and have the advantage of hemodynamic benefits in sinus rhythm. In such patients, the dual-chamber device would make sense.

Younger patients who are highly active may have problems with more than one lead. Having multiple leads in younger patients can lead to risk for lead fractures and lead dislodgements. Furthermore, for younger individuals with the potential for requiring multiple devices over their lifetime, it would make sense to minimize the number of implantable leads. Nevertheless, such individuals may be at high risk for inappropriate shocks and an atrial lead may be advantageous. Atrial leads do not necessarily reduce the risk of inappropriate shocks, especially if they are caused by sinus tachycardia.

## SUMMARY

Dual-chamber ICDs offer some specific advantages and programming flexibility that single-chamber ICDs simply cannot. The ICD of choice for the patient who has an indication for an ICD but does not need CRT is a dual-chamber ICD.

## REFERENCES

1. Epstein AE, DiMarco JP, Ellenbogen KA, et al. ACC/AHA/HRS 2008 Guidelines for Device-Based Therapy of Cardiac Rhythm Abnormalities: a report of the American College of Cardiology/American Heart Association Task Force on Practice Guidelines (Writing Committee to Revise the ACC/AHA/NASPE 2002 Guideline Update for Implantation of Cardiac Pacemakers and Antiarrhythmia Devices): developed in collaboration with the American Association for Thoracic Surgery and Society of Thoracic Surgeons. Circulation 2008;117(21):e350–408.

2. Moss AJ, Hall WJ, Cannom DS, et al. Improved survival with an implanted defibrillator in patients with coronary disease at high risk for ventricular arrhythmia. Multicenter Automatic Defibrillator Implantation Trial Investigators. N Engl J Med 1996;335(26):1933–40.

3. Moss AJ, Zareba W, Hall WJ, et al. Prophylactic implantation of a defibrillator in patients with myocardial infarction and reduced ejection fraction. N Engl J Med 2002;346(12):877–83.

4. Bardy GH, Lee KL, Mark DB, et al. Amiodarone or an implantable cardioverter-defibrillator for congestive heart failure. N Engl J Med 2005;352(3):225–37.

5. A comparison of antiarrhythmic-drug therapy with implantable defibrillators in patients resuscitated from near-fatal ventricular arrhythmias. The Antiarrhythmics versus Implantable Defibrillators (AVID) Investigators. N Engl J Med 1997;337(22):1576–83.

6. Lawrence D, Von Bergen N, Law IH, et al. Inappropriate ICD discharges in single-chamber versus dual-chamber devices in the pediatric and young adult population. J Cardiovasc Electrophysiol 2009;20(3):287–90.

7. Kutalek SP, Sharma AD, McWilliams MJ, et al. Effect of pacing for soft indications on mortality and heart failure in the dual chamber and VVI implantable defibrillator (DAVID) trial. Pacing Clin Electrophysiol 2008;31(7):828–37.

8. Melzer C, Bohm M, Bondke HJ, et al. Chronotropic incompetence in patients with an implantable cardioverter defibrillator: prevalence and predicting factors. Pacing Clin Electrophysiol 2005;28(10):1025–31.

9. Proclemer A, Della Bella P, Facchin D, et al. Indications for dual-chamber cardioverter defibrillators at implant and at 1 year follow-up: a retrospective analysis in the single-chamber defibrillator era. Europace 2001;3(2):132–5.

10. Lamas GA, Orav EJ, Stambler BS, et al. Quality of life and clinical outcomes in elderly patients treated with ventricular pacing as compared with dual-chamber pacing. Pacemaker Selection in the Elderly Investigators. N Engl J Med 1998;338(16):1097–104.

11. Olshansky B, Day JD, Moore S, et al. Is dual-chamber programming inferior to single-chamber programming in an implantable cardioverter-defibrillator? Results of the INTRINSIC RV (Inhibition of Unnecessary RV Pacing With AVSH in ICDs) study. Circulation 2007;115(1):9–16.

12. Olshansky B, Day J, McGuire M, et al. Inhibition of unnecessary RV pacing with AV Search Hysteresis in ICDs (INTRINSIC RV): design and clinical protocol. Pacing Clin Electrophysiol 2005;28(1):62–6.

13. Olshansky B, Stolen K, Jones P, et al. Arrhythmia rate distribution and tachyarrhythmia therapy in an ICD population. Heart Rhythm 2009;6:S127.

14. Saxon LA, Hayes DL, Gilliam FR, et al. Long-term outcome after ICD and CRT implantation and influence of remote device follow-up: the ALTITUDE survival study. Circulation 2010;122(23):2359–67.

15. Daubert JP, Zareba W, Cannom DS, et al. Inappropriate implantable cardioverter-defibrillator shocks in MADIT II: frequency, mechanisms, predictors, and survival impact. J Am Coll Cardiol 2008;51(14):1357–65.

16. Poole JE, Johnson GW, Hellkamp AS, et al. Prognostic importance of defibrillator shocks in patients with heart failure. N Engl J Med 2008;359(10):1009–17.

17. Theuns DA, Rivero-Ayerza M, Goedhart DM, et al. Morphology discrimination in implantable cardioverter-defibrillators: consistency of template match percentage during atrial tachyarrhythmias at different heart rates. Europace 2008;10(9):1060–6.

18. Luthje L, Vollmann D, Rosenfeld M, et al. Electrogram configuration and detection of supraventricular tachycardias by a morphology discrimination algorithm in single chamber ICDs. Pacing Clin Electrophysiol 2005;28(6):555–60.

19. Theuns DA, Rivero-Ayerza M, Goedhart DM, et al. Evaluation of morphology discrimination for ventricular tachycardia diagnosis in implantable cardioverter-defibrillators. Heart Rhythm 2006;3(11):1332–8.

20. Friedman PA, McClelland RL, Bamlet WR, et al. Dual-chamber versus single-chamber detection enhancements for implantable defibrillator rhythm diagnosis: the detect supraventricular tachycardia study. Circulation 2006;113(25):2871–9.

21. Volosin KJ, Exner DV, Wathen MS, et al. Combining shock reduction strategies to enhance ICD therapy: a role for computer modeling. J Cardiovasc Electrophysiol 2011;22(3):280–9.

22. Wilkoff BL, Kuhlkamp V, Volosin K, et al. Critical analysis of dual-chamber implantable cardioverter-defibrillator arrhythmia detection: results and technical considerations. Circulation 2001;103(3):381–6.

23. Gold MR, Shorofsky SR, Thompson JA, et al. Advanced rhythm discrimination for implantable cardioverter defibrillators using electrogram vector timing and correlation. J Cardiovasc Electrophysiol 2002;13(11):1092–7.

24. Kouakam C, Kacet S, Hazard JR, et al. Performance of a dual-chamber implantable defibrillator algorithm for discrimination of ventricular from supraventricular tachycardia. Europace 2004;6(1):32–42.

25. Theuns DA, Rivero-Ayerza M, Boersma E, et al. Prevention of inappropriate therapy in implantable defibrillators: a meta-analysis of clinical trials comparing single-chamber and dual-chamber arrhythmia discrimination algorithms. Int J Cardiol 2008;125(3):352–7.

26. Theuns DA, Klootwijk AP, Goedhart DM, et al. Prevention of inappropriate therapy in implantable cardioverter-defibrillators: results of a prospective, randomized study of tachyarrhythmia detection algorithms. J Am Coll Cardiol 2004;44(12):2362–7.

27. Li HG, Thakur RK, Yee R, et al. Ventriculoatrial conduction in patients with implantable cardioverter defibrillators: implications for tachycardia discrimination by dual chamber sensing. Pacing Clin Electrophysiol 1994;17(12 Pt 1):2304–6.

28. Jodko L, Kornacewicz-Jach Z, Kazmierczak J, et al. Inappropriate cardioverter-defibrillator discharge continues to be a major problem in clinical practice. Cardiol J 2009;16(5):432–9.

29. Anselme F, Mletzko R, Bowes R, et al. Prevention of inappropriate shocks in ICD recipients: a review of 10,000 tachycardia episodes. Pacing Clin Electrophysiol 2007;30(Suppl 1):S128–33.

30. Wilkoff BL, Williamson BD, Stern RS, et al. Strategic programming of detection and therapy parameters in implantable cardioverter-defibrillators reduces shocks in primary prevention patients: results from the PREPARE (Primary Prevention Parameters Evaluation) study. J Am Coll Cardiol 2008;52(7):541–50.

31. Wilkoff BL, Cook JR, Epstein AE, et al. Dual-chamber pacing or ventricular backup pacing in patients with an implantable defibrillator: the Dual Chamber and VVI Implantable Defibrillator (DAVID) trial. JAMA 2002;288(24):3115–23.

32. Glotzer TV, Hellkamp AS, Zimmerman J, et al. Atrial high rate episodes detected by pacemaker diagnostics predict death and stroke: report of the Atrial Diagnostics Ancillary Study of the MOde Selection Trial (MOST). Circulation 2003;107(12):1614–9.

33. Glotzer TV, Daoud EG, Wyse DG, et al. The relationship between daily atrial tachyarrhythmia burden from implantable device diagnostics and stroke risk: the TRENDS study. Circ Arrhythm Electrophysiol 2009;2(5):474–80.

34. Ziegler PD, Glotzer TV, Daoud EG, et al. Incidence of newly detected atrial arrhythmias via implantable devices in patients with a history of thromboembolic events. Stroke 2010;41(2):256–60.

35. Sweeney MO, Bank AJ, Nsah E, et al. Minimizing ventricular pacing to reduce atrial fibrillation in sinus-node disease. N Engl J Med 2007;357(10): 1000–8.

36. Yu CM, Chan JY, Zhang Q, et al. Biventricular pacing in patients with bradycardia and normal ejection fraction. N Engl J Med 2009;361(22): 2123–34.

37. Lamas GA, Lee KL, Sweeney MO, et al. Ventricular pacing or dual-chamber pacing for sinus-node dysfunction. N Engl J Med 2002;346(24): 1854–62.

38. Sweeney MO, Hellkamp AS. Heart failure during cardiac pacing. Circulation 2006;113(17):2082–8.

39. Steinberg JS, Fischer A, Wang P, et al. The clinical implications of cumulative right ventricular pacing in the multicenter automatic defibrillator trial II. J Cardiovasc Electrophysiol 2005;16(4):359–65.

40. Barsheshet A, Moss AJ, McNitt S, et al. Long-term implications of cumulative right ventricular pacing among patients with an implantable cardioverter-defibrillator. Heart Rhythm 2011;8(2): 212–8.

41. Smit MD, Van Dessel PF, Nieuwland W, et al. Right ventricular pacing and the risk of heart failure in implantable cardioverter-defibrillator patients. Heart Rhythm 2006;3(12):1397–403.

42. Olshansky B, Day JD, Lerew DR, et al. Eliminating right ventricular pacing may not be best for patients requiring implantable cardioverter-defibrillators. Heart Rhythm 2007;4(7):886–91.

43. Wilkoff BL, Kudenchuk PJ, Buxton AE, et al. The DAVID (Dual Chamber and VVI Implantable Defibrillator) II trial. J Am Coll Cardiol 2009;53(10):872–80.

44. Almendral J, Arribas F, Wolpert C, et al. Dual-chamber defibrillators reduce clinically significant adverse events compared with single-chamber devices: results from the DATAS (Dual chamber and Atrial Tachyarrhythmias Adverse events Study) trial. Europace 2008;10(5):528–35.

45. Sweeney MO, Ellenbogen KA, Tang AS, et al. Atrial pacing or ventricular backup-only pacing in implantable cardioverter-defibrillator patients. Heart Rhythm 2010;7(11):1552–60.

46. Olshansky B, Day J, McGuire M, et al. Reduction of right ventricular pacing in patients with dual-chamber ICDs. Pacing Clin Electrophysiol 2006; 29(3):237–43.

47. Sharma AD, Rizo-Patron C, Hallstrom AP, et al. Percent right ventricular pacing predicts outcomes in the DAVID trial. Heart Rhythm 2005;2(8):830–4.

48. Ricci RP, Quesada A, Almendral J, et al. Dual-chamber implantable cardioverter defibrillators reduce clinical adverse events related to atrial fibrillation when compared with single-chamber defibrillators: a subanalysis of the DATAS trial. Europace 2009;11(5):587–93.

49. Sweeney MO, Ellenbogen KA, Tang AS, et al. Severe atrioventricular decoupling, uncoupling, and ventriculoatrial coupling during enhanced atrial pacing: incidence, mechanisms, and implications for minimizing right ventricular pacing in ICD patients. J Cardiovasc Electrophysiol 2008;19(11):1175–80.

50. Sweeney MO, Ruetz LL, Belk P, et al. Bradycardia pacing-induced short-long-short sequences at the onset of ventricular tachyarrhythmias: a possible mechanism of proarrhythmia? J Am Coll Cardiol 2007;50(7):614–22.

51. Himmrich E, Przibille O, Zellerhoff C, et al. Proarrhythmic effect of pacemaker stimulation in patients with implanted cardioverter-defibrillators. Circulation 2003;108(2):192–7.

52. Eberhardt F, Bode F, Bonnemeier H, et al. Long term complications in single and dual chamber pacing are influenced by surgical experience and patient morbidity. Heart 2005;91(4):500–6.

53. Aggarwal RK, Connelly DT, Ray SG, et al. Early complications of permanent pacemaker implantation: no difference between dual and single chamber systems. Br Heart J 1995;73(6):571–5.

54. Mueller X, Sadeghi H, Kappenberger L. Complications after single versus dual chamber pacemaker implantation. Pacing Clin Electrophysiol 1990; 13(6):711–4.

55. Dewland T, Pellegrini C, Youngfei W, et al. Dual chamber ICD selection is associated with racial and socioeconomic disparities and increased complication rates among patients enrolled in the NCDR ICD Registry. Circulation 2008;118:S834–5.

56. Al-Khatib SM, Hellkamp A, Curtis J, et al. Non-evidence-based ICD implantations in the United States. JAMA 2011;305(1):43–9.

57. Lee DS, Krahn AD, Healey JS, et al. Evaluation of early complications related to De Novo cardioverter defibrillator implantation insights from the Ontario ICD database. J Am Coll Cardiol 2010;55(8):774–82.

58. Krahn AD, Lee DS, Birnie D, et al. Predictors of short-term complications after implantable cardioverter-defibrillator replacement: results from the Ontario ICD database. Circ Arrhythm Electrophysiol 2011; 4(2):136–42.

59. Goldberger Z, Elbel B, McPherson CA, et al. Cost advantage of dual-chamber versus single-chamber cardioverter-defibrillator implantation. J Am Coll Cardiol 2005;46(5):850–7.

60. Mond HG, Whitlock RM. The Australian and New Zealand cardiac pacing and implantable cardioverter-defibrillator survey: calendar year 2009. Heart Lung Circ 2011;20(2):99–104.

61. Olshansky B, Day J, Stolen K, et al. Electrophysiologists prefer dual-chamber implantable cardioverter defibrillator programming even when right ventricular pacing is likely. J Card Fail 2005;11:S147.

62. Sticherling C, Zabel M, Spencker S, et al. Comparison of a novel, single-lead atrial sensing system with a dual-chamber implantable cardioverter-defibrillator system in patients without antibradycardia pacing indications: results of a randomized study. Circ Arrhythm Electrophysiol 2011;4(1): 56–63.

# Evaluation of the Young Patient Resuscitated from Ventricular Fibrillation

Rajesh N. Subbiah, MBBS, PhD[a,b], Peter Leong-Sit, MD[c],
Lorne J. Gula, MD[c], Allan C. Skanes, MD[c],
James A. White, MD[c], Raymond Yee, MD[c],
George J. Klein, MD[c], Andrew D. Krahn, MD[c,*]

**KEYWORDS**

- Sudden cardiac death • Sudden cardiac arrest
- Ventricular fibrillation • Genetic

Sudden cardiac death is defined by the World Health Organization as death occurring within the first 24 hours after the onset of symptoms. A more specific and probably more accurate definition of sudden death is a nontraumatic death that occurs within an hour of the onset of acute symptoms or during sleep.[1] Autopsy studies have shown that approximately one-third of sudden deaths have noncardiac causes,[2] with the remainder attributed to heart disease and classified as sudden cardiac arrest (SCA). Pre-existing heart disease may be recognized, but the time and mode of death are unexpected. Despite improvements in first response and resuscitation delivery, survival after SCA remains in the range of 4% to 5%.[3,4]

Most cases of SCA result from ventricular tachycardia, ventricular fibrillation, profound bradycardia, or pulseless electrical activity.[5,6] Considerable variability in the reported incidence of SCA exists, with an incidence of less than 10 per 100,000 person-years in young healthy individuals (age <35 years) to more than 50 per 10,000 person-years in patients with structural heart disease.[7] The overall burden of disease amounts to an estimated 1 case per 1000 person-years and is more common in men and with increasing age.[8] Young adults (defined arbitrarily as age <35 years) with SCA typically present with ventricular fibrillation and represent a specific group that is the focus of this review. A specific causative diagnosis is highly desirable in these individuals and may also be of value for the risk stratification of relatives. Investigations aimed at this goal require a comprehensive and systematic approach that enables prompt identification of reversible or attributable causes, provides for identification of specific phenotype and genotype of inherited causes, and ideally leads to tailored therapy (**Fig. 1**).

## INITIAL ASSESSMENT

Patients with SCA are often first assessed in the early postresuscitation state. This assessment is often difficult because the patients may be intubated and ventilated with bystanders no longer available for questioning. Despite these

Funding sources: Dr Krahn is a Career Investigator of the Heart and Stroke Foundation of Ontario. Supported by the Heart and Stroke Foundation of Ontario (T6730).
Disclosures: the authors had full access to the data and take full responsibility for its integrity. All authors have read and agreed to the article as written. The authors have no conflicts of interest to declare.
[a] Department of Cardiology, St Vincent's Hospital, Darlinghurst, Sydney, New South Wales 2010, Australia
[b] University of New South Wales, Sydney, New South Wales 2052, Australia
[c] Division of Cardiology, University of Western Ontario, 339 Windermere Road, London, ON N6A 5A5, Canada
* Corresponding author. Arrhythmia Service, London Health Sciences Centre, 339 Windermere Road, London, ON N6A 5A5, Canada.
E-mail address: akrahn@uwo.ca

Card Electrophysiol Clin 3 (2011) 593–608
doi:10.1016/j.ccep.2011.08.005
1877-9182/11/$ – see front matter © 2011 Elsevier Inc. All rights reserved.

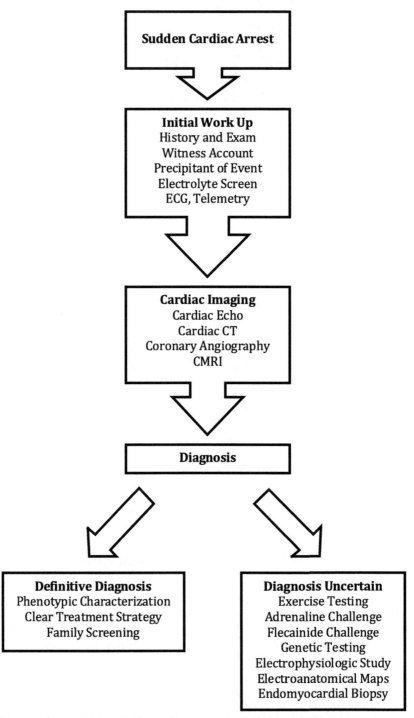

**Fig. 1.** Flow diagram of investigations in the cardiac arrest survivor. See text for discussion.

challenges, a careful history may be highly valuable. Close review of emergency medical assessments, accounts of the sequence of events by witnesses, and analysis of ambulance telemetry and ECG recordings can all provide important information. It is important to access this information rapidly because witness recollection and resuscitation materials, such as rhythm strips, are commonly misplaced and may not migrate to the permanent medical record. A previous history of known heart disease, chest pain, palpitations, syncope, or drug ingestion or a family history of sudden death may provide key historical correlates that may guide further investigations. Detailed information regarding a family history of unexplained drowning, single-vehicle accidents, sudden infant death syndrome, or epilepsy provides clues that point toward inherited conditions such as long QT syndrome (LQTS).

ECG interpretation may be challenging in the postresuscitation period with nonspecific changes or changes related to induced hypothermia in the intensive care setting for neuroprotection. Serial ECGs and cardiac telemetry recordings (including those performed up to several days post cardiac arrest) as well as ECGs obtained from patients at any stage before the event may be useful. **Table 1** details several recognized arrhythmia syndromes and related ECG findings that may be identified.

Physiologic or situational triggers for cardiac arrest may be suggestive of a specific cause. Physical exertion may trigger events in coronary artery disease[9–11] but has also been implicated in arrhythmogenic right ventricular cardiomyopathy (ARVC), LQTS (in particular, types 1 and 2), catecholaminergic polymorphic ventricular tachycardia (CPVT), and hypertrophic cardiomyopathy (HCM).[12–14] Events occurring at rest or during sleep are typically observed in Brugada syndrome and LQT3. A febrile illness may precipitate events in Brugada syndrome[15] and drugs that affect repolarization can worsen or unmask the phenotype of Brugada syndrome or LQTS (summarized at www.qtdrugs.org and www.brugadadrugs.org). A recent febrile illness should also raise suspicion of myocarditis as a potential myocardial insult that may trigger malignant ventricular arrhythmias.

## BASELINE BLOOD WORK

Comprehensive screening blood work is routinely performed to exclude significant electrolyte or metabolic disturbances that may precipitate arrhythmia or unmask an indolent phenotype of an existing arrhythmia syndrome. In some instances, electrolyte or metabolic changes can mimic the ECG changes typically seen in arrhythmia syndromes[16,17]; therefore, caution is suggested in the interpretation of such findings before the correction of these disturbances. Recreational drug and toxin screening within the serum or urine is also an essential part of the work-up, especially in patients who are considered at risk. Although minor elevation in serum cardiac markers may be attributable to global myocardial hypoperfusion during cardiac arrest, more substantial elevations in these markers should still prompt consideration of ischemic or nonischemic (ie, inflammatory) injury as a potential contributor to the patient's clinical presentation.

## BASELINE ELECTROCARDIOGRAM
### Myocardial Ischemia

The majority of SCAs in the general population can be attributed to underlying coronary artery disease,[18,19] either due to acute coronary ischemia or as a result of arrhythmia associated with regions of prior myocardial injury and scarring. The former is more likely to result in polymorphic ventricular tachycardia or ventricular fibrillation whereas the latter typically presents with monomorphic ventricular tachycardia. A thorough review of ECGs and telemetry rhythm strips, especially before the arrest, is therefore fundamental to differentiation of arrhythmia causes. Although coronary artery disease is a common contributor of arrhythmic events in the general population, it becomes a less likely precipitant of arrhythmia in younger individuals. Nonetheless, fixed or coronary spasm–related myocardial ischemia should be actively excluded, especially if typical ischemic ECG changes of ST elevation or ST depression preceding or after the cardiac arrest are identified. Use of high lateral and posterior chest leads should be considered

**Table 1**
**ECG correlates of inherited causes of cardiac arrest**

| Arrhythmia Syndrome | ECG Correlates |
|---|---|
| Brugada syndrome | Coved ST elevation $V_1$–$V_3$ |
| Long QT syndrome | Prolonged QTc interval >460 ms in women or >440 ms in men ST-T–wave changes Torsades de pointes |
| Short QT syndrome | QTc interval <360 ms |
| Arrhythmogenic right ventricular dysplasia | Epsilon waves T-wave inversion in precordial leads RBBB |
| Catecholaminergic polymorphic ventricular tachycardia | Polymorphic ventricular tachycardia Bidirectional ventricular tachycardia |
| Hypertrophic cardiomyopathy | Increased voltage Widespread QRS and ST-T changes |

in the acute setting if clinical suspicion is high for ischemic injury and the standard 12-lead ECG is normal or nonspecific. Ischemic ECG changes should prompt early consideration of invasive coronary angiography and should be correlated with serial cardiac markers and regional reductions in left ventricular function by transthoracic echocardiography. In the setting of acute injury patterns on ECG and associated regional wall motion abnormalities, transient coronary vasospasm should be considered in those revealing otherwise normal coronary angiography. In the absence of acute ischemic ECG changes, a noninvasive coronary CT angiography may then be considered as an alternative to invasive angiography to exclude anomalous coronary asteries or acquired coronary artery disease.[20]

## Pre-Excitation

An ECG should be examined for pre-excitation, especially in young adults presenting with ventricular fibrillation given the increased incidence of SCA in patients with a rapidly conducting accessory pathway.[20–22] Cardiac electrophysiology studies definitively assess the properties of the accessory pathway and propensity for ventricular fibrillation. The use of exercise stress testing and demonstration of intermittent pre-excitation may also be helpful in assessing the refractory period of the accessory pathway.[20–22]

## QRS Morphology and Epsilon Waves

Analysis of QRS morphology can provide clues to underlying substrate for SCA. T-wave inversion in the anteroseptal precordial leads ($V_1$, $V_2$, and $V_3$) is probably one of the most common ECG manifestations of ARVC,[23,24] although less frequently an epsilon wave (**Fig. 2**) or late potential, signifying delayed myocardial conduction and probable underlying scar/substrate for ventricular arrhythmias, may be observed.[23–25] Areas of myocardial necrosis, scar, or ischemia result in inhomogenous ventricular depolarization and present a substrate for reentrant ventricular arrhythmias. This may manifest as additional notching (R' or S') or fragmentation of the QRS complexes on surface ECG.

Quantitatively defined fragmentation of the QRS complexes based on specific scoring algorithms is associated with increased mortality and arrhythmic events in patients with implantable defibrillators. Patients with HCM typically have ECG changes of hypertrophy characterized by both tall R waves, and ST-T–wave abnormalities.[26] Abnormal axis or bundle branch block, especially in young patients, may indicate underlying congenital heart disease or undiagnosed cardiomyopathy.

## Early Repolarization Changes

Identification of abnormalities of early repolarization may provide insights into substrate for SCA. Typically, early repolarization manifests by J-point elevation or notching of the terminal QRS.[27,28] It is considered a normal variant in most patients but is present in more malignant conditions, such as Brugada syndrome, SCA-associated early repolarization syndromes, hypothermia, hypercalcemia, brain injury, and hypervagotonia.[29–31] Haissaguerre and colleagues[32] recently described early repolarization syndromes associated with SCA, with manifest J-point elevation, usually with notching of the terminal QRS in 2 contiguous lateral or inferior leads.[33] This is distinct from Brugada syndrome and ARVC that predominantly involve the right precordial leads $V_1$–$V_3$.

## QT Assessment and T-Wave Morphology

The QT interval should be measured in all SCA survivors and corrected for rate using the Bazett formula.[34] The Bazett formula overcorrects with heart rates greater than 110 beats per minute and undercorrects with heart rates less than 60 beats per minute. The Framingham correction may be preferable in these circumstances.[35] There is no specific lead that is consistently best to measure the QT interval. Traditionally, leads II and $V_5$ are used. The authors recommend careful assessment of all 12 leads, and, if possible, previous ECGs of patients when examining for subtle changes that could provide a clue to the mechanism of cardiac arrest. QT interval prolongation after SCA is common but is usually secondary to ischemia or metabolic or other factors. Some degree of QT prolongation is often evident in patients with non–ST-elevation myocardial infarction or anoxic brain injury.[36–38] The presence of QT prolongation in this clinical context requires careful identification of extrinsic factors with analysis of prearrest ECGs or review of ECGs several days or even weeks post event. As alluded to previously, transient repolarization changes and QT prolongation may be seen during induced hypothermia that resolves with warming.[39] Serial ECGs or review of archived ECGs from family members are likely to demonstrate the absence of underlying repolarization abnormalities.

Not only is QT prolongation a measure of increased risk of SCA, but also the more prolonged the QT interval, the higher the risk of SCA.[40–42] Even in patients with acute myocardial infarction, the QT interval can predict increased risk of SCA.[43] In the context of a prolonged QT interval, there are specific ST-T–wave changes

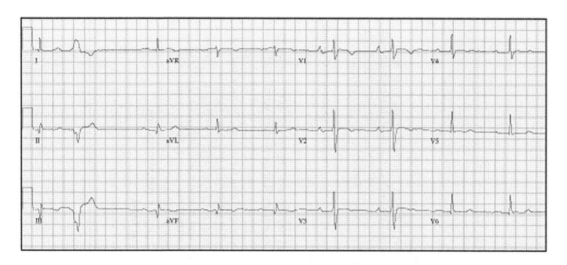

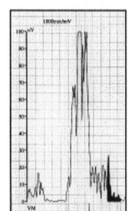
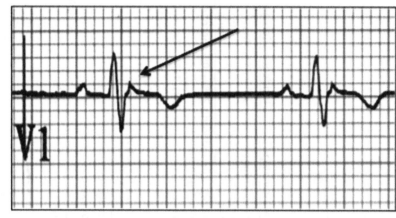

**Fig. 2.** ECG and SAECG in a 37-year-old man with cardiac arrest caused attributed to underlying ARVC. The resting ECG (*upper panel*) shows anterior precordial T-wave inversion, along with prolonged terminal activation in the S wave in $V_1$ and $V_2$. A single right ventricular premature ventricular contraction is also noted. The SAECG (*lower left*) shows fragmented late activation, termed late potentials. The lower right panel from a separate patient demonstrates a low-amplitude, high-frequency, late depolarization that is seldom seen in ARVC, termed an epsilon wave (*arrow*).

that point to a specific genotype of LQTS.[44] **Table 2** details the spectrum of LQTSs.

Short QT syndrome (SQTS) is rare but should also be excluded when other causes of QT shortening have been excluded, such as hyperthermia, hyperkalemia, hypercalcemia, digoxin toxicity, and acidosis.[45] A QTc interval less than 360 ms in men and less than 370 ms in women is considered abnormal.[46] Further data, including consistent QT shortening and a molecular correlate, need to be pursued before establishing a diagnosis.

## ASSESSMENT OF CARDIAC FUNCTION

The left ventricular ejection fraction has been shown to be the strongest predictor of cardiovascular mortality in patients with ischemic and nonischemic cardiomyopathy.[47,48] Typically this is measured by echocardiography but can also be measured using cardiovascular MRI, gated nuclear imaging, or invasive contrast ventriculography. In patients with left ventricular dysfunction, reductions in the ejection fraction have been correlated with a higher the risk of primary or recurrent SCA, with an estimated 21% increased risk of SCA for every 5% decrease in the ejection fraction.[49,50] In young SCA survivors, functional assessments of ventricular function may permit identification of an explanatory substrate for ventricular fibrillation and also help risk stratification, if present. The initial echocardiogram may demonstrate significant reductions in global systolic function due to myocardial stunning related to resuscitative injury or metabolic

**Table 2**
The long QT syndromes

| LQT Type | Genotype | Characteristic QT Morphology | Clinical Phenotype | Incidence | Comments |
|---|---|---|---|---|---|
| 1 | KCNQ1 | Broad-based, symmetric T wave | Adrenergic triggers (swimming, emotion, or exercise) | 30%–35% | Most common but least severe. Homozygotes have severe phenotype with congenital deafness (Jervell and Lange-Nielsen syndrome). β-Blockers efficacious |
| 2 | KCNH2/HERG | Bifid T wave | Commonly drug induced. Auditory stimuli | 25%–30% | Second most common. β-Blockers largely efficacious |
| 3 | SCN5A | Delayed-onset/asymmetric T wave | Rest/sleep | 5%–10% | Little β-blocker effect. May respond to sodium channel blockers |
| 4 | ANK2 | | Exercise | <1% | |
| 5 | KCNE1 | | Exercise and emotion | <1% | Homozygotes have severe phenotype with congenital deafness (Jervell and Lange-Nielsen syndrome) |
| 6 | KCNE2 | | Rest, drugs, or exercise | <1% | |
| 7 | KCNJ2 | Prominent U waves with pseudo-QT prolongation | Rest or exercise | <1% | Linked to Andersen-Tawil syndrome. Periodic paralysis, skeletal muscle deformity and hypokalemia |
| 8 | CACNA1C | Prominent and widely split T-U waves. Prolonged terminal T-wave slope and minimal QT prolongation | Exercise | <1% | Timothy syndrome. Congenital heart disease, autism, syndactyly, and immune deficiency. Early-onset, malignant arrhythmic course. Some response to calcium channel blockers |
| 9 | CAV3 | | Rest or sleep | <1% | Possible limb-girdle myodystrophy link |
| 10 | SCN4B | | Exercise | <0.1% | Atrioventricular block |
| 11 | AKAP9 | | Exercise | <0.1% | |
| 12 | SNTA1 | Bifid | Rest | <0.1% | |

derangement. Repeat echocardiography several days after cardiac arrest is, therefore, recommended because reversibility of this left ventricular dysfunction is common in this context.[51] Persistent reduction or delayed recovery, however, of systolic function may represent the presence of acute myocarditis[52,53] and early consideration should be given to cardiovascular MRI for its optimal detection. Other features that should prompt consideration of myocarditis are any history of preceding febrile illness, known inflammatory connective tissue disease, significant troponin rise, elevated inflammatory markers, and global repolarization changes seen on the ECG.

Echocardiography is also useful in assessing right ventricular dimensions and function in young SCA survivors. The spectrum of findings could range from severe right heart failure and high pulmonary pressures in the context of a massive pulmonary embolus to right ventricular dysfunction and regional or global wall motion abnormalities that may signal the presence of ARVC.[54]

## CARDIOVASCULAR MRI

Cardiovascular magnetic resonance (CMR) imaging is a highly valuable clinical tool for the diagnosis of cardiovascular disease in survivors of SCA. CMR in SCA survivors aims to assess cardiac morphology and function, identify the presence of acute myocardial injury, and characterize the presence and extent of prior myocardial disease that has led to either scar accumulation or fatty replacement. The spectrum of diseases detectable using a comprehensive CMR tissue characterization protocol, inclusive of T1-weighted (fat) imaging, T2-weighted (edema) imaging, and postcontrast delayed enhancement (scar) imaging includes the following: acute and healed ischemic injury, acute and healed inflammatory injury (ie, viral, sarcoidosis, autoimmune, or drug induced), HCM, infiltrative cardiomyopathies (amyloid and Fabry disease), and ARVC.[55] With respect to ARVC, emphasis is currently placed on the more objective findings of right ventricular remodeling and functional impairment.[54] More subjective findings of regional wall motion abnormalities and fat infiltration (based on T1-weighted imaging) require expert interpretation by highly trained and experienced CMR interpreters to avoid risk of overinterpretation.[56–58] A normal CMR study does not exclude the diagnosis of ARVC.

Although cine CMR imaging may identify structural abnormalities less well appreciated by transthoracic echocardiography, the incremental value of CMR is best appreciated from its capacity to characterize tissue level pathology. T2-weighted imaging identifies regional or global abnormalities in tissue water content that can be used for the detection of acute myocardial ischemia and acute inflammatory injury (ie, myocarditis).[59,60] Respective increases in tissue water may persist for weeks after initial injury and, therefore, may still provide diagnostic usefulness late after arrhythmia presentation. Injury leading to tissue necrosis is also detectable through the use of postcontrast delayed enhancement imaging. This technique identifies the extent of acute myocyte necrosis as well as mature myocardial scar, the latter is a recognized marker of future arrhythmic events in patients with prior myocardial infarction, dilated cardiomyopathy, HCM, and cardiac sarcoid.[61–66] **Fig. 3** demonstrates the usefulness of these 2 CMR techniques for the detection of otherwise unrecognized acute ischemic injury in a young patient presenting with SCA and normal coronary arteries.

Rarely, intramyocardial tumor may be identified as a cause for ventricular arrhythmia in the young and is optimally evaluated using CMR. Finally, coronary MRA techniques have improved substantially and may now reliably offer adequate exclusion of anomalous coronary anatomy without exposure to ionizing radiation. Overall, CMR remains the gold standard for the noninvasive evaluation of myocardial tissue pathology and is the imaging modality of choice in patients with unexplained cardiac arrest.

## CORONARY ANGIOGRAPHY

Invasive coronary angiography is indicated in the vast majority of patients who are SCA survivors. The rare exception is young patients with a clearly identifiable arrhythmia syndrome in whom a coronary CT scan may suffice to exclude coronary artery disease or anomalies. Coronary artery spasm is a challenging diagnosis to make unless there is ECG evidence supported by angiographic findings. The role of provocative testing is controversial but should be considered in all patients with unexplained cardiac arrest, in particular smokers.[53,67–71] The identification of significant coronary artery disease that requires revascularization or anomalous coronary arteries provides a potential target for treatment, although risk of recurrent SCA needs to be re-evaluated before discharge of the patient. This is typically a complex decision that is driven by imperfect understanding of the residual risk, with left ventricular function and completeness of revascularization strongly influencing prognosis. The presence

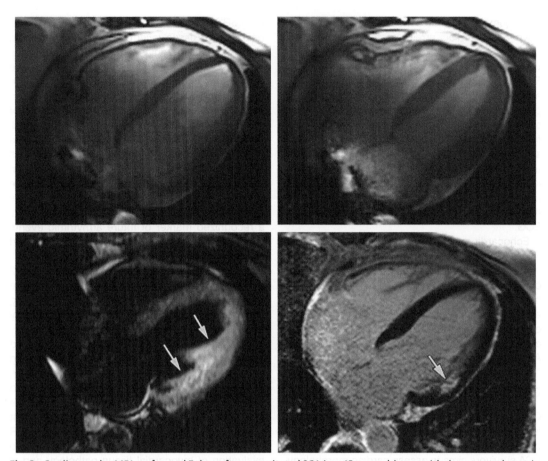

**Fig. 3.** Cardiovascular MRI performed 5 days after resuscitated SCA in a 43-year-old man with documented ventricular fibrillation, normal echocardiography, and normal invasive coronary angiography. Cine imaging in the 4-chamber orientation (*upper left and right panels*) demonstrates normal systolic function. T2-weighted (edema) imaging (*lower left panel*) shows markedly increased signal throughout the lateral wall, consistent with recent myocardial ischemia in the circumflex vascular territory (*arrows*). Matched delayed enhancement imaging (*lower right panel*) shows a small, focal subendocardial myocardial infarction centralized at the core of this region (*arrow*).

of significant reduction in ejection fraction may negate the need for further risk stratification, because implantable cardioverter defibrillator (ICD) therapy may still be indicated.

In addition to left ventriculography for assessment of ejection fraction, right ventriculography can be performed. Hypokinesis of the right ventricle or aneurysmal wall motion abnormalities may be demonstrated in patients with ARVC.[72] With the more widespread availability of cardiac MRI, right ventriculography is used less often to assess the right ventricle.

## EXERCISE TESTING

Treadmill or bicycle exercise testing is a useful physiologic assessor in cardiac arrest survivors who have demonstrated absence of ischemic or structural heart disease. It is often overlooked

because coronary angiography is performed early in the investigation cascade. Exercise testing may unmask evidence of exercise-induced arrhythmia, such as polymorphic ventricular tachycardia in CPVT and QT prolongation in LQTS (**Fig. 4**). Identification of abnormalities should prompt further testing, including genetic evaluation. Phenotypic screening of relatives may then be possible with exercise testing.

## SIGNAL-AVERAGED ECG

Signal averaged of the ECG (SAECG) facilitates the detection of low-amplitude late potentials seen in the terminal portion of the QRS complex (**Fig. 5**). These late potentials signify areas of slow and abnormal ventricular conduction potentially caused by myocardial infarction or fibrosis and serve as a substrate for re-entry.[73] There are

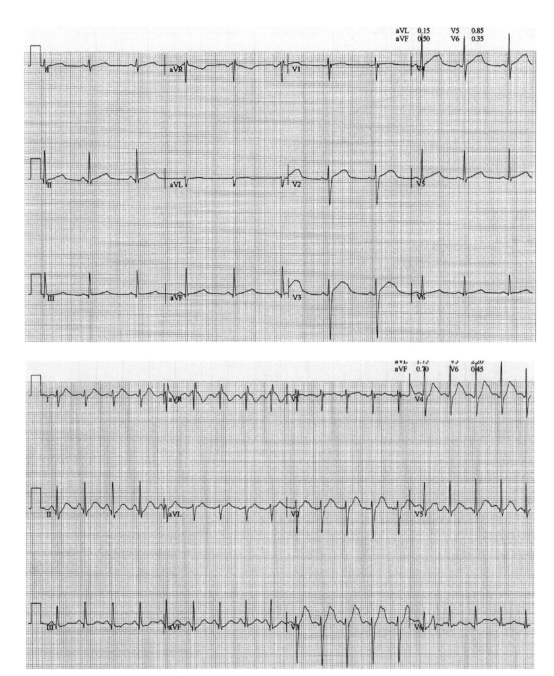

**Fig. 4.** Resting and exercise ECGs in a 32-year-old woman with previous cardiac arrest. The resting ECG shows a QT interval at the upper limit of normal, with unusual T-wave morphology with a late peaked and even notched T wave. Early in exercise, failed shortening of the QT interval with abnormal T-wave morphology confirms the diagnosis of LQTS, subsequently confirmed with genetic testing.

several processing systems for ECG analysis, with frequency-domain analysis preferable to time-domain analysis in patients with bundle branch block.[74] Several parameters are examined when analyzing the SAECG, which is considered abnormal if at least 2 of the following criteria are fulfilled: (1) a filtered QRS greater than or equal

to 114 ms, (2) a root mean square voltage less than or equal to 25 mV in the terminal 40 ms of the QRS, and (3) low-amplitude signal (<40 mV) duration greater than 40 ms. Although the arrhythmia or its sequelae are already manifest in a SCA survivor, identification of an abnormal SAECG should prompt consideration of an occult

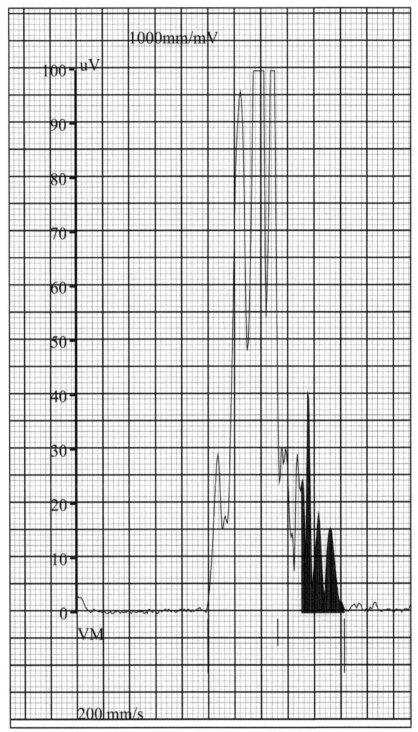

**Fig. 5.** SAECG of a cardiac arrest survivor with suspicious T-wave inversion in the anterior precordial leads that was attributed to cerebral anoxia. The presence of late potentials pointed to an underlying myopathic process, which was confirmed with subsequent cardiac MRI as ARVC. See text for discussion of interpretation.

myocardial process, such as ARVC, myocarditis, sarcoidosis, or amyloidosis, when myocardial infarction has been excluded. Recent data suggest that a single positive criterion is more sensitive than 2 in detection of patients with ARVC, without loss of specificity.[75]

## CARDIAC ELECTROPHYSIOLOGY TESTING

Electrophysiological studies (EPSs) have been used to identify patients with a substrate for ventricular arrhythmias that are at high risk of SCA. Inducible sustained monomorphic ventricular tachycardia with up to 3 ventricular extrastimuli at 2 drive cycle lengths is considered abnormal and associated with high risk of SCA. A low risk of SCA cannot be inferred, however, by the absence of inducible ventricular tachycardia. EPS also provides few prognostic data in patients with nonischemic cardiomyopathy. EPS has limited value in guiding therapeutic interventions in SCA survivors, because ICD is indicated in all survivors in the absence of specific contraindications. Thus, it is performed in few cases, largely selected because diagnostic uncertainty remains after extensive testing (as outlined previously).

The failure to induce ventricular tachycardia does not obviate ICD in patients with ARVC or other less common causes of cardiac arrest. EPS in conjunction with voltage mapping, however, can corroborate evidence of scar from imaging studies to support the diagnosis in ARVC and may identify patients at high risk of recurrent arrhythmia. EPS and ablation are indicated in patients with ventricular pre-excitation.

## PHARMACOLOGIC CHALLENGE

The diagnostic features of arrhythmic syndromes are often intermittent, subtle, or absent on the resting ECG. Challenging or stressing the dominant ion channel abnormality or the specific mechanism of the arrhythmia with pharmacologic agents can unmask the latent ECG abnormalities. Epinephrine infusion has been used in the clinical evaluation of LQTS. Two infusion protocols have been developed—the epinephrine bolus followed by infusion and the graded epinephrine infusion.[76,77] The latter is better tolerated and may be associated with lower incidence of false-positive responses. The graded epinephrine infusion is commenced at 0.05 μg/kg/min, doubling every 5 minutes to 0.2 μg/kg/min, and the QT interval is measured at each increment and at 5 and 10 minutes after the infusion. An absolute increase in QT interval of at least 30 ms at low-dose epinephrine infusion ($\leq$0.1 μg/kg/min) is

considered abnormal and provides a presumptive diagnosis of LQT1.[76] The result of epinephrine challenge should not be inferred from exercise testing and vice versa, because epinephrine infusion results in greater QT shortening for a given increase in heart rate compared with exercise testing. Epinephrine infusion can also been used to unmask CPVT.[53]

Epinephrine infusion should be stopped in the event of a systolic blood pressure over 200 mm Hg, nonsustained ventricular tachycardia or polymorphic ventricular tachycardia, frequent (>10) premature ventricular contractions per minute, T-wave alternans, or patient intolerance. Appropriate resuscitation equipment, including intravenous β-blocker, should be available, despite the reported safety of epinephrine challenge.

Provocative pharmacologic testing with intravenous class IC sodium channel blockers (ajmaline, 1 mg/kg; flecainide, 2 mg/kg, maximum 150 mg; or procainamide, 15 mg/kg, maximum 1 g, depending on availability) is used to unmask or amplify the ST changes in patients with Brugada syndrome.[78–80] The development of typical type 1 Brugada ECG pattern ($\geq$2-mm J-point elevation and coved-type ST-T–segment elevation in leads $V_1$ and $V_2$) is considered positive. Monitoring should be continued until normalization of the ECG. Placing the precordial leads at higher intercostal space increases the sensitivity of detecting typical Brugada ECG pattern compared with conventional 12-lead ECG (**Fig. 6**). Isoproterenol may be used to suppress ventricular arrhythmias in patients with Brugada syndrome.

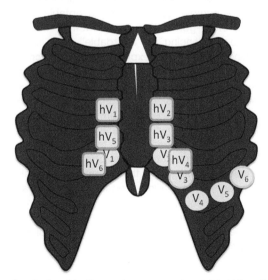

**Fig. 6.** Graphic illustrating conventional ($V_1$–$V_6$) and high (h$V_1$–h$V_6$) precordial lead positioning. The high leads increase the yield of detecting a type 1 Brugada pattern during sodium channel blocker infusion.

## GENETIC TESTING

Genetic testing can be a useful modality in the work-up of SCA survivors, in particular young adults with ventricular fibrillation, when structural disease has been excluded. There is a clear association between genetic abnormalities and sudden cardiac death in patients with inheritable ion channel defects, such as Brugada syndrome and LQTS (see **Table 2**). Genetic testing of individuals who are suspected of having an ion channel abnormality driven by the results of clinical testing provides the opportunity to establish a genotype-phenotype correlate, improve the yield of screening relatives, and guide treatment options. In patients without a suspected ion channel defect, there is evidence that a family history of cardiac arrest or sudden death in the context of acute ischemia increases the risk for first-degree relatives, independent of cardiac risk factors.[73,81–83] The specific genetic mechanism of this observation and resultant opportunity for genetic testing have not been completely elucidated, although genome-wide association studies point to multiple factors, including influences on thrombosis, inflammation, and cardiac ion channels.[84–87]

An inheritable arrhythmogenic disease is probably a more encompassing description of genetically mediated SCA syndromes and includes Brugada syndrome, LQTS, SQTS, CPVT, ARVC, and HCM. Diagnostic yield of genetic testing beyond ion channel defects is on the whole lower, but this does not rule out its use. Commercial genetic testing companies are increasingly offering panels based on genetic screening of a large number of genes at acceptable costs using next-generation sequencing. Whole-exome sequencing at "affordable" cost is also imminent, in effect exploring the transcribed portion of the entire DNA sequence. This will greatly enhance the ability to access and screen contributory genes, but in turn greatly increase the complexity of interpretation, because multiple variants of unknown significance are likely to emerge that will be difficult to interpret in the context of a limited or absent phenotype. This is a rapidly evolving field that warrants discussion between the immediate bedside physician and a local or regional expert when a genetic contribution is suspected. A genetic test is optimally pursued with a specific search based on phenotypic clues.

## ENDOMYOCARDIAL BIOPSY

In rare cases, endomyocardial biopsy guided by the results of other diagnostic modalities may be helpful in the diagnosis of sarcoidosis, myocarditis, ARVC, or cardiac masses. Cardiac MRI should direct the biopsy, assisting in targeting tissue likely affected by the observed changes.

## IDIOPATHIC VENTRICULAR FIBRILLATION

The diagnosis of idiopathic ventricular fibrillation is made when no other cause is found. The Canadian Cardia Arrest Survivors with Preserved Ejections Fractions Registry (CASPER) has demonstrated that despite systematic screening tests, approximately half of cardiac arrest patients without overt heart disease remain undiagnosed or idiopathic. Historically, Brugada syndrome, early repolarization, and even LQTS resided in this category until the hallmarks were recognized and their physiologic basis began to be understood. Such is the case for a recently described familial cause of sudden death and cardiac arrest in Dutch families with no known phenotypic test, linked to a haplotype in the DPP6 gene that may present with the short coupled variant of torsades de pointes.[88] There are several contenders for a diagnosis in this cohort, including coronary spasm, occult sarcoidosis, and latent forms of all of the known cardiac arrest–related conditions (described previously), in particular early repolarization and SQTS, because they remain without validated provocation tests. As registries expand and diagnostic technologies in ICDs improve, more of these patients will obtain a diagnosis.

## IMPLICATIONS FOR THERAPY

The ICD has in some respects distracted from the key quest to explain the mechanism of ventricular fibrillation in the young cardiac arrest population and deliver cause-specific therapy. Although the majority of survivors of cardiac arrest warrants an ICD as a safety net, there is a clear role for establishing a mechanistic diagnosis to prevent recurrence, which may in future obviate an ICD. Such a strategy was inferred by a recent case series of type-1 LQTS patients who suffered a cardiac arrest and were treated with β-blockers, typically highly effective in this population. All patients received an ICD, but no patient compliant with the β-blocker had recurrent arrest.[89] An accompanying editorial speculated on the merits of the ICD implant in this predominantly young population, in whom ICDs are not without concern.[90] The majority of underlying causes (as outlined previously) has specific therapy, such as β-blockers, pacing, calcium channel blockers, or lifestyle recommendations, that reduces recurrence.

## SUMMARY

There is considerable prognostic, therapeutic, and psychological importance in identifying the cause of ventricular fibrillation. Although the majority of cardiac arrests conforms to stereotypical patterns of structural coronary and myocardial diseases, a minority remain elusive to standard testing and require further provocative testing and advanced imaging, revealing latent forms of structural disease and primary electrical diseases. Even so, a significant proportion of these remain undiagnosed. Until understanding of these causes leads to definitive disease-specific treatment, protection with an ICD is generally warranted. Ongoing studies are needed in both genetic and electrophysiologic fields to expand understanding in this area, ideally leading to optimal therapy and prevention strategies.

## REFERENCES

1. Winkle RA. Clinical efficacy of antiarrhythmic drugs in prevention of sudden coronary death. Ann N Y Acad Sci 1982;382:247–57.

2. Leach IH, Blundell JW, Rowley JM, et al. Acute ischaemic lesions in death due to ischaemic heart disease. An autopsy study of 333 cases of out-of-hospital death. Eur Heart J 1995;16(9): 1181–5.

3. Huikuri HV, Castellanos A, Myerburg RJ. Sudden death due to cardiac arrhythmias. N Engl J Med 2001;345(20):1473–82.

4. Myerburg RJ. Sudden cardiac death: exploring the limits of our knowledge. J Cardiovasc Electrophysiol 2001;12(3):369–81.

5. Myerburg RJ, Interian A Jr, Mitrani RM, et al. Frequency of sudden cardiac death and profiles of risk. Am J Cardiol 1997;80(5B):10F–9F.

6. Zipes DP, Wellens HJ. Sudden cardiac death. Circulation 1998;98(21):2334–51.

7. de Vreede-Swagemakers JJ, Gorgels AP, Dubois-Arbouw WI, et al. Out-of-hospital cardiac arrest in the 1990's: a population-based study in the Maastricht area on incidence, characteristics and survival. J Am Coll Cardiol 1997;30(6):1500–5.

8. Straus SM, Bleumink GS, Dieleman JP, et al. The incidence of sudden cardiac death in the general population. J Clin Epidemiol 2004;57 (1):98–102.

9. Ciampricotti R, Taverne R, El Gamal M. Clinical and angiographic observations on resuscitated victims of exercise-related sudden ischemic death. Am J Cardiol 1991;68(1):47–50.

10. Albert CM, Mittleman MA, Chae CU, et al. Triggering of sudden death from cardiac causes by vigorous exertion. N Engl J Med 2000;343(19):1355–61.

11. Mittleman MA, Maclure M, Tofler GH, et al. Triggering of acute myocardial infarction by heavy physical exertion. Protection against triggering by regular exertion. Determinants of Myocardial Infarction Onset Study Investigators. N Engl J Med 1993; 329(23):1677–83.

12. Schwartz PJ, Zaza A, Locati E, et al. Stress and sudden death. The case of the long QT syndrome. Circulation 1991;83(Suppl 4):II71–80.

13. Priori SG, Aliot E, Blomstrom-Lundqvist C, et al. Task force on sudden cardiac death of the European Society of cardiology. Eur Heart J 2001;22(16): 1374–450.

14. Spooner PM, Albert C, Benjamin EJ, et al. Sudden cardiac death, genes, and arrhythmogenesis: consideration of new population and mechanistic approaches from a national heart, lung, and blood institute workshop, part I. Circulation 2001;103(19): 2361–4.

15. Keller DI, Rougier JS, Kucera JP, et al. Brugada syndrome and fever: genetic and molecular characterization of patients carrying SCN5A mutations. Cardiovasc Res 2005;67(3):510–9.

16. Tamene A, Sattiraju S, Wang K, et al. Brugada-like electrocardiography pattern induced by severe hyponatraemia. Europace 2010;12(6):905–7.

17. Mok NS, Tong CK, Yuen HC. Concomitant-acquired Long QT and Brugada syndromes associated with indapamide-induced hypokalemia and hyponatremia. Pacing Clin Electrophysiol 2008; 31(6):772–5.

18. Chugh SS, Jui J, Gunson K, et al. Current burden of sudden cardiac death: multiple source surveillance versus retrospective death certificate-based review in a large U.S. community. J Am Coll Cardiol 2004; 44(6):1268–75.

19. Chugh SS, Senashova O, Watts A, et al. Postmortem molecular screening in unexplained sudden death. J Am Coll Cardiol 2004;43(9):1625–9.

20. Srinivasan KG, Gaikwad A, Kannan BR, et al. Congenital coronary artery anomalies: diagnosis with 64 slice multidetector row computed tomography coronary angiography: a single-centre study. J Med Imaging Radiat Oncol 2008;52(2):148–54.

21. Klein GJ, Yee R, Sharma AD. Longitudinal electrophysiologic assessment of asymptomatic patients with the Wolff-Parkinson-White electrocardiographic pattern. N Engl J Med 1989;320(19):1229–33.

22. Santinelli V, Radinovic A, Manguso F, et al. Asymptomatic ventricular preexcitation: a long-term prospective follow-up study of 293 adult patients. Circ Arrhythm Electrophysiol 2009;2(2):102–7.

23. Jain R, Dalal D, Daly A, et al. Electrocardiographic features of arrhythmogenic right ventricular dysplasia. Circulation 2009;120(6):477–87.

24. Nasir K, Bomma C, Tandri H, et al. Electrocardiographic features of arrhythmogenic right ventricular

dysplasia/cardiomyopathy according to disease severity: a need to broaden diagnostic criteria. Circulation 2004;110(12):1527–34.

25. Nava A, Folino AF, Bauce B, et al. Signal-averaged electrocardiogram in patients with arrhythmogenic right ventricular cardiomyopathy and ventricular arrhythmias. Eur Heart J 2000;21(1):58–65.

26. Fananapazir L, Tracy CM, Leon MB, et al. Electrophysiologic abnormalities in patients with hypertrophic cardiomyopathy. A consecutive analysis in 155 patients. Circulation 1989;80(5):1259–68.

27. Klatsky AL, Oehm R, Cooper RA, et al. The early repolarization normal variant electrocardiogram: correlates and consequences. Am J Med 2003;115(3):171–7.

28. Mehta M, Jain AC, Mehta A. Early repolarization. Clin Cardiol 1999;22(2):59–65.

29. Marcus RR, Kalisetti D, Raxwal V, et al. Early repolarization in patients with spinal cord injury: prevalence and clinical significance. J Spinal Cord Med 2002; 25(1):33–8 [discussion: 39].

30. Antzelevitch C, Yan GX. J wave syndromes. Heart Rhythm 2010;7(4):549–58.

31. Brunson CE, Abbud E, Osman K, et al. Osborn (J) wave appearance on the electrocardiogram in relation to potassium transfer and myocardial metabolism during hypothermia. J Investig Med 2005; 53(8):434–7.

32. Haissaguerre M, Derval N, Sacher F, et al. Sudden cardiac arrest associated with early repolarization. N Engl J Med 2008;358(19):2016–23.

33. Tikkanen JT, Anttonen O, Junttila MJ, et al. Long-term outcome associated with early repolarization on electrocardiography. N Engl J Med 2009; 361(26):2529–37.

34. Bazett HC. An analyisis of time relations of electrocardiograms. Heart 1920;7:353–70.

35. Sagie A, Larson MG, Goldberg RJ, et al. An improved method for adjusting the QT interval for heart rate (the Framingham Heart Study). Am J Cardiol 1992;70(7):797–801.

36. Chauhan VS, Tang AS. Dynamic changes of QT interval and QT dispersion in non-Q-wave and Q-wave myocardial infarction. J Electrocardiol 2001; 34(2):109–17.

37. Molnar J, Rosenthal JE, Weiss JS, et al. QT interval dispersion in healthy subjects and survivors of sudden cardiac death: circadian variation in a twenty-four-hour assessment. Am J Cardiol 1997;79(9):1190–3.

38. Drory Y, Ouaknine G, Kosary IZ, et al. Electrocardiographic findings in brain death; description and presumed mechanism. Chest 1975;67(4):425–32.

39. Mattu A, Brady WJ, Perron AD. Electrocardiographic manifestations of hypothermia. Am J Emerg Med 2002;20(4):314–26.

40. Moss AJ, Zareba W, Kaufman ES, et al. Increased risk of arrhythmic events in long-QT syndrome with mutations in the pore region of the human ether-a-go-go-related gene potassium channel. Circulation 2002;105(7):794–9.

41. Goldenberg I, Moss AJ, Bradley J, et al. Long-QT syndrome after age 40. Circulation 2008;117(17): 2192–201.

42. Goldenberg I, Zareba W, Moss AJ. Long QT Syndrome. Curr Probl Cardiol 2008;33(11):629–94.

43. Schwartz PJ, Wolf S. QT interval prolongation as predictor of sudden death in patients with myocardial infarction. Circulation 1978;57(6):1074–7.

44. Zhang L, Timothy KW, Vincent GM, et al. Spectrum of ST-T-wave patterns and repolarization parameters in congenital long-QT syndrome: ECG findings identify genotypes. Circulation 2000;102(23):2849–55.

45. Garberoglio L, Giustetto C, Wolpert C, et al. Is acquired short QT due to digitalis intoxication responsible for malignant ventricular arrhythmias? J Electrocardiol 2007;40(1):43–6.

46. Gollob MH, Redpath CJ, Roberts JD. The short QT syndrome: proposed diagnostic criteria. J Am Coll Cardiol 2011;57(7):802–12.

47. Huikuri HV, Tapanainen JM, Lindgren K, et al. Prediction of sudden cardiac death after myocardial infarction in the beta-blocking era. J Am Coll Cardiol 2003;42(4):652–8.

48. Huikuri HV, Makikallio TH, Raatikainen MJ, et al. Prediction of sudden cardiac death: appraisal of the studies and methods assessing the risk of sudden arrhythmic death. Circulation 2003;108(1): 110–5.

49. Solomon SD, Anavekar N, Skali H, et al. Influence of ejection fraction on cardiovascular outcomes in a broad spectrum of heart failure patients. Circulation 2005;112(24):3738–44.

50. Solomon SD, Zelenkofske S, McMurray JJ, et al. Sudden death in patients with myocardial infarction and left ventricular dysfunction, heart failure, or both. N Engl J Med 2005;352(25):2581–8.

51. Kern KB, Hilwig RW, Rhee KH, et al. Myocardial dysfunction after resuscitation from cardiac arrest: an example of global myocardial stunning. J Am Coll Cardiol 1996;28(1):232–40.

52. Phillips M, Robinowitz M, Higgins JR, et al. Sudden cardiac death in Air Force recruits. A 20-year review. JAMA 1986;256(19):2696–9.

53. Krahn AD, Healey JS, Chauhan V, et al. Systematic assessment of patients with unexplained cardiac arrest: cardiac arrest survivors with preserved ejection fraction registry (CASPER). Circulation 2009; 120(4):278–85.

54. Marcus FI, McKenna WJ, Sherrill D, et al. Diagnosis of arrhythmogenic right ventricular cardiomyopathy/dysplasia. Proposed modification of the task force criteria. Circulation 2010;121(13):1533–41.

55. White JA, Patel MR. The role of cardiovascular MRI in heart failure and the cardiomyopathies. Cardiol Clin 2007;25(1):71–95, vi.

56. Jain A, Tandri H, Calkins H, et al. Role of cardiovascular magnetic resonance imaging in arrhythmogenic right ventricular dysplasia. J Cardiovasc Magn Reson 2008;10(1):32.

57. Tandri H, Calkins H, Nasir K, et al. Magnetic resonance imaging findings in patients meeting task force criteria for arrhythmogenic right ventricular dysplasia. J Cardiovasc Electrophysiol 2003;14(5):476–82.

58. Bluemke DA, Krupinski EA, Ovitt T, et al. MR Imaging of arrhythmogenic right ventricular cardiomyopathy: morphologic findings and interobserver reliability. Cardiology 2003;99(3):153–62.

59. Eitel I, Friedrich MG. T2-weighted cardiovascular magnetic resonance in acute cardiac disease. J Cardiovasc Magn Reson 2011;13:13.

60. Friedrich MG, Sechtem U, Schulz-Menger J, et al. Cardiovascular magnetic resonance in myocarditis: a JACC white paper. J Am Coll Cardiol 2009; 53(17):1475–87.

61. Nazarian S, Bluemke DA, Lardo AC, et al. Magnetic resonance assessment of the substrate for inducible ventricular tachycardia in nonischemic cardiomyopathy. Circulation 2005;112(18):2821–5.

62. Bogun FM, Desjardins B, Good E, et al. Delayed-enhanced magnetic resonance imaging in nonischemic cardiomyopathy: utility for identifying the ventricular arrhythmia substrate. J Am Coll Cardiol 2009;53(13):1138–45.

63. Roes SD, Borleffs CJ, van der Geest RJ, et al. Infarct tissue heterogeneity assessed with contrast-enhanced MRI predicts spontaneous ventricular arrhythmia in patients with ischemic cardiomyopathy and implantable cardioverter-defibrillator. Circ Cardiovasc Imaging 2009;2(3):183–90.

64. Assomull RG, Prasad SK, Lyne J, et al. Cardiovascular magnetic resonance, fibrosis, and prognosis in dilated cardiomyopathy. J Am Coll Cardiol 2006; 48(10):1977–85.

65. O'Hanlon R, Grasso A, Roughton M, et al. Prognostic significance of myocardial fibrosis in hypertrophic cardiomyopathy. J Am Coll Cardiol 2010;56(11):867–74.

66. Patel MR, Cawley PJ, Heitner JF, et al. Detection of myocardial damage in patients with sarcoidosis. Circulation 2009;120(20):1969–77.

67. Brembilla-Perrot B, Miljoen H, Houriez P, et al. Causes and prognosis of cardiac arrest in a population admitted to a general hospital; a diagnostic and therapeutic problem. Resuscitation 2003;58(3): 319–27.

68. MacAlpin RN. Cardiac arrest and sudden unexpected death in variant angina: complications of coronary spasm that can occur in the absence of severe organic coronary stenosis. Am Heart J 1993; 125(4):1011–7.

69. Adams JN, Denver MA, Rae AP. Coronary artery spasm leading to life threatening arrhythmias. Heart 1998;80(1):89–90.

70. Krahn AD, Gollob M, Yee R, et al. Diagnosis of unexplained cardiac arrest: role of adrenaline and procainamide infusion. Circulation 2005;112(15):2228–34.

71. Takagi Y, Yasuda S, Tsunoda R, et al. Clinical characteristics and long-term prognosis of vasospastic angina patients who survived out-of-hospital cardiac arrest: multicenter registry study of the Japanese Coronary Spasm Association. Circ Arrhythm Electrophysiol 2011;4(3):295–302.

72. Indik JH, Wichter T, Gear K, et al. Quantitative assessment of angiographic right ventricular wall motion in arrhythmogenic right ventricular dysplasia/cardiomyopathy (ARVD/C). J Cardiovasc Electrophysiol 2008; 19(1):39–45.

73. Josephson ME, Simson MB, Harken AH, et al. The incidence and clinical significance of epicardial late potentials in patients with recurrent sustained ventricular tachycardia and coronary artery disease. Circulation 1982;66(6):1199–204.

74. Lindsay BD, Ambos HD, Schechtman KB, et al. Improved selection of patients for programmed ventricular stimulation by frequency analysis of signal-averaged electrocardiograms. Circulation 1986;73(4): 675–83.

75. Kamath GS, Zareba W, Delaney J, et al. Value of the signal-averaged electrocardiogram in arrhythmogenic right ventricular cardiomyopathy/dysplasia. Heart Rhythm 2011;8(2):256–62.

76. Vyas H, Hejlik J, Ackerman MJ. Epinephrine QT stress testing in the evaluation of congenital long-QT syndrome: diagnostic accuracy of the paradoxical QT response. Circulation 2006; 113(11):1385–92.

77. Shimizu W, Noda T, Takaki H, et al. Epinephrine unmasks latent mutation carriers with LQT1 form of congenital long-QT syndrome. J Am Coll Cardiol 2003;41(4):633–42.

78. Rolf S, Bruns HJ, Wichter T, et al. The ajmaline challenge in Brugada syndrome: diagnostic impact, safety, and recommended protocol. Eur Heart J 2003;24(12):1104–12.

79. Sangwatanaroj S, Prechawat S, Sunsaneewitayakul B, et al. New electrocardiographic leads and the procainamide test for the detection of the Brugada sign in sudden unexplained death syndrome survivors and their relatives. Eur Heart J 2001;22(24):2290–6.

80. Shimizu W, Antzelevitch C, Suyama K, et al. Effect of sodium channel blockers on ST segment, QRS duration, and corrected QT interval in patients with Brugada syndrome. J Cardiovasc Electrophysiol 2000; 11(12):1320–9.

81. Friedlander Y, Siscovick DS, Weinmann S, et al. Family history as a risk factor for primary cardiac arrest. Circulation 1998;97(2):155–60.

82. Dekker LR, Bezzina CR, Henriques JP, et al. Familial sudden death is an important risk factor for primary ventricular fibrillation: a case-control study in acute

myocardial infarction patients. Circulation 2006; 114(11):1140–5.

83. Kaikkonen KS, Kortelainen ML, Linna E, et al. Family history and the risk of sudden cardiac death as a manifestation of an acute coronary event. Circulation 2006;114(14):1462–7.

84. Albert CM, MacRae CA, Chasman DI, et al. Common variants in cardiac ion channel genes are associated with sudden cardiac death. Circ Arrhythm Electrophysiol 2010;3(3):222–9.

85. Gavin MC, Newton-Cheh C, Gaziano JM, et al. A common variant in the Beta-2 adrenergic receptor and risk of sudden cardiac death. Heart Rhythm 2011;8(5):704–10.

86. Hernesniemi JA, Karhunen PJ, Oksala N, et al. Interleukin 18 gene promoter polymorphism: a link between hypertension and pre-hospital sudden cardiac death: the Helsinki Sudden Death Study. Eur Heart J 2009;30(23):2939–46.

87. Bezzina CR, Pazoki R, Bardai A, et al. Genome-wide association study identifies a susceptibility locus at 21q21 for ventricular fibrillation in acute myocardial infarction. Nat Genet 2010;42(8): 688–91.

88. Alders M, Koopmann TT, Christiaans I, et al. Haplotype-sharing analysis implicates chromosome 7q36 harboring DPP6 in familial idiopathic ventricular fibrillation. Am J Hum Genet 2009; 84(4):468–76.

89. Vincent GM, Schwartz PJ, Denjoy I, et al. High efficacy of beta-blockers in long-QT syndrome type 1: contribution of noncompliance and QT-prolonging drugs to the occurrence of beta-blocker treatment "failures". Circulation 2009;119 (2):215–21.

90. Viskin S, Halkin A. Treating the long-QT syndrome in the era of implantable defibrillators. Circulation 2009;119(2):204–6.

# Sudden Cardiac Death After Heart Transplantation

Daniel J. Cantillon, MD

**KEYWORDS**

- Cardiac transplantation • Bradyarrhythmia
- Sudden cardiac death

Pioneering surgical innovation and medical immunosuppressive therapy in the 1970s and 1980s greatly enhanced survival for patients after cardiac transplantation.[1] The first cardiac transplant surgery was performed in 1967 by the South African surgeon Dr Christiaan Barnard,[2] and the patient survived for only 18 days. Later surgical innovations include the now classic biatrial technique, introduced by Drs Lower and Shumway,[3,4] and the bicaval technique, which was first introduced in 1989.[5,6] Medical and surgical advancements have now extended median survival beyond 10 years, creating steady growth in the number of cardiac recipients despite a leveling off in the number of actual transplant surgeries performed annually.[7] Despite improved survival, bradyarrhythmias and tachyarrhythmias occur in up to 40% and 66% of cardiac transplant recipients, respectively.[8] Sudden death estimates over 5 years range between 9.7% and 58%, with reported outcomes varying widely among centers.[9–14] Electrophysiologists are increasingly called on to treat arrhythmias and provide risk stratification for sudden cardiac death in this population.

## SUDDEN CARDIAC DEATH OVERVIEW

In the patient population with heart failure, bradyarrhythmias are estimated to account for 10% or less of sudden death, and almost all are attributed to ventricular tachyarrhythmias.[15] This ratio is opposite in the cardiac transplant population. According to data from the University of California, Los Angeles (UCLA), sudden death occurred in 41 of 116 transplant recipients (35%) who died over a mean 76-month follow-up, and the terminal arrhythmia was most commonly asystole (n = 14, 34%), followed by pulseless electrical activity (n = 8, 20%), and, least commonly, ventricular fibrillation (n = 4, 10%) (**Fig. 1**).[14] In an autopsy study of 74 transplant recipient deaths by Chantranuwat and colleagues,[10] no anatomic cause, including a lack of acute coronary arteriopathy, or acute cellular or antibody-mediated rejection was identified as the proximate cause of death in approximately a third of the patients.

## BRADYARRHYTHMIAS

Pacemaker-requiring bradyarrhythmias complicate between 7% and 10% of contemporary transplants but was historically as high as 40%.[16–19] For decades, the cause and clinical significance of bradyarrhythmias in this population was poorly understood. More recently, dedicated research in this population has created a better understanding of the associated factors and triggers. As listed in **Table 1**, factors associated with bradyarrhythmias among cardiac transplant recipients are best understood categorically as (1) preoperative factors, (2) operative considerations, and (3) acquired posttransplant conditions conferring increased risk. Systematic consideration of these factors enables the consulting electrophysiologist to identify all relevant issues when treating a transplant recipient, particularly when implantable cardiac devices are involved.

Disclosures: The author reports consulting/honoraria from Medtronic (modest).
Cardiac Electrophysiology and Pacing, Heart and Vascular Institute, Department of Cardiovascular Medicine, Cleveland Clinic, 9500 Euclid Avenue Desk J2-2, Cleveland, OH 44195, USA
*E-mail address:* cantild@ccf.org

Card Electrophysiol Clin 3 (2011) 609–616
doi:10.1016/j.ccep.2011.08.004

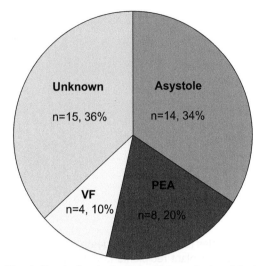

**Fig. 1.** Terminal arrhythmia in 41 transplant recipients with sudden cardiac death. PEA, pulseless electrical activity; VF, ventricular fibrillation. (*Data from* Vaseghi M, Lellouche N, Ritter H, et al. Mode and mechanisms of death after orthotopic heart transplantation. Heart Rhythm 2009;6:503–9.)

## Preoperative Amiodarone Usage

The dominant preoperative factor associated with postoperative bradyarrhythmias is the use of amiodarone,[20] a class III antiarrhythmic drug with a half-life of 40 to 55 days commonly used in patients with pretransplant heart failure to treat both ventricular and atrial tachyarrhythmias. The drug's effect on α- and β-adrenergic receptors and sodium, potassium, and calcium channels simultaneously prolongs action potential duration, tissue refractory periods, as well as slowing atrioventricular (AV) nodal conduction and sinoatrial automaticity. This effect persists after cardiac transplantation in a dose-dependent manner because of the drug's

long half-life, causing many of the early postoperative bradyarrhythmias, particularly sinus node dysfunction.[20] Patients receiving a permanent pacemaker for early sinus node dysfunction in the setting of heavy preoperative amiodarone less commonly require pacing at 6-month follow-up in the device clinic.[19,20] Despite this well-known phenomenon, implanting a permanent pacemaker is often unavoidable because the sinus node dysfunction can limit early postoperative rehabilitation efforts. When preoperative amiodarone use is identified as the principal culprit, functional assessments (ie, observed heart rate response to patient activity or even formal exercise testing) are useful to guide the decision on implanting a permanent pacemaker. Early sinus node dysfunction after cardiac transplant surgery is the most common bradyarrhythmia encountered overall and has been demonstrated to be benign without adverse effects on long-term survival.[8,19–21]

## Surgical Technique

Technical aspects of cardiac transplantation are decided on and applied by surgeons in the operating room. Understanding the approaches used by contemporary transplant surgeons is important for the consulting electrophysiologist. In this section, the classic biatrial and newer bicaval techniques are compared with an emphasis on the implications in managing postoperative bradyarrhythmias and the outcomes associated with each technique.

The classic biatrial surgical technique involves a recipient atriotomy with extension into the high posterior right atrium, across the posterior interatrial septum and the left atrial posterior cuff containing the pulmonary venous antrum. The resultant cardiectomy leaves behind a contiguous cuff of both right and left recipient atrial tissue. Similarly, the donor heart is prepared by excising the posterior right and left atria. Subsequent surgical anastomosis to the recipient atrial remnants is made in a running suture line involving atrial-to-atrial connection of both chambers. The end result is relatively larger atrial chambers with atriotomy scar/suture lines running in close proximity to the epicardial sinus node in the high posterior right atrium along the border between the original recipient atrial remnants and the newly anastomosed donor heart. The recipient's right atrial remnant often includes original sinus node tissue, producing a dissociated ghost P wave detected on a surface electrocardiogram (ECG). Early postoperative sinus node dysfunction attributed to transient injury or inflammation associated with surgical technique is the most common cause

**Table 1**
**Factors associated with bradyarrhythmias in the cardiac transplant population**

| Preoperative | Operative | Postoperative (Acquired) |
|---|---|---|
| Amiodarone use | Donor heart ischemic time | Cellular/ antibody-mediated rejection |
| Recipient age | Surgical technique (biatrial > bicaval) | Cardiac allograft vasculopathy |
| Donor age | — | — |

of early preoperative bradyarrhythmias and confers a benign prognosis.[8,18–21]

The bicaval technique involves transection at the level of the mid–ascending aorta, the main pulmonary artery, the mid–superior vena cava, and the low right atrium. The recipient's heart is nearly completely removed. Only a small remnant of the recipient's posterior left atrium, sufficient to retain the pulmonary venous antrum, is left behind. The architecture of the transplanted donor heart, consequently, is largely preserved because the anastomosis is made at the great vessels, superior/inferior vena cava (hence bicaval), and the posterior cuff of the recipient left atrial remnant containing the pulmonary venous antrum. The sinus node remains largely unperturbed.

Multiple studies[19,22,23] and a meta-analysis[24] now confirm a lower incidence of pacemaker-requiring bradyarrhythmias among patients with a bicaval cardiac transplant, in addition to lower atrial filling pressures; less tricuspid regurgitation; and, possibly, even lower overall mortality when compared with the biatrial technique.[25] However, the survival advantage of a bicaval technique remains controversial. Arguing against this finding is a 2008 published analysis of the United Network for Organ Sharing/Organ Procurement and Transplantation Network (UNOS/OPTN) registry demonstrating that the apparent higher mortality at 24% versus 18% at 5 years with biatrial transplant disappeared after correction for confounding variables.[1]

In a 10-year, multivariable analysis of the UNOS/OPTN registry published in 2010, the bicaval technique was strongly protective against pacemaker-requiring bradyarrhythmias (odds ratio, 0.33;

confidence interval [CI], 0.29–0.36; $P<.001$), and there was an alarming increased mortality (17.7% vs 13.8% at 5 years, $P<.001$) among patients without a pacemaker that persisted despite multivariable adjustment and propensity-matched analysis (adjusted hazard ratio, 0.84; CI, 0.8–0.88; $P<.001$, for permanent pacemaker recipients) (**Fig. 2**).[26] From this analysis alone, one cannot conclude that pacemakers improve survival, given the possibility for unidentified confounding variables present in registry data sets. Nonetheless, the plausible and disturbing implication is that late-onset bradyarrhythmias may go unrecognized when patients are not in hospital or monitored by telemetry. Although not definitive, the analysis certainly underscores the importance of careful postdischarge follow-up with attention to warning signs such as syncopal events and/or posttransplant-acquired conditions conferring increase risk, particularly those resulting in His-Purkinje disease, or intermittent high-grade bradyarrhythmias detected by ambulatory Holter or event monitoring recommended in response to patient symptoms such as dizziness, presyncope, or palpitations. However, the role of each of these as risk stratification tools has not yet been prospectively validated.

Although advantages of the bicaval technique for arrhythmia have been clearly highlighted, disadvantages include a more technically demanding procedure associated with longer donor heart ischemic time.[25] Thus, both techniques are applied according to the surgeon's training and experience and patient-specific considerations. The electrophysiologist's task is to apply knowledge of the given technique to postoperative arrhythmia management.

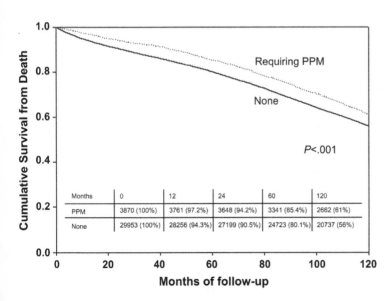

Fig. 2. Survival from all-cause mortality stratified by pacemaker status among 33,824 pacemaker recipients adjusted for donor/recipient age, donor heart ischemic time, UNOS listing status, graft rejection requiring treatment, and other common medical comorbidities. (*From* Cantillon DJ, Tarakji KG, Hu T, et al. Long-term outcomes and clinical predictors for pacemaker-requiring bradyarrhythmias after cardiac transplantation: analysis of the UNOS/OPTN cardiac transplant database. Heart Rhythm 2010;7: 1569; with permission.)

| Months | 0 | 12 | 24 | 60 | 120 |
|---|---|---|---|---|---|
| PPM | 3870 (100%) | 3761 (97.2%) | 3648 (94.2%) | 3341 (85.4%) | 2662 (61%) |
| None | 29953 (100%) | 28256 (94.3%) | 27199 (90.5%) | 24723 (80.1%) | 20737 (56%) |

## Donor Heart Ischemic Time

Prolonged deprivation of blood flow and oxygen to cardiac tissues is associated with ischemic injury and cell death and has the potential to affect electrically important structures such as the sinus node, AV node, or His-Purkinje system. Longer donor heart ischemic times have been associated with a higher rate of bradyarrhythmias.[8,19] However, in the 2010 UNOS/OPTN analysis, donor heart ischemic time was not associated with pacemaker-requiring bradyarrhythmias in a multivariable analysis.[26] Inability to detect such an effect in this analysis argues against donor heart ischemic time serving as a dominant mechanism in the overall transplant population, although it is still perhaps important in individual patients with particularly long ischemic times resulting from a complex or technically difficult surgery.

## Donor and Recipient Age

Increasing age is an association for bradyarrhythmias in both heart failure and cardiac transplant populations.[19] Although this association was present in the larger UNOS/OPTN database, it is uniformly weak for both donor and recipient age.[26] This suggests that senescent degeneration of electrically important cardiac tissues is probably a contributing factor rather than a root cause for the development of bradyarrhythmias. Simply put, older hearts may be more sensitive to the other injurious mechanisms described.

## Cellular and Antibody-Mediated Rejection

Cellular rejection has been associated with abrupt-onset bradyarrhythmias and sudden death, by virtue of disease involving the His bundle and septal fibers.[9,17] However, analysis of the Cleveland Clinic and the UNOS/OPTN database did not associate cellular rejection, antibody-mediated rejection, or any allograft rejection requiring treatment with the development of pacemaker-requiring bradyarrhythmias at the population level.[19,26] Although this finding remains controversial, it is plausible that the often patchy nature of allograft rejection is capable of causing advanced arrhythmias in individual patients, but the involvement of critical electrically conductive limbs remains uncommon overall.

## Cardiac Allograft Vasculopathy

Cardiac allograft vasculopathy has been previously associated with sudden death[11-13] and is characterized by both immune-mediated and nonimmune-mediated endothelial injury patterns resulting in progressive luminal coronary stenosis in the transplanted heart, typically diagnosed by conventional angiography.[27] This condition can occur both in a slowly progressive or rapidly accelerated time frame.[12,27] Allograft vasculopathy can result in myocardial ischemia, infarction, and ventricular systolic dysfunction.[12] According to The International Society for Heart and Lung Transplant data, allograft vasculopathy represents a leading cause of late graft failure and retransplantation worldwide.[7] It is the reason many transplant centers perform routine coronary angiography on their patients at follow-up.

**Fig. 3** demonstrates the classic before and after angiographic appearance in similar right anterior oblique caudal projections obtained 1 year apart of a 59-year-old Cleveland Clinic transplant recipient with allograft vasculopathy who abruptly suffered a bradycardic arrest while hospitalized 2 years after transplant. This particular patient had presented with what his referring physicians had dubbed as "posttussive syncope." **Fig. 4** shows the patient's ECG on admission, which demonstrates advanced His-Purkinje disease. **Fig. 5** depicts the inpatient telemetry tracing from the patient's bradycardic arrest. Significant P-P interval prolongation is followed by nonconducted atrial premature complexes and then asystole requiring cardiopulmonary resuscitation. Before this event, the patient's telemetry had only demonstrated sinus rhythm with blocked atrial premature complexes.

Despite compelling case scenarios documented in the literature,[11-13,27] the aggregate Cleveland Clinic and UNOS/OPTN data do not associate allograft vasculopathy with pacemaker-requiring bradyarrhythmias at the larger population level.[19,26] Once again, this underscores the importance of the consulting electrophysiologist considering patient-specific arrhythmia mechanisms and triggers in the previously outlined approach. Clinical features such as syncope, His-Purkinje disease, and intermittent high-grade block may intuitively suggest higher risk. However, there are absolutely no data to support any of these as predictors of future events or conferring incrementally increased risk.

## VENTRICULAR TACHYARRHYTHMIAS

Ventricular tachyarrhythmias are uncommon in transplant recipients but have been previously associated with both cellular rejection and allograft vasculopathy.[13,28-30] In the Cleveland Clinic data, nonfatal ventricular tachyarrhythmias greater than 30 seconds duration or requiring external shock occurred in just more than 1% of 1309 cardiac transplant recipients.[19] Data from UCLA

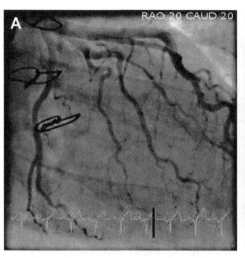 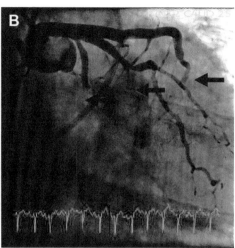

## 1 week post-transplant        20 months later

**Fig. 3.** Comparable right anterior oblique caudal angiographic views obtained from a 59-year-old male patient who developed cardiac allograft vasculopathy and later suffered a bradycardic arrest. (*A*) Normal coronary circulation. (*B*) Interval occlusions in the left circumflex artery, the inferior subdivision of a large diagonal branch, and the left anterior descending artery (marked with *arrows* from left to right, respectively), in addition to severe diffuse luminal narrowing throughout the coronary circulation.

suggest that fatal ventricular tachyarrhythmias account for only 10% of sudden cardiac death in their transplant population.[14] There are few data concerning the incremental risk associated with left ventricular systolic dysfunction, the presence of nonsustained ventricular tachycardia, or other risk-stratifying modalities, such as electrophysiologic study, T-wave alternans, or heart rate variability in this population. Heart rate variability is abnormal by virtue of obligatory surgical vagal denervation in cardiac transplant recipients.

Some centers, including the Cleveland Clinic, apply primary prevention implantable cardioverter-defibrillator (ICD) criteria from the heart failure population to the cardiac transplant population and effectively regard allograft vasculopathy as a disease equivalent to atheromatous coronary artery disease, including the associated left ventricular systolic

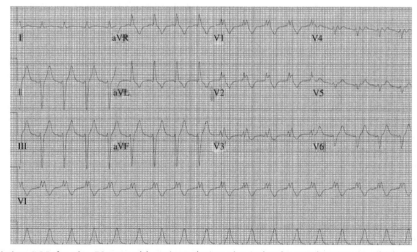

**Fig. 4.** Admitting ECG for the 59-year-old patient during the index hospitalization in which he suffered the bradycardic arrest demonstrates sinus rhythm with first-degree AV block, right bundle branch block, and left anterior hemiblock (so-called trifascicular block).

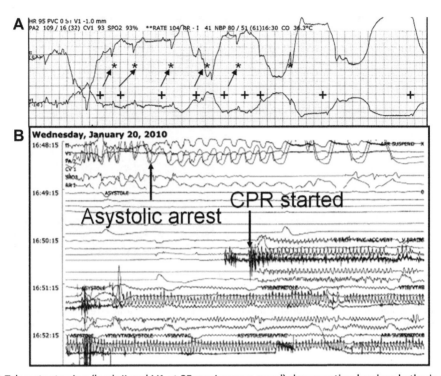

**Fig. 5.** (A) Telemetry tracing (leads II and V1 at 25 mm/s paper speed) documenting bradyarrhythmia onset. The baseline undulation sway is attributed to patient motion. QRS complexes are marked with an asterisk (*) in top lead II and P waves with a plus (+) in bottom lead V1, with AV conduction depicted by arrows. Findings suggest P-P slowing interrupted by nonconducted atrial premature complexes and then asystole. (B) Zoomed-out telemetry view demonstrating asystolic onset corresponding to that shown in (A) followed by low-frequency undulations attributed to agonal respiration, followed by a complete flat line until cardiopulmonary resuscitation was started by nursing staff approximately 1.5 minutes later.

dysfunction. The latter condition not only occurs in transplanted hearts but also can be present in the donor heart at the time it is implanted into the recipient's body. For this reason, many centers routinely perform coronary angiography. There are few data to support any of these approaches, and future research is needed.

## PACEMAKER OUTCOMES

The Cleveland Clinic and UNOS/OPTN registry data demonstrate that cardiac transplant pacemaker recipients enjoy an excellent, if not superior, prognosis.[19,26] This finding remains important because early theoretical concerns for higher cardiac device infection rates in this immunocompromised population have historically resulted in hesitation to implant pacemakers. In the Cleveland Clinic analysis, the cardiac device infection rate requiring extraction in this population was approximately 1%.[19] Thus, when a pacemaker is appropriately indicated, there are no grounds to withhold therapy on this basis.

## SUMMARY

Sudden deaths among cardiac transplant recipients are most commonly related to bradyarrhythmias, yet most bradyarrhythmias in this population are benign. This paradox makes indications for cardiac implantable devices, notably pacemakers, challenging and requires understanding of the unique considerations in this population. In short, lethal events are more commonly late onset and often occur with little warning. Early postoperative bradyarrhythmias tend to be more benign sinus node dysfunction relating to either preoperative amiodarone or transient injury/inflammation adjacent to the sinus node from right atriotomy. The use of the contemporary bicaval surgical technique has greatly reduced the incidence of pacemaker-requiring bradyarrhythmias. Acquired conditions after transplant, such as allograft rejection and/or vasculopathy, remain controversial but do likely play an important role in the late-occurring events. Further research is specifically needed in this subpopulation. Pacemaker implantation in the transplant population is associated with favorable outcomes. Acquired left ventricular dysfunction in the transplant population, regardless of cause, remains poorly understood as it pertains to the development of ventricular tachyarrhythmias and ICD indications.

## FUTURE DIRECTIONS

Additional research is needed to define the role for risk stratification modalities such as ambulatory Holter monitoring; event monitoring; and, possibly, implantable loop recorders. Identifying patients to target for arrhythmia surveillance, such as those with syncope, His-Purkinje disease, or acquired posttransplant conditions such as allograft vasculopathy or persistent rejection, is also needed. The subset of patients with acquired ventricular systolic dysfunction after transplant remains particularly understudied.

## REFERENCES

1. Weiss ES, Nwakanma LU, Russell SB, et al. Outcomes in bicaval versus biatrial techniques in heart transplantation: an analysis of the UNOS database. J Heart Lung Transplant 2008;27(2):178–83.
2. Barnard C. Reflections on the first heart transplant. S Afr Med J 1987;72(11):XIX–XX.
3. Lower RR, Shumway NE. Studies of orthotopic homotransplantation of the canine heart. Surg Forum 1960;11:18–9.
4. Shumway NE, Lower R, Stofer RC. Transplantation of the heart. Adv Surg 1966;2:265–84.
5. Miniati DN, Robbins RC. Techniques in orthotopic cardiac transplantation: a review. Cardiol Rev 2001;9: 131–6.
6. Lia KK, Bolman RM. Operative techniques in orthotopic heart transplantation. Semin Thorac Cardiovasc Surg 2004;16:370–7.
7. Taylor DO, Stehlik J, Edwards LB, et al. Registry of the International Society for Heart and Lung Transplantation: twenty-sixth official adult heart transplant report. J Heart Lung Transplant 2009;28(10):1007–22.
8. Jacquet L, Ziady G, Stein K, et al. Cardiac rhythm disturbances early after orthotopic heart transplantation: prevalence and clinical importance of the observed abnormalities. J Am Coll Cardiol 1990; 16:832–7.
9. Leonelli FM, Dunn JK, Young JB, et al. Natural history, determinants, and clinical relevance of conduction abnormalities following orthotopic heart transplantation. Am J Cardiol 1996;77(1):47–51.
10. Chantranuwat C, Blakey JD, Kobashigawa JA, et al. Sudden, unexpected death in cardiac transplant recipients: an autopsy study. J Heart Lung Transplant 2004;23(6):683–9.
11. Grinstead WC, Smart FW, Pratt CM, et al. Sudden death caused by bradycardia and asystole in a heart

12. Marzoa-Rivas R, Perez-Alvarez L, Paniagua-Martin MJ, et al. Sudden cardiac death of two heart transplant patients with correctly functioning implantable cardioverter defibrillators. J Heart Lung Transplant 2009; 28(4):412–4.
13. Patel VS, Lim M, Massin EK, et al. Sudden cardiac death in cardiac transplant recipients. Circulation 1996;94(9S):II273–7.
14. Vaseghi M, Lellouche N, Ritter H, et al. Mode and mechanisms of death after orthotopic heart transplantation. Heart Rhythm 2009;6(4):503–9.
15. Zipes DP, Camm AJ, Borggreffe MA, et al. AHA/ACC/ESC 2006 guidelines for management of patients with ventricular arrhythmias and the prevention of sudden cardiac death. Circulation 2006;114: e385–484.
16. DiBiase A, Tse TM, Schnittger I, et al. Frequency and mechanism of bradycardia in cardiac transplant recipients and need for pacemakers. Am J Cardiol 1991;67:1385–9.
17. Blanche C, Czer LS, Fishbein MC, et al. Permanent pacemaker for rejection episodes after heart transplantation: a poor prognostic sign. Ann Thorac Surg 1995;60:1263–6.
18. Rothman SA, Jeevanandam V, Combs WG, et al. Eliminating bradyarrhythmias after orthotopic heart transplantation. Circulation 1996;94(2):278–82.
19. Cantillon DJ, Gorodeski EZ, Caccamo M, et al. Long-term outcomes and clinical predictors for pacing after cardiac transplantation. J Heart Lung Transplant 2009;28:791–8.
20. Scott CD, Dark JH, McComb JM. Sinus node function after cardiac transplantation. J Am Coll Cardiol 1994;24(5):1334–41.
21. Heinz G, Hirschl M, Buxbaum P, et al. Sinus node dysfunction after orthotopic heart transplant: postoperative incidence and long-term implications. Pacing Clin Electrophysiol 1992;15:731–7.
22. Meyer SR, Modry DL, Bainey K, et al. Declining need for permanent pacemaker insertion with the bicaval technique of orthotopic heart transplantation. Can J Cardiol 2005;21:159–63.
23. Kratochwill C, Schmid S, Koller-Strametz J, et al. Decrease in pacemaker incidence after orthotopic cardiac transplantation: a review. Cardiol Rev 2001;9:131–6.
24. Schnoor M, Schafer T, Luhmann D, et al. Bicaval versus standard technique in orthotopic heart transplantation: a systematic review and meta-analysis. J Thorac Cardiovasc Surg 2007;134:1322–31.
25. Jacob S, Sellke F. Is bicaval orthotopic heart transplantation superior to the biatrial technique? Interact Cardiovasc Thorac Surg 2009;9(2):333–42.
26. Cantillon DJ, Tarakji KG, Hu T, et al. Long-term outcomes and clinical predictors for pacemaker-requiring

bradyarrhythmias after cardiac transplantation: analysis of the UNOS/OPTN database. Heart Rhythm 2010;7:1567–71.

27. Weis M, von Scheidt W. Cardiac allograft vasculopathy: a review. Circulation 1997;96(6):2069–77.

28. Alexopoulos D, Yusuf S, Bostock J, et al. Ventricular arrhythmias in long term survivors of orthotopic and heterotopic cardiac transplantation. Br Heart J 1988; 59(6):648–52.

29. Park JK, Hsu DT, Hordof AJ, et al. Arrhythmias in pediatric heart transplant recipients: prevalence and association with death, coronary artery disease and rejection. J Heart Lung Transplant 1993;12(6): 956–64.

30. Uretsky BF, Kormos RL, Zerbe TR, et al. Cardiac events after heart transplantation: incidence and predictive value of coronary arteriography. J Heart Lung Transplant 1992;11(2):S45–51.

# Device Recalls: What's an Electrophysiologist to Do?

Laura Perrotta, MD*, Giuseppe Ricciardi, MD,
Paolo Pieragnoli, MD, Luigi Padeletti, MD

## KEYWORDS

• ICDs • Recall • Advisory • Psychological impact • Devices

Large randomized trials for primary[1–3] and secondary prevention[4,5] of sudden cardiac death in at-risk patients have shown that implantable cardiac defibrillators (ICDs) reduce mortality, resulting in more than 150,000 implants worldwide per year. Despite enhancements in device technology and manufacturing processes, a sharp increase in manufacturer recalls has occurred recently,[6–9] and the management of alerts and advisories involving ICDs has become part of current clinical practice. ICD recalls present several issues, with a major concern for physicians being how to deal with patients implanted with these devices. The competing risks of device failure and complication associated with device replacement must be carefully assessed for each patient; therefore, having reliable data on device failure rate is crucial.

Despite boards of experts from professional societies proposing a set of guidelines for the management of patients implanted with devices potentially affected by malfunctions,[10–12] the lack of clinical data on this topic still leave unanswered questions on what could be the best strategy. After the death of a young patient with hypertrophic cardiomyopathy who received a Ventak Prizm II DR ICD (Boston Scientific Corporation, formerly Guidant, Natick, MA, USA), Boston Scientific issued a notification to physicians and patients about a potential short circuit that might have affected that device (model 1861) manufactured on or before April 16, 2002, and about a potential

deterioration in the wire insulator within the lead connector block in the Renewal I (model H135) and Renewal II (model H155) cardiac resynchronization defibrillators manufactured on or before August 26, 2004.[13] On July 1, 2005, the FDA classified Boston Scientific's notifications as class I recalls (ie, device defect that has the likelihood of causing serious adverse health outcomes or death), indicating that the device had to be replaced and returned to the company for testing.

Manufacturers recently established a framework to enhance the quality control process associated with devices impacted by advisories, in adherence to the recommendations of the Guidance for the Heart Rhythm Society (HRS) and the obligations of the International regulatory environment. When a device is returned to a manufacturer, laboratory technicians and engineers assess overall device function and perform analysis through a series of diagnostic tests that verify the performance of defibrillation, pacing, sensing, memory, and recording functions. Test results are compared with original manufacturing records and design intent. The companies should inform regulatory bodies of each significant event that poses a potential risk to patient health, and periodically publish a performance report indicating the overall incidence of malfunctions in each product.

Additionally, all of the existing information provided by the companies and scientific societies is aimed at aiding health care practitioners make specific monitoring and treatment decisions for

Disclosures: Laura Perrotta, Giuseppe Ricciardi, and Paolo Pieragnoli have no disclosures to report; Luigi Padeletti is a consultant for Medtronic, Inc, St Jude Medical, Sorin Group, and Boston Scientific Corporation.
Department of Heart and Vessels, University of Florence, Viale Morgagni, 85, 50134 Florence, Italy
* Corresponding author.
*E-mail address:* laura_perrotta81@hotmail.com

Card Electrophysiol Clin 3 (2011) 617–622
doi:10.1016/j.ccep.2011.08.012
1877-9182/11/$ – see front matter © 2011 Elsevier Inc. All rights reserved.

their patients. The whole communication framework that was established after the first advisory in 2005 is therefore oriented toward increasing physician awareness of the real risks associated with malfunctions in devices affected by advisories, and guiding them in the choice of replacing or retaining the devices. Therefore, postexplant reports sent to physicians after laboratory analysis, and product reports issued by medical device industry and recent publications may have contributed to physician's subsequent decisions.

## RECOMMENDATIONS FOR CLINICIANS MANAGING DEVICE ADVISORY NOTICES: U.S. FOOD AND DRUG ADMINISTRATION AND HRS

The decision process should take into account estimates of the possible malfunction rate, the likely effect of the issue on specific patients (eg, pacemaker dependency), and the individual center's procedural risk associated with replacement.

The U.S. Food and Drug Administration (FDA)[14] and HRS[10] established guidelines for advisories. The FDA uses the term *recall* to describe "an action taken to address a problem with a medical device that violates FDA law. Recalls occur when a medical device is defective, when it could be a risk to health, or when it is both defective and a risk to health."[14] The FDA classifies medical device recalls as either class I, class II, or class III, representing the potential risk to public health. A class I recall indicates a high risk of serious adverse health consequences or death, and a class III indicates a low risk. This classification process usually occurs after the company has issued its recall.

The HRS advocates use of the term *advisory* as opposed to recall, because it is more neutral and less emotive. HRS also recommends some changes in FDA nomenclature, such as replacing the term *recall* with advisory; changing the term "class I recall" to "class I advisory notice or class I safety alert," indicating that a replacement should be considered because of the reasonable probability that the malfunction could result in death or significant harm; and changing class II and III recalls (non–life-threatening malfunctions or potential malfunctions) to "advisory notice or safety alerts."[10]

When an advisory is issued, patients with an affected device must be contacted and the physicians must consider the best management strategy based on the key points described by HRS (**Table 1**).[10]

## CURRENT PRACTICE AND OUTCOME OF PATIENTS WITH A RECALLED DEVICE

Although the HRS and FDA[10,14] proposed guidelines for the management of patients with a recalled device, the response to an advisory is still variable among different centers. Physicians have adopted various strategies, such as replacing all the recalled device; replacing a few devices; and not replacing any. Maisel[15] reported that the percentage of ICDs replaced in response to advisory ranged from 6% to 45% among centers (average, 17.1%).

Gould and Krahn[6] conducted one of the first larger multicenter analysis on device recall in Canada. Between October 2004 and October 2005, 17 Canadian implanting centers were surveyed; of 2915 patients with a recall device, 533 (18.3%) underwent elective replacement. The complication rate associated with the replacement was 8.1% (43 patients), whereas major complications requiring reoperation were observed in 31 patients (5.8%), including two deaths. This rate of

---

**Table 1**
**Key points in physicians' decision-making process regarding device advisories**

| Related to Device/Lead Malfunction | Related to Patient Characteristic |
|---|---|
| Mechanism of malfunction known and potentially recurrent | Pacemaker dependency |
| The risk of malfunction is likely to lead to patient death or serious harm | ICD for secondary prevention for sudden cardiac death |
| The risk of replacement is less than, or at least not substantially greater than, the risk of device malfunction | ICD for primary prevention of sudden cardiac death, with a recorded sustained ventricular arrhythmia treated successfully by the ICD |
| | Device approaching elective replacement indicator |

*Data from* Carlson MD, Wilkoff BL, Maisel WH, et al. Recommendations from the heart rhythm society task force on device performance policies and guidelines endorsed by the ACCF, the AHA and the International Coalition of Pacing and Electrophysiology Organizations (COPE). Heart Rhythm 2006;3(10):1250–73.

complications was higher than the stated risk of failure (comparing the number of failures with the number of devices implanted) associated with advisories for that period, ranging from 0.009% to 2.6%. Subsequent single-center studies reported lower complication rates, with Kapa and colleagues[16] at the Mayo Clinic reporting 0.62%, Costea and colleagues[9] reporting 4.1%, and Moore and colleagues[17] reporting 2.1%. Most of the published data concerning advisories analyzed the management of recalled device generators, whereas fewer studies investigated lead advisories.

In 1994, the Telectronics Accufix active fixation pacing leads (Accufix Research Institute, Parker CO, USA) were recalled[18] because of a reported fracture and protrusion of the J retention wire, causing right atrium perforation or embolization to the pulmonary circulation. A review from Kay and colleagues[18] showed that 5299 leads were extracted (13% affected by the recall), but the risk of complications associated with lead extraction was higher than that associated with leaving the recalled lead in place, especially in elderly patients because major complications increased with age, whereas the risk of lead fracture and heart injury was lower in elderly patients.

A recent three-center study[19] analyzed 1023 patients implanted with Medtronic Sprint Fidelis implantable cardioverter-defibrillator leads and compared them with 1668 patients who received Medtronic Sprint Quattro leads (Medtronic, Inc, Minneapolis, MN, USA). The Fidelis lead began to fracture soon after it was introduced in 2004, causing primarily inappropriate shocks and few reported deaths.[20] The failure rate for Fidelis leads observed in this multicenter study was 2.81% per year compared with 0.43% per year for Quattro; it was higher in younger patients, women, patients with hypertrophic cardiomyopathy, and patients with arrhythmogenic right ventricular dysplasia or channelopathies.

These findings underline the importance of accurate patient risk stratification based on clinical evaluation when replacing an advisory lead, because higher complication rates are associated with lead extraction.

### The Italian Experience

Between July 2005 and October 2009, 3185 ICDs were recalled in 247 Italian Centers, including 843 Prizm (151 centers) and 2342 Renewal models (164 centers).[21]

Of the 843 potentially affected Prizm ICD devices, 139 (16.5%) were explanted (median time from implant, 4 years) and returned for laboratory analysis. Testing showed that none exhibited the failure described in the communication. The remaining devices were monitored according to Boston Scientific's original patient management recommendations (ie, normal follow-up at 3-month intervals) until their explant for normal end of life. These devices were not returned to Boston Scientific for analysis.

Of the 2342 Renewal devices potentially affected, 458 (19.6%) were explanted (median time from implant, 3 years) and returned for analysis. One device (0.21%) showed the malfunction described in the advisory, provoked by tests. Seven devices not explanted at the time of the advisory were explanted later before elective replacement indication (ERI) after they exhibited the failure mode described in the communication (0.29%). No adverse patient symptoms were reported. Additionally, 76 of these devices were explanted for normal ERI (3.24%) and 10 were explanted because they exhibited a different failure (0.42%).

To date, physicians have not reported any deaths to the company as being potentially associated with the device failure described in the advisory for Prizm and Renewal devices. Moreover, no additional communications (ie, product experience) associated with these failures were reported during the follow-up of these devices until year 2009. Therefore, in the hypothesis of an accurate and complete reporting to the company of any adverse occurrence, and in the absence of other forms of underestimation (ie, patient death for unexplained causes, potentially related to the failure), the total incidence over a 4-year time frame of the failure event would have been equal to 0 of 843 (0%) for Prizm and 8 of 2342 (0.34%) for Renewal.

Only 18.7% of devices impacted by recall have been explanted according to indications. Among the 247 Italian centers, a mean of 13 ICDs per site were impacted by recall. The authors divided the centers according to the number of recalled devices and found that 19 centers had more than 30 (7.69%), 74 had between 10 and 30 (29.96%), and 154 had fewer than 10 (62.35%). No significant differences were observed in the proportion of explant procedures among the three groups ($P = .092$).

The data analyzed from the Italian centers showed that only a limited percentage of devices affected by recall (18%) were definitely explanted following the indications stated into the advisory update communication. This final decision was left to the patient after discussion with the implanting physician. The proportion of explanted devices was 16.8%, similar the findings of Costea and colleagues[9] and Amin and colleagues,[22] whose findings ranged between 15% and 20%. Thus, in common clinical practice, the choice of more frequent follow-up has prevailed over that of an immediate device explant.

No additional data on patient outcomes (ie, mortality, including death cause) were available for the patients that were followed up without explant, preventing a general conclusion on patient safety for the entire set of devices impacted by the communication. Nevertheless, physicians did not ask to verify if these deaths were related to device malfunctioning in any of the patients who died.

The failure rates that resulted from the authors' data analysis (0% for Prizm and 0.34% for Renewal) were inferior to those already found or projected along the device lifetime globally, as reported in the company's most recent Product Performance Report (0.72% for Prizm and 1.83% for Renewal). In absence of underestimation of the events, a lower incidence than expected could resize the dimension of the problem, justifying the decision of both patient and physician to not explant the device and to increase the frequency of follow-up visits.

## PATIENTS' POINT OF VIEW (PSYCHOLOGICAL IMPACTS)

The impact of ICD advisories on patient well-being and patient-centered outcomes, such as symptoms, anxiety, distress, and quality of life, has been largely neglected, even though it is a key aspect for a patient's active and responsible involvement in the decision-making process.

Previous studies showed that ICD implantation is associated with psychological distress, manifesting as anxiety and depression in 13% to 38% of patients implanted with an ICD.[23–25] Awareness of the potential risk of malfunction could increase patients' anxiety and alter their psychological status, but data from the few studies on patient-centered outcome are not uniform.

Pedersen and colleagues[26] examined the impact of ICD advisories on patient-centered outcomes via a systematic literature review. They identified six studies,[27–32] four of which used a case-control design and two that were prospective, with sample sizes ranging from 30 to 86 patients. All advisories were class I, class II, or a combination. The assessment of patient-centered outcome was not uniform across the studies, using different scales to examining patients' overall perception of the ICD recall. A considerable variability was also seen between the time that the advisory notification was received and when the assessment of patient-centered outcomes was performed, ranging from 1 to 24 months. As a result, evidence of an impact on device advisories was mixed, with two prospective studies showing an increase in anxiety over time, whereas none of the larger case-control studies found a difference in patient-centered outcomes between cases and controls.

In a subgroup analysis, Undavia and colleagues[31] showed that patients with devices that had a class I recall had a slightly worse overall quality of life compared with those with devices with a class II recall. Therefore, a class I advisory may have a more severe psychological impact than a class II advisory, given that a class I recall is potentially associated with a greater likelihood of life-threatening malfunction.

In all of the studies, patients had more confidence in and preferred learning about the recalls from their physicians rather than from media and device manufacturers. Thus, good physician-patient communication along with a level of trust and an established rapport may play an important role in alleviating concerns and anxiety in patients with devices subject to an ICD recall.

A challenge for physicians and health care professionals in relation to future ICD advisories will be to inform patients before the media does, because patients believe that the information is more accurate when it is provided by their physician than the media.[33]

In addition, to increase knowledge regarding the psychological impact of recalls in the future, standardized instruments to assess patient-centered outcomes should be included in ICD registries and incorporated into standard clinical care for each patient.

## FUTURE PERSPECTIVE: DEVELOPMENT OF DECISION MODELS AND REMOTE MONITORING

A high degree of variability remains in patient management strategies.[7] Quantitative information and specific models to drive decisions are still needed and should be the main issue to address in the next years. One possible way to obtain information is the development of validated decision models, which can provide indicators of the benefit of a specific strategy or highlight trade-offs among different decisions. These models may indicate risk of serious complications associated with device replacement based on a set of variables (ie, patient age, disease, device type) compared with the device's expected failure rate usually reported in the advisory communications.

Amin and colleagues[34] recently developed a Markov decision model using a simulation of a two-armed clinical trial to assess the benefit of immediate device replacement compared with continued monitoring. They found that the most powerful variables in the decision-making process were the estimated device failure rates indicated in the advisory and the mortality rates associated with device replacements, whereas the remaining generator life and the patient's age and sex had little influence. Gula and colleagues[35] found similar data using another Markov model. Even in this analysis, the main factor indicating the best strategy for generator replacement was the estimated risk of device failure. This finding should be sufficient to confer a survival advantage to a replacement strategy.

A novel approach used by Priori and colleagues[36] introduced the concept of the "number needed to replace," which is the number of advisory devices that would be need to be replaced to save one life. It was calculated considering four parameters: (1) the expected annual sudden cardiac death rate, (2) the residual device life, (3) the difference in failure rate between the advisory device and the replacement device, and (4) the mortality risk associated with the replacement procedure. The data suggested an advantage to replacing a recalled device when a high failure rate ($\geq$1%), high arrhythmic risk ($\geq$25%), and pacemaker dependency are present.

Recently Amin and colleagues[22] compared the common practice with device advisories at the Virginia University Medical Center with the best patient management strategy predicted by a decision analysis model. They observed that physicians replace more devices than are indicated by the decision model; in particular, a relevant proportion of device replacements are ICDs rather than pacemakers, because of a higher perceived risk of malfunction by the physician or higher reported patient anxiety. Despite being considered important tools, these models still rely on the accuracy of the estimated failure rates provided by device companies, which are based on bench-testing data and may differ from real-life observed data. Therefore, these decision models should be adequately supported by the future development of clinical studies to be implemented in patients affected by device recalls. Data from recently introduced remote monitoring systems can address the need for continuous and automatic monitoring of specific device parameters and contribute to reducing the need to replace the device.

Finally, patient-centered outcomes, such as symptoms, anxiety, distress, and quality of life, which were mainly neglected recent research,[26] should be included in future studies to unveil important aspects related to patient's perception of device recalls, with the goal of increasing active and responsible patient involvement in the decision-making process. Media have an important role in how physicians and patients perceive a recall, and therefore efforts must be made to increase awareness on this topic and avoid decisions based only on personal perceived risks generated by unfavorable press releases. Health care professionals should be adequately informed of all aspects related to a device recall, trained in recall management, and able to inform patients and involve them in an accurate and transparent decision-making process that can ultimately minimize risk, reduce expenses of unnecessary replacement procedures, diminish patient anxiety, and preserve quality of life.

## REFERENCES

1. Moss AJ, Zareba W, Hall WJ, et al, Multicenter Automatic Defibrillator Implantation Trial II Investigators. Prophylactic implantation of a defibrillator in patients with myocardial infarction and reduced ejection fraction. N Engl J Med 2002;346:877–83.

2. Bristow MR, Saxon LA, Boehmer J, et al, Comparison of Medical Therapy, Pacing, and Defibrillation in Heart Failure (COMPANION) Investigators. Cardiac resynchronization therapy with or without an implantable defibrillator in advanced chronic heart failure. N Engl J Med 2004;350:2140–50.

3. Bardy GH, Lee KL, Mark DB, et al, Sudden Cardiac Death in Heart Failure Trial (SCD-HeFT) Investigators. Amiodarone or an implantable cardioverter-defibrillator for congestive heart failure. N Engl J Med 2005;352:225–37.

4. Connolly SJ, Gent M, Roberts RS, et al. Canadian Implantable Defibrillator Study (CIDS): a randomized trial of the implantable cardioverter defibrillator against amiodarone. Circulation 2000;101:1297–302.

5. The Antiarrhythmics versus Implantable Defibrillators (AVID) Investigators. A comparison of antiarrhythmic drug therapy with implantable defibrillators in patients resuscitated from near-fatal ventricular arrhythmias. N Engl J Med 1997;337:1576–83.

6. Gould PA, Krahn AD, Canadian Heart Rhythm Society Working Group on Device Advisories. Complications associated with implantable cardioverter-defibrillator replacement in response to device advisories. JAMA 2006;295(16):1907–11.

7. Maisel WH. Pacemaker and ICD generator reliability: meta-analysis of device registries. JAMA 2006;295: 1929–34.

8. Wilkoff BL. Pacemaker and ICD malfunction – an incomplete picture. JAMA 2006;295:1944–6.

9. Costea A, Rardon DP, Padanilam B, et al. Complications associated with generator replacement in response to device advisories. J Cardiovasc Electrophysiol 2008;19(3):266–9.

10. Carlson MD, Wilkoff BL, Maisel WH, et al. Recommendations from the Heart Rhythm society task force on device performance policies and guidelines endorsed by the ACCF, the AHA and the International Coalition of Pacing and Electrophysiology Organizations (COPE). Heart Rhythm 2006;3(10):1250–73.

11. Santini M, Brachmann J, Cappato R, et al. Recommendations of the European Cardiac Arrhythmia Society on device failures and complications. Pacing Clin Electrophysiol 2006;29:653–69.

12. Auricchio A, Gropp M, Ludgate S, et al. Writing committee for the European heart rhythm association guidance document on cardiac rhythm management produce performance. Europace 2006;8:313–22.

13. Boston Scientific announces physician communications related to products in its CRM group. Medscape Today Web site. Available at: http://www.medscape.com/pages/editorial/pressreleases/pr-crm-bostonsci5. Accessed June 24, 2011.

14. Recent medical device recalls. U.S. Food and Drug Administration Web site. Available at: http://www.fda.gov/cdrh/recalls/learn.html. Accessed June 24, 2011.

15. Maisel WH. Physician management of pacemaker and implantable cardioverter defibrillator advisories. Pacing Clin Electrophysiol 2004;27(4):437–42.

16. Kapa S, Hyberger L, Rea RF, et al. Complication risk with pulse generator change: implications when reacting to a device advisory or recall. Pacing Clin Electrophysiol 2007;30:730–3.

17. Moore JW III, Barrington W, Bazaz R, et al. Complications of replacing implantable devices in response to advisories: a single center experience. Int J Cardiol 2009;134(1):42–6.

18. Kay GN, Brinker JA, Kawanishi DT, et al. Risks of spontaneous injury and extraction of an active fixation pacemaker lead: report of the Accufix Multicenter Clinical Study and Worldwide Registry. Circulation 1999;100(23):2344–52.

19. Hauser RG, Maisel WH, Friedman PA, et al. Longevity of Sprint Fidelis implantable cardioverter-defibrillator leads and risk factors for failure: implications for patient management. Circulation 2011; 123(4):358–63.

20. Hauser RG, Kallinen LM, Almquist AK, et al. Early failure of a small-diameter high-voltage implantable cardioverter-defibrillator lead. Heart Rhythm 2007; 4(7):892–6.

21. Perrotta L, Pieragnoli P, Ricciardi G, et al. Multicenter experience with implantable defibrillators subject to recall. Pacing Clin Electrophysiol 2011;34(8): 998–1002.

22. Amin MS, Wood MA, Shepard RK, et al. Clinical judgment versus decision analysis for managing device advisories. Pacing Clin Electrophysiol 2008; 31:1236–40.

23. Sears SF Jr, Conti JB. Quality of life and psychological functioning of ICD patients. Heart 2002;87(5): 488–93.

24. Heller SS, Ormont MA, Lidagoster L, et al. Psychosocial outcome after ICD implantation: a current perspective. Pacing Clin Electrophysiol 1998;21(6): 1207–15.

25. Sears SF Jr, Todaro JF, Lewis TS, et al. Examining the psychosocial impact of implantable cardioverter defibrillators: a literature review. Clin Cardiol 1999; 22(7):481–9.

26. Pedersen SS, van den Berg M, Theuns DA. A viewpoint on the impact of device advisories on patient-centered outcomes. Pacing Clin Electrophysiol 2009;32(8):1006–11.

27. van den Broek KC, Denollet J, Nyklíček I, et al. Psychological reaction to potential malfunctioning of implantable defibrillators. Pacing Clin Electrophysiol 2006;29(9):953–6.

28. Cuculi F, Herzig W, Kobza R, et al. Psychological distress in patients with ICD recall. Pacing Clin Electrophysiol 2006;29(11):1261–5.

29. Gibson DP, Kuntz KK, Levenson JL, et al. Decision-making, emotional distress, and quality of life in patients affected by the recall of their implantable cardioverter defibrillator. Europace 2008;10(5): 540–4.

30. Sneed NV, Finch NJ, Leman RB. The impact of device recall on patients and family members of patients with automatic implantable cardioverter defibrillators. Heart Lung 1994;23(4):317–22.

31. Undavia M, Goldstein NE, Cohen P, et al. Impact of implantable cardioverter-defibrillator recalls on patients' anxiety, depression, and quality of life. Pacing Clin Electrophysiol 2008;31(11):1411–8.

32. Birnie DH, Sears SF, Green MS, et al. No long-term psychological morbidity living with an implantable cardioverter defibrillator under advisory: the Medtronic Marquis experience. Europace 2009;11(1):26–30.

33. Stutts LA, Conti JB, Aranda JM Jr, et al. Patient evaluation of ICD recall communication strategies: a vignette study. Pacing Clin Electrophysiol 2007; 30(9):1105–11.

34. Amin MS, Matchar DB, Wood MA, et al. Management of recalled pacemakers and implantable cardioverter-defibrillators: a decision analysis model. JAMA 2006;296(4):412–20.

35. Gula LJ, Massel D, Krahn AD, et al. Survival rates as a guide to implanted cardioverter-defibrillator replacement strategies for device recalls–adding statistical insight to clinical intuition. Am Heart J 2007;153(2):253–9.

36. Priori SG, Auricchio A, Nisam S, et al. To replace or not to replace: a systematic approach to respond to device advisories. J Cardiovasc Electrophysiol 2009;20(2):164–70.

# Device-Detected Atrial Fibrillation: Perils and Pitfalls

Tahmeed Contractor, MD[a], Mehul B. Patel, MD[b],
Ranjan K. Thakur, MD, MPH, MBA, FHRS[a],*

## KEYWORDS

- Atrial fibrillation • Atrial high rate events • Stroke
- Implantable heart rhythm devices

Atrial fibrillation (AF) is the most common sustained arrhythmia encountered in clinical practice, and has an estimated prevalence as high as 9% in elderly people.[1] The risk of stroke is increased 5-fold in patients with nonrheumatic AF and 17-fold in patients with rheumatic AF.[2,3] One of the foremost goals of managing AF is the reduction of thromboembolic strokes and systemic embolism. Implantable heart rhythm devices, such as implantable cardioverter-defibrillators (ICDs), cardiac resynchronization therapy (CRT) devices (pacemakers [CRT-P] and defibrillators [CRT-D]), and permanent pacemakers (PPMs) are increasingly being used worldwide. These devices are capable of sensing intrinsic atrial activity and often detect spontaneous atrial high rate events (AHREs) in asymptomatic patients. Barring any spurious causes, AHREs seen by these devices are supposedly tantamount to having AF or atrial flutter (AFL), because several studies have documented a correlation between AHRE and electrocardiogram (ECG)-documented episodes of AF/AFL with a high degree of sensitivity and specificity. However, the critical duration, frequency, or overall burden of AHRE that increases stroke risk is still unknown, and thus the threshold level of AHREs that warrants anticoagulation is still unclear. This article reviews the current literature on the risk of stroke with device-detected AHREs and raises questions that need further clarification.

## AF AS A RISK FACTOR FOR STROKE

AF is a major, independent risk factor for stroke, and accounts for 10% of all ischemic strokes.[4] Almost 25% of strokes in patients aged 80 to 89 years are secondary to AF, with the propensity of AF to cause strokes increasing with age.[2] In the United States alone, AF causes approximately 75,000 strokes per year.[5] Because of the large size of emboli compared with other sources, AF-related strokes tend to be more severe, and therefore have a greater impact on morbidity and mortality.[6,7] Over the past few decades, warfarin has remained the only anticoagulant that has significantly reduced stroke burden in AF.[8] Perceived bleeding risks, need for monitoring International Normalized Ratio (INR), narrow therapeutic window, and drug and dietary interactions are some reasons why warfarin is not prescribed in many high-risk patients with AF, especially more than 65 years of age.[9,10] However, new treatment alternatives are emerging. Newer oral anticoagulants, such as dabigatran and rivaroxaban, are equally efficacious, with a lower risk of intracranial hemorrhage, and obviate the need for anticoagulation monitoring.[11,12] Left atrial appendage occlusion devices, such as the WATCHMAN device (Atritech, Minneapolis, MN, USA), are also being evaluated for stroke reduction in nonvalvular AF and may replace the need for long-term anticoagulation, at least in some

[a] Department of Cardiology, Lehigh Valley Health Network, 1240 South Cedar Crest Boulevard, Allentown, PA 18103, USA
[b] Department of Clinical Cardiac Electrophysiology, The Bay Pines Veterans Affairs Health Care System, University of South Florida, Tampa 10000 Bay Pines Boulevard, Bay Pines, FL 33744, USA
* Corresponding author.
E-mail address: thakur@msu.edu

Card Electrophysiol Clin 3 (2011) 623–630
doi:10.1016/j.ccep.2011.07.003
1877-9182/11/$ – see front matter © 2011 Elsevier Inc. All rights reserved.

patients.[13] Availability of these alternative options may make thromboembolic prophylaxis possible in more patients.

Alongside better treatment methods, advanced diagnostic modalities, such as transtelephonic ECG monitoring, mobile cardiac outpatient telemetry, and implantable loop recorders, are more effective in diagnosing AF, especially paroxysmal AF.[14,15] These advanced techniques have detected paroxysmal AF in up to 25% patients with cryptogenic stroke.[15] The risk of ischemic stroke with paroxysmal AF is similar to that with permanent AF, and can be significantly reduced with anticoagulation.[16,17] However, the degree or duration of paroxysmal AF that increases the risk of stroke is still unknown.

### AHREs and AF

Devices such as ICDs, CRT devices, and dual-chamber PPMs provide a wealth of information on atrial and ventricular sensed and paced events. The critical atrial rate that must be exceeded to trigger labeling it an AHRE can be programmed, allowing these devices to accurately report their frequency, duration, and overall burden compared with sensed or paced atrial rhythm. Several studies

have documented a positive correlation between PPM-identified AHREs and ECG-documented episodes of AF or AFL with a high degree of sensitivity and specificity.[18,19] However, the correlation is imperfect because oversensing (eg, far-field sensing, double counting, T-wave oversensing in sinus tachycardia) can lead to false-positive reporting of AF (**Fig. 1**), and undersensing (eg, P-wave sensitivity set too low or too high) can lead to underdetection of AF (**Fig. 2**).

AHREs have been found in nearly 50% of dual-chamber PPM recipients with or without known AF.[20,21] Subsequent studies that excluded patients with known AF reported AHREs in approximately 30% of PPM recipients.[18,22] A similar incidence (approximately 25%) has been found in CRT device recipients, and patients with these events showed less echocardiograph response to CRT and a greater number of adverse cardiac outcomes, such as appropriate/inappropriate ICD shocks and hospitalizations for heart failure.[23,24] Risk factors for developing AHREs include a previous history of AF,[25] underlying sinus node dysfunction,[21] and right ventricular pacing.[22,26] In the Mode Selection Trial (MOST), AF increased by 1% for every 1% increase in right ventricular pacing.[26] Similarly, Cheung and colleagues[22] found that in PPM recipients with

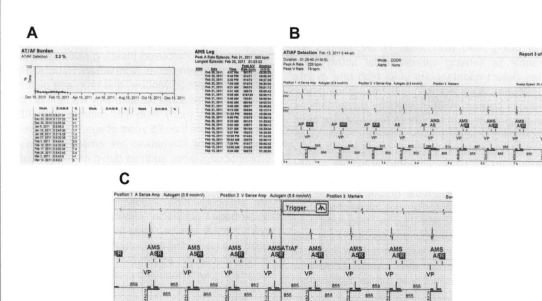

**Fig. 1.** Pacemaker interrogation strips from a patient with a dual-chamber pacemaker shows far-field sensing of R waves leading to inappropriate detection of atrial tachycardia (AT)/AF. (A) Overall AF burden of 2.2% and weekly burden from 0% to 5%. A typical episode of automatic mode switch (AMS) occurred on February 13, 2011 at 6:44 AM, lasting 1 hour, 28 minutes, and 50 seconds (*bottom, right column*). (B) Atrial and ventricular pacing for the first three cycles. V pacing is followed by far-field R wave sensing falling in the refractory period (AR). After an AS-VP event, AP-VP is again far-field sensed in the atrium and leads to AMS and VVI pacing, leading to double-counting of atrial activity (far-field paced R waves and intrinsic atrial activity), leading to detection of AT/AF (C). AF, atrial fibrillation; AMS, automated mode switch; AP, atrial paced; AR, atrial refratory period; AS, atrial sensed; AT, atrial tachycardia; R, refractory period; VP, ventricular paced; VS, ventricular sensed.

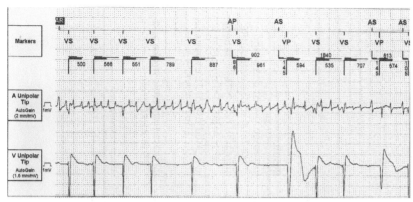

**Fig. 2.** Pacemaker interrogation strip from a patient with a dual-chamber pacemaker shows AF undersensing. AF is present in the atrial channel, whereas the ventricular channel shows a well-controlled, irregular rhythm. The marker channel at the top clearly shows appropriate sensing of ventricular activity, whereas atrial activity is undersensed. AP, atrial paced; AR, atrial refratory period; AS, atrial sensed; VP, ventricular paced; VS, ventricular sensed; VVI, ventricle paced, ventricle sensed, inhibitory.

a cumulative right ventricular pacing of 50% or greater, the risk of AF was doubled (hazard ratio [HR], 2.2; 95% CI, 1.0–4.7; $P = .04$).

The duration of AHREs varies considerably. For example, Cheung and colleagues[22] found that 60% of the population had an AHRE duration of more than 1 hour, and in 16%, the AHRE episode lasted more than 1 week. Brief episodes may precede longer episodes, because almost 50% of patients with an AHRE lasting less than 1 hour had subsequent episodes lasting 1 hour or longer. However, some of the early-onset, brief episodes in the immediate postimplant phase may be secondary to the temporary proarrhythmic state caused by the inflammatory effect of atrial lead implantation. An analysis of the Silent Atrial Fibrillation Detection With Stored EGMs (SAFE) registry showed that almost 25% of AHREs occurred within the first 30 days after PPM implantation without subsequent recurrence.[27]

Several studies have attempted to estimate the approximate duration of an AHRE that correlates with clinician-documented AF. When a cutoff of 5 minutes and a rate of greater than 250 beats per minute (bpm) is chosen to signify a significant AHRE, a strong correlation is seen between pacemaker-identified AHREs and clinically confirmed AF.[19] Similarly, a subanalysis of the MOST population, which used more than 220 bpm for 5 minutes to indicate significant AHREs, found a high correlation with clinically detected AF (HR, 5.93; $P = .0001$).[28] Shorter cutoffs lead to overdetection, commonly from far-field R and T wave oversensing.[29]

That the AHRE events are AF or AFL and not spuriously labeled is critical to corroborate, because of the clinical implications. Because

of the limited memory allocated for intracardiac ECGs, pacing devices may store only limited ECG data to corroborate that the events labeled as AHRE or AHRE-triggered automatic mode switch (AMS) events are AF or AFL. Because most AHRE episodes are asymptomatic and found incidentally on device interrogation, symptom correlation is usually absent.[19] Atrial undersensing can lead to nondetection of low amplitude atrial signals, and thus underestimate AF burden, whereas oversensing issues can lead to erroneous overestimation of AF burden.

In the absence of correlation with stored ECGs, the diagnosis may be impossible to confirm and one must make decisions about therapeutic interventions. For example, Kohno and colleagues[30] recently reported that a cumulative increase in atrial pacing and the use of an atrial overdrive pacing algorithm might be closely associated with spurious AHRE detection. Using caution when confirming that the device-detected AHRE represents true AF or AFL is even more important in the era of remote monitoring, when potentially every AHRE (meeting predefined atrial rate and duration criteria) leading to an AMS can be reported to the pacemaker clinic.

## AHREs and Thromboembolism

Recent studies that have assessed the risk of thromboembolism associated with AHRE detected in pacing devices are shown in **Table 1**. Initial evidence of increased risk came from a subanalysis of 312 patients enrolled in MOST,[28] which was a randomized trial of dual-chamber, rate-modulated pacing versus single-changer, ventricular rate-modulated pacing in patients

**Table 1**
Clinical studies evaluating risk of thromboembolism with device-detected atrial high rate episodes

| Study | Year | No. of Subjects | Design | Population | Significant AHRE Definition | Results |
|---|---|---|---|---|---|---|
| Glotzer et al[28] | 2003 | 312 | RCT subanalysis | Dual-chamber pacemaker recipients | Atrial rate ≥220 bpm lasting ≥5 min | Increased risk of death and nonfatal stroke with AHRE |
| Capucci et al[31] | 2005 | 725 | Prospective, Observational | Dual-chamber pacemaker recipients | AF for 5 m or 1 d | Increased risk of TE in patients with AHRE>1 d duration |
| TRENDS study[32] | 2009 | 2486 | Prospective, Observational | Pacemaker/defibrillator recipients with an equal or greater stroke risk factor | Atrial rate ≥175 bpm lasting ≥20 s | Increased risk of TE in patients with AHRE ≥5.5 h |
| ASSERT study[33,34] | 2010 | 2580 | Randomized trial | Pacemaker/defibrillator recipients with hypertension and ≥65 years of age | Atrial rate ≥190 bpm lasting ≥6 min | Increased ischemic stroke and TE in AHRE group |

*Abbreviations:* AHRE, atrial high rate events; AF, atrial fibrillation; ASSERT, asymptomatic atrial fibrillation and stroke evaluation in pacemaker patients and the atrial fibrillation reduction atrial pacing trial; bpm, beats per minute; RCT, randomized controlled trial; TE, thromboembolism.

with sinus node dysfunction.[26] In this subanalysis, an AHRE was defined as an atrial rate of 220 bpm or more lasting at least 5 minutes. Over a median follow-up of 27 months, AHREs were observed in 51% of the population, and were an independent predictor of mortality (HR, 2.48; $P$ = .009) and nonfatal stroke (HR, 2.79; $P$ = .001). The MOST study subanalysis concluded that AHREs detected through pacemakers in patients with sinus node dysfunction can identify those who are more than twice as likely to die or have a stroke and six times as likely to develop AF compared with similar patients without AHRE. However, this study was conducted in patients with early-generation pacemakers that had limited device memory and diagnostic capability to accurately assess duration and rate of the AHRE.

Subsequently, Capucci and colleagues[31] conducted a larger, prospective, multicenter observational study in patients who received PPMs for bradycardia. A total of 725 patients were monitored for arterial embolic events (including stroke, transient ischemic attack, and peripheral arterial embolism) over a median follow-up of 22 months. An AHRE duration of more than 5 minutes was considered significant in this study. Using a Cox proportional hazard model, the association between two different AHRE durations (>5 minutes and 1 day) and thromboembolism was assessed. Although a higher incidence of arterial embolism was found in patients with an AHRE duration of more than 1 day ($P$ = .03), a similar increase was not found in patients with an AHRE duration of longer than 5 minutes. The exact AHRE duration associated with stroke risk could not be estimated from this study, because patients with AHRE duration ranging from 5 minutes to 24 hours were included in the same group, and these patients were not further stratified. Thus, the risk of thromboembolism and the need for anticoagulation in patients with an AHRE duration of more than 5 minutes remained unclear.

The TRENDS study was a prospective observational study conducted in ICD, CRT, or PPM recipients with a CHADS2 score of 1 or greater.[32] A total of 2486 patients with at least 30 days of device data were followed up for a mean of 1.4 years. An atrial rate of greater than 175 bpm lasting 20 seconds or longer was used to define an AHRE. AHRE burden, defined as the longest AHRE duration in a 30-day period, was divided into three subsets: zero, low (<5.5 hours), and high (≥5.5 hours). The annual risk of thromboembolism or transient ischemic events was significantly greater in the high-burden subset when compared with the zero/low-burden subsets

(2.4% vs 1.1%). After adjusting for stroke risk factors and antithrombotic treatment, the HR for thromboembolic events in the high-burden group compared with the zero-burden group did not reach statistical significance (HR, 2.20; CI, 0.96–3.8; $P$ = .06). A significant limitation of this study was the low event rate (1.3%) in the study population compared with the observed rate (4%) in patients with a similar CHADS2 score (ie, >2). This limitation precluded further stratification of the population into increasing AHRE burden levels. Although this study provided some indication suggesting an increased risk of thromboembolism in patients with a high AHRE burden, further clarification was required.

The Asymptomatic AF and Stroke Evaluation in Pacemaker Patients and the AF Reduction Atrial Pacing Trial (ASSERT) assessed dual-chamber PPM or ICD recipients with hypertension aged 65 years or older.[33] Unlike prior studies, patients with known atrial tachycardia (AT)/AF or on warfarin or other anticoagulant therapy were excluded. A total of 2580 patients from 136 centers were followed for approximately three years. In this study, AHRE was defined as an episode of device-detected atrial rate greater than 190 bpm, lasting longer than 6 minutes, which was found in a third of the population. The risk of ischemic stroke and systemic embolism was significantly higher in the AHRE group than the non-AHRE group (relative risk, 2.49; CI, 1.28–4.84; $P$ = .007).[34] This risk remained significantly higher in the AHRE group in subsequent analyses after excluding those with surface ECG-detected AF (thus isolating device-detected AF), controlling for stroke risk factors and limiting comparison with the high-risk group (ie, CHADS2 ≥2). Although this study did not substratify groups based on AHRE burden to define a specific AHRE threshold value that increases stroke risk, it removed confounding from other clinical factors and thus gave a better assessment of risk of ischemic stroke from device-detected AHRE.

## Unanswered Questions

Although device-detected AHRE implies AF/AFL and, potentially, increased risk of thromboembolism, many questions remain unanswered:

1. How should device-detected AF be defined? The definition of AHRE, which is a surrogate marker of paroxysmal AF, differs among different trials, and the best definition for this remains unclear. Atrial rate and duration are two parameters that characterize an AHRE. Initial studies indicate that a rate of greater than 250 bpm and a duration of more than

5 minutes correlates best with clinician confirmed AF. The ASSERT trial used a slightly lower rate (190 bpm) for AHRE, and it is possible that results of ASSERT would have differed had investigators used a different definition of AHRE. Requiring a longer duration of high atrial rate for cutoff, may lead to underestimating the AF burden, although the converse may lead to overestimation. Therefore, what is the optimal atrial rate and duration to define an AHRE?

2. What is the best atrial sensitivity setting to prevent undersensing or oversensing? The interplay between atrial sensitivity setting and atrial and far-field signal size measured by the device may lead to oversensing or undersensing of AHREs and can significantly change the recorded AHRE burden in a given patient. Sometimes, increasing atrial sensitivity (lower threshold value) can lead to a paradoxical undersensing of AF because of inappropriate atrial noise reversion.[35]

3. What is the critical AHRE burden that warrants therapeutic intervention? The threshold burden beyond which thromboembolic risk is increased remains undefined. Stroke risk is likely related to both, the longest duration of AHRE and total AHRE burden; these issues need further study.

4. Should patients with device-detected AHREs be routinely anticoagulated? Based on the result of the ASSERT trial, it seems appropriate to anticoagulate high-risk patients with significant AHREs (as defined by an atrial rate of >190 bpm and duration >6 minutes). Ghali and colleagues[36] have observed that clinicians initiate anticoagulation in device-detected AHRE if they had a prior history of AF or a significant burden. No studies have looked at outcomes after anticoagulation in device-detected AHRE.

5. Should device recipients be actively monitored for AHREs via continuous remote monitoring systems? The CONNECT (Clinical Evaluation of Remote Notification to Reduce Time to Clinical Decision) Trial showed that wireless remote monitoring with predefined automatic alerts significantly reduced the time to a clinical decision in response to the alert, compared with standard in-office follow-up.[37] Other studies of remote monitoring also show beneficial outcomes.[38,39] The IMPACT study is a randomized single-blinded control study that includes ICD and CRT-D device recipients.[40] It will compare the benefit of using BIOTRONIK home monitory technology to detect AF/AFL with a predefined anticoagulation plan compared with conventional device follow-up in the clinic and physician-initiated anticoagulation, as per the discretion of the treating physician. Similar to ASSERT, this study also excludes patients with known AF or those already on anticoagulation.

## SUMMARY

AF is an important risk factor for stroke and thromboembolism, and AF-related stroke has a high morbidity and mortality. Device-detected AHREs are usually tantamount to having clinical AF, but many exceptions exist. Although the risk of stroke with clinical AF is well known, the thromboembolic risk of device-detected AHREs is unclear because studies have used differing criteria of atrial rate and duration for defining AHREs. Recently, the ASSERT study showed an increased risk of stroke in patients with device-detected AHREs, even in the absence of a previous history of clinical AF. However, an accurate definition of what constitutes a significant device-detected AHREs, a threshold AHRE burden level that confers a stroke risk and thus the need for anticoagulation, and the ideal monitoring strategy, such as continuous remote monitoring versus periodic surveillance in the device clinic, are some areas that need further study.

## REFERENCES

1. Go AS, Hylek EM, Phillips KA, et al. Prevalence of diagnosed atrial fibrillation in adults: national implications for rhythm management and stroke prevention: the Anticoagulation and Risk Factors in Atrial Fibrillation (ATRIA) Study. JAMA 2001;285:2370–5.

2. Wolf PA, Abbott RD, Kannel WB. Atrial fibrillation as an independent risk factor for stroke: the Framingham Study. Stroke 1991;22:983–8.

3. Wolf PA, Dawber TR, Thomas HE Jr, et al. Epidemiologic assessment of chronic atrial fibrillation and risk of stroke: the Framingham study. Neurology 1978;28:973–7.

4. Hart RG, Pearce LA, Rothbart RM, et al. Stroke with intermittent atrial fibrillation: incidence and predictors during aspirin therapy. Stroke Prevention in Atrial Fibrillation Investigators. J Am Coll Cardiol 2000;35:183–7.

5. Chugh SS, Blackshear JL, Shen WK, et al. Epidemiology and natural history of atrial fibrillation: clinical implications. J Am Coll Cardiol 2001;37:371–8.

6. Harrison MJ, Marshall J. Atrial fibrillation, TIAs and completed strokes. Stroke 1984;15:441–2.

7. Anderson DC, Kappelle LJ, Eliasziw M, et al. Occurrence of hemispheric and retinal ischemia in atrial

fibrillation compared with carotid stenosis. Stroke 2002;33:1963–7.

8. Morley J, Marinchak R, Rials SJ, et al. Atrial fibrillation, anticoagulation, and stroke. Am J Cardiol 1996;77:38A–44A.

9. Beyth RJ, Antani MR, Covinsky KE, et al. Why isn't warfarin prescribed to patients with nonrheumatic atrial fibrillation? J Gen Intern Med 1996;11:721–8.

10. O'Hare JA, Ul-Iman N, Geoghegan M. Non-anticoagulation in atrial fibrillation. Ir J Med Sci 1994;163: 448–50.

11. Connolly SJ, Ezekowitz MD, Yusuf S, et al. Dabigatran versus warfarin in patients with atrial fibrillation. N Engl J Med 2009;361:1139–51.

12. Ehrens I, Lip GY, Peters K. What do the RE-LY, AVERROES and ROCKET-AF trials tell us for stroke prevention in atrial fibrillation. Thromb Haemost 2011;105:574–8.

13. Holmes DR, Reddy VY, Turi ZG, et al. Percutaneous closure of the left atrial appendage versus warfarin therapy for prevention of stroke in patients with atrial fibrillation: a randomized non-inferiority trial. Lancet 2009;374:534–42.

14. Gaillard N, Deltour S, Vilotijevic B, et al. Detection of paroxysmal atrial fibrillation with transtelephonic EKG in TIA or stroke patients. Neurology 2010;74: 1666–70.

15. Tayal AH, Tian M, Kelly KM, et al. Atrial fibrillation detected by mobile cardiac outpatient telemetry in cryptogenic TIA or stroke. Neurology 2008;71: 1696–701.

16. Hohnloser SH, Pajitnev D, Pogue J, et al. Incidence of stroke in paroxysmal versus sustained atrial fibrillation in patients taking oral anticoagulation or combined antiplatelet therapy: an ACTIVE W Substudy. J Am Coll Cardiol 2007;50:2156–61.

17. Friberg L, Hammar N, Rosenqvist M. Stroke in paroxysmal atrial fibrillation: report from the Stockholm Cohort of Atrial Fibrillation. Eur Heart J 2010; 31:967–75.

18. Schuchert A, Lepage S, Ostrander JJ, et al. Automatic analysis of pacemaker diagnostic data in the identification of atrial tachyarrhythmias in patients with no prior history of them. Europace 2005;7:242–7.

19. Pollak WM, Simmons JD, Interian A Jr, et al. Clinical utility of intraatrial pacemaker stored electrograms to diagnose atrial fibrillation and flutter. Pacing Clin Electrophysiol 2001;24:424–9.

20. Defaye P, Dournaux F, Mouton E. Prevalence of supraventricular arrhythmias from the automated analysis of data stored in the DDD pacemakers of 617 patients: the AIDA study. The AIDA Multicenter Study Group. Automatic Interpretation for Diagnosis Assistance. Pacing Clin Electrophysiol 1998;21:250–5.

21. Gillis AM, Morck M. Atrial fibrillation after DDDR pacemaker implantation. J Cardiovasc Electrophysiol 2002;13:542–7.

22. Cheung JW, Keating RJ, Stein KM, et al. Newly detected atrial fibrillation following dual chamber pacemaker implantation. J Cardiovasc Electrophysiol 2006;17:1323–8.

23. Borleffs CJ, Ypenburg C, van Bommel RJ, et al. Clinical importance of new-onset atrial fibrillation after cardiac resynchronization therapy. Heart Rhythm 2009;6:305–10.

24. Leclercq C, Padeletti L, Cihák R, et al. Incidence of paroxysmal atrial tachycardias in patients treated with cardiac resynchronization therapy and continuously monitored by device diagnostics. Europace 2010;12:71–7.

25. Orlov MV, Ghali JK, Araghi-Niknam M, et al. Asymptomatic atrial fibrillation in pacemaker recipients: incidence, progression, and determinants based on the atrial high rate trial. Pacing Clin Electrophysiol 2007;30:404–11.

26. Sweeney MO, Hellkamp AS, Ellenbogen KA, et al. Adverse effect of ventricular pacing on heart failure and atrial fibrillation among patients with normal baseline QRS duration in a clinical trial of pacemaker therapy for sinus node dysfunction. Circulation 2003;107:2932–7.

27. Mittal S, Stein K, Gilliam FR III, et al. Frequency, duration, and predictors of newly-diagnosed atrial fibrillation following dual-chamber pacemaker implantation in patients without a previous history of atrial fibrillation. Am J Cardiol 2008;102:450–3.

28. Glotzer TV, Hellkamp AS, Zimmerman J, et al. Atrial high rate episodes detected by pacemaker diagnostics predict death and stroke: report of the Atrial Diagnostics Ancillary Study of the MOde Selection Trial (MOST). Circulation 2003;107:1614–9.

29. Seidl K, Meisel E, VanAgt E, et al. Is the atrial high rate episode diagnostic feature reliable in detecting paroxysmal episodes of atrial tachyarrhythmias? Pacing Clin Electrophysiol 1998;21:694–700.

30. Kohno R, Abe H, Oginosawa Y, et al. Reliability and characteristics of atrial tachyarrhythmias detection in dual chamber pacemakers. Circ J 2011;75(5): 1090–7.

31. Capucci A, Santini M, Padeletti L, et al. Monitored atrial fibrillation duration predicts arterial embolic events in patients suffering from bradycardia and atrial fibrillation implanted with antitachycardia pacemakers. J Am Coll Cardiol 2005;46:1913–20.

32. Glotzer TV, Daoud EG, Wyse DG, et al. The relationship between daily atrial tachyarrhythmia burden from implantable device diagnostics and stroke risk: the TRENDS study. Circ Arrhythm Electrophysiol 2009;2:474–80.

33. Hohnloser SH, Capucci A, Fain E, et al. Asymptomatic atrial fibrillation and stroke evaluation in pacemaker patients and the atrial fibrillation reduction atrial pacing trial (ASSERT). Am Heart J 2006;152: 442–7.

34. ASSERT: Device-detected atrial tachyarrhythmias are common, raise stroke risk. Available at: http://www.theheart.org/article/1153461.do. Accessed March 24, 2011.

35. Kolb C, Halbfass P, Zrenner B, et al. Paradoxical atrial undersensing due to inappropriate atrial noise reversion of atrial fibrillation in dual-chamber pacemakers. J Cardiovasc Electrophysiol 2005;16:696–700.

36. Ghali JK, Orlov MV, Araghi-Niknam M, et al. The influence of symptoms and device detected atrial tachyarrhythmias on medical management: insights from A-HIRATE. Pacing Clin Electrophysiol 2007;30:850–7.

37. Crossley GH, Boyle A, Vitense H, et al. The CONNECT (Clinical Evaluation of Remote Notification to Reduce Time to Clinical Decision) Trial: the value of wireless remote monitoring with automatic clinician alerts. J Am Coll Cardiol 2011;57:1181–9.

38. Varma N, Epstein AE, Irimpen A, et al, for the TRUST Investigators. Efficacy and safety of automatic remote monitoring for implantable cardioverter-defibrillator follow-up: the Lumos-T Safety Reduces Routine Office Device Follow-Up (TRUST) trial. Circulation 2010;122:325–32.

39. Crossley GH, Chen J, Choucair W, et al. Clinical benefits of remote versus transtelephonic monitoring of implanted pacemakers. J Am Coll Cardiol 2009; 54:2012–9.

40. Ip J, Waldo AL, Lip GY, et al. Multicenter randomized study of anticoagulation guided by remote rhythm monitoring in patients with implantable cardioverter-defibrillator and CRT-D devices: rationale, design, and clinical characteristics of the initially enrolled cohort the IMPACT study. Am Heart J 2009;158: 364–70.

# Anticoagulation Therapy for Atrial Fibrillation in Patients with Implanted Cardiac Arrhythmia Devices

John H. Ip, MD[a],*, Jonathan L. Halperin, MD[b]

## KEYWORDS

- Atrial fibrillation • Implantable cardioverter–defibrillator
- Cardiac resynchronization device • Remote monitoring
- Oral anticoagulation

Atrial fibrillation (AF) is the most common arrhythmia requiring medical treatment, with the lifetime risk of developing AF approximately 25% in the general population.[1] Atrial fibrillation and atrial flutter (AFl) are common cardiac arrhythmias associated with an increased incidence of stroke in patients with additional risk factors. About 1 in 6 strokes is attributable to AF, and this fraction increases with age such that AF is the likely cause of over 25% of strokes in patients over 70 years old. Although oral anticoagulation (OAC) therapy reduces the risk of stroke, OAC therapy is usually initiated after AF is documented on an electrocardiogram (ECG) or after an ischemic event occurs.

## THE INTERACTION BETWEEN HEART FAILURE AND AF

Heart failure (HF) afflicts approximately 5 million Americans and ranks among the most important factors contributing to morbidity and mortality. HF and AF are inextricably linked in that patients with either disorder are at substantially increased risk of developing the other. Furthermore, the combination of the two carries a substantially poorer prognosis than either alone.[2] In the Framingham Heart Study, HF increased the risk of AF 4.5-fold in men and 5.9-fold in women.[3,4] The Euro Heart survey, conducted in 24 European countries in 2000 and 2001, found that approximately 45% of patients with HF presented with AF.[3] The prevalence of AF ranges from 10% to 20% in patients with mild HF and up to 50% in patients with more severe HF. The Atrial Fibrillation Investigators reported an annual risk of stroke of 1.03% per year in patients with AF who had no underlying cardiovascular disease, but the risk increased to 3.6% per year in the presence of HF.[5] In the stroke prevention in atrial fibrillation-I trial, clinical HF within 3 months was associated with a 2.5-fold greater risk of stroke among in patients with nonvalvular AF.[6]

Disclosures: The authors receive consulting fees from Biotronik, Incorporated as cochairmen of the Steering Committee for the impact of biotronik home monitoring guided anticoagulation on stroke risk in patients with implanted defibrillator clinical trial.

a Ingham Regional Medical Center, Michigan State University, Lansing, MI, USA
b The Cardiovascular Institute, Mount Sinai School of Medicine, Mount Sinai Medical Center, One Gustave L. Levy Place, New York, NY 10029, USA
* Corresponding author. Thoracic & Cardiovascular Healthcare Foundation, Suite 425, 405 West Greenlawn, Lansing, MI 48910.
E-mail address: jip@tciheart.com

Card Electrophysiol Clin 3 (2011) 631–639
doi:10.1016/j.ccep.2011.08.006
1877-9182/11/$ – see front matter © 2011 Published by Elsevier Inc.

## STROKE RISK STRATIFICATION IN PATIENTS WITH AF

In addition to HF, several other risk factors increase the risk of stroke in patients with AF. These include advanced age, diabetes mellitus, hypertension and, most importantly, previous thromboembolism (ischemic stroke or transient ischemic attack [TIA]). The most widely adopted risk stratification scheme is the CHADS$_2$ score (**Table 1**), which provides a practical method for estimation of risk of stroke in patients with non-valvular AF based on these risk factors to guide selection of patients for OAC therapy (**Table 2**).[7] Other stroke risk stratification systems, most notably the CHA$_2$DS$_2$VASc score, incorporate such additional variables as gender and various manifestations of atherosclerotic vascular disease to enhance discrimination of patients at higher or lower risk when classified as at intermediate risk according to the CHADS$_2$ schema.

## ORAL ANTICOAGULATION TO PREVENT STROKE IN PATIENTS WITH AF

The efficacy of OAC therapy to reduce the risk of stroke in patients with AF is well established on the basis of multiple randomized trials.[5,6,8] Multiple clinical practice guidelines[8] recommend anticoagulation for patients with AF at risk, and a vitamin K antagonist (VKA) such as warfarin is the conventional approach.[9] Available VKA agents are highly effective for prevention of ischemic events, but their narrow therapeutic index and numerous drug and food interactions require routine monitoring and frequent dose adjustment to maintain anticoagulation intensity, making sustained therapy challenging for many patients and resulting in a search for alternative agents that are equally effective but more convenient to administer over time.[10]

Based on the results of the large randomized evaluation of long term anticoagulant therapy

**Table 2**
**Annual risk of stroke based on CHADS$_2$ score**

| CHADS$_2$ Score | Risk of Stroke (% per year) |
| --- | --- |
| 0 | 1.9 |
| 1 | 2.8 |
| 2 | 4.0 |
| 3 | 5.9 |
| 4 | 8.5 |
| 5 | 12.5 |
| 6 | 18.2 |

trial,[11] the oral direct thrombin inhibitor dabigatran etexilate was approved by the US Food and Drug Administration (FDA) in 2010 for prevention of stroke in patients with nonvalvular AF. In this trial, 18,113 patients with AF and at least 1 additional stroke risk factor were randomly assigned to receive 1 of 2 doses of dabigatran etexilate (110 mg or 150 mg twice daily) in a blinded fashion or warfarin (dose-adjusted to target international normalized ratio [INR] 2.0–3.0) in an unblinded fashion. The primary efficacy outcome was all stroke or systemic embolism. Dabigatran etexilate, 110 mg twice daily, was associated with a primary event rate similar to that with warfarin, while the rate of major hemorrhage was lower with dabigatran. Compared with warfarin, dabigatran etexilate 150 mg twice daily was associated with a lower rate of stroke and systemic embolism but a similar rate of major bleeding. Importantly, rates of hemorrhagic stroke, the most feared complication of OAC therapy, were substantially lower with either fixed dose of dabigatran than with warfarin. Three additional new fixed-dose OAC agents, rivaroxaban, apixaban, and edoxaban, are in late stages of clinical development for prevention of stroke in patients with AF and are expected to face regulatory review within the next year or two.[11–14]

## ASYMPTOMATIC AF AND THE RISK OF STROKE

A major limitation of the current approach to stroke prevention in patients with AF is that episodes of paroxysmal AF are often asymptomatic. Among patients with AF-related stroke in the Framingham Heart Study, the arrhythmia was newly diagnosed in 24%. In a study of patients taking antiarrhythmic drug therapy, biweekly monitoring by even limited 30-second electrocardiogram (ECG) recordings revealed asymptomatic episodes of AF in nearly 20%,[15] and the actual incidence is undoubtedly higher. Even patients with symptomatic episodes

**Table 1**
**CHADS$_2$ risk score assessment**

| Risk Factor | Number of Points Assigned |
| --- | --- |
| C—congestive heart failure | 1 |
| H—hypertension | 1 |
| A—age 75 or older | 1 |
| D—diabetes mellitus | 1 |
| S—previous stroke or transient ischemic attack | 2 |

of AF typically have additional episodes that are asymptomatic.[16,17] When adjusted for clinical risk factors, patients with paroxysmal AF face a risk of stroke comparable to those with persistent AF.[18] Yet it is inherently difficult to detect, characterize, and quantify asymptomatic paroxysmal AF.

## AF DETECTION BY IMPLANTED ARRHYTHMIA DEVICES

Implanted cardiac pacemakers[19] and defibrillators[20] have been developed with AF/AFI detection algorithms that improve the likelihood of detecting AF/AFI compared with intermittent, office-based ECG recordings. Technological advances in the design of implanted dual-chamber cardioverter–defibrillators (ICDs) and cardiac resynchronization-defibrillators (CRT-Ds) allow immediate detection and verification of AF/AFI by automatic transmission of intracardiac electrograms (IEGM) to the clinician.[21] Advances in implanted dual-chamber cardiac device technology provide a method for more comprehensive detection of asymptomatic paroxysmal AF[16,17] and could facilitate earlier prophylactic OAC treatment compared with conventional periodic office-based evaluation. Many device-detected episodes of atrial high-rate activity (ARHE) are of short duration, lasting just a few seconds or minutes. These dual-chamber pacemaker, ICD and CRT-D devices provide real-time remote monitoring of the IEGM,[21] making it possible to detect virtually every AHRE and to accurately measure the burden of AF (proportion of time AF is present). Several groups have characterized the incidence and burden of symptomatic and asymptomatic AF in patients with implanted pacemakers.[22,23] While prolonged, symptomatic episodes of AF (lasting several days) carry a substantial risk of stroke, the clinical significance of more abbreviated episodes has not been fully established. Furthermore, the ability to detect episodes of asymptomatic AF by dual-chamber ICD or CRT-D devices begs the question of whether therapeutic action based on AHRE information might reduce the risk of stroke. Although ongoing trials may verify that remote monitoring is a superior strategy for diagnosis of AF/AFI to guide thromboembolism prophylaxis, available data are insufficient to form the basis for recommendations to guide antithrombotic therapy in patients with implanted arrhythmia devices. In short, it is not yet clear whether initiation of OAC therapy based on remote rhythm monitoring can reduce the risk of stroke.

## DEVICE-DETECTED ATRIAL TACHYARRHYTHMIA AND STROKE RISK

The Mode Selection Trial (MOST) was the first prospective study to show a relationship between device-detected AHRE and stroke risk. This 6-year randomized, multicenter trial compared ventricular rate-responsive (VVIR) pacing with dual-chamber rate-responsive (DDDR) pacing in patients with bradycardia.[24] A secondary analysis of data from 312 patients found that more than half (51.3%) had at least 1 AHRE (atrial rate >220 beats per minute for 10 consecutive beats) of at least 5 minutes duration over a median follow-up of 27 months. Death or nonfatal stroke occurred in 20.6% of patients with AHRE compared with 10.5% of those without AHRE. By multivariate analysis, the presence of any AHRE was an independent predictor of both mortality and stroke (hazard ratio, 2.79, $P = .0011$). The analysis was limited by small sample size and the fact that the majority of patients had symptomatic supraventricular tachyarrhythmias before enrollment.

The more recent TRENDS study provides additional information about the relationship between device-based ARHE burden and stroke risk.[25] This observational study enrolled 3045 patients with at least 1 stroke risk factor and a dual-chamber pacemaker or ICD. The devices recorded the onset and duration of each AHRE episode; AHRE burden was defined as the longest AHRE on any day during a 30-day period. The mean baseline $CHADS_2$ score was 2.2 plus or minus 1.2; 20% of patients were taking OAC therapy at enrollment. Patents were divided into subgroups with zero, low (<5.5 h/d), and high ($\geq$5.5 h/d) AHRE burden. During a mean follow-up of 1.4 years, the annualized risk of thromboembolism in 2486 patients with at least 30 consecutive days of device-based rhythm data was 1.1% for those with zero, 1.1% with low, and 2.4% with high AHRE burdens. By multivariate analysis compared with the zero burden subgroup, the adjusted hazard ratios for thromboembolism in the low and high burden groups were 0.98 ($P = .97$) and 2.20 ($P = .06$), respectively.

The Asymptomatic AF and Stroke Evaluation in Pacemaker Patients and the AF Reduction Atrial Pacing Trial (ASSERT) is seeking additional information about the risk of stroke in patients with device-detected AHRE.[26] This trial enrolled patients over 65 years of age with a history of hypertension and dual-chamber pacemaker or ICD for standard indications. Those with a history of AF or receiving OAC therapy were excluded. The investigators enrolled 2582 patients with a mean $CHADS_2$ score of 2.4 and followed them for a mean of 2.8 years, during which time 7.5% of patients initiated OAC therapy. AHRE as defined on the basis of atrial rate greater than 190 beats per minute and duration greater than 6 minutes. By 3 months after enrollment, 10% of patients displayed at least 1 AHRE, and this increased to 36% by the end of follow-up. The presence of at least 1 AHRE in the first 3 months was associated with a 2.5-fold greater risk of subsequent stroke or systemic embolism. Among patients with a $CHADS_2$ score greater than 2 at entry, the risk of thromboembolism in those without AHRE in the first 3 months was 0.7% per year, compared with 2.1% per year for those developing AHRE (relative risk, 2.7, $P<.001$).

## REMOTE ATRIAL RHYTHM MONITORING TO GUIDE THERAPY

The IMPACT trial is an international, multicenter, single-blind, parallel-group randomized investigation of remote monitoring coupled with a predefined OAC plan for patients with implanted dual-chamber ICD or CRT devices.[26] Enrolled subjects are randomly assigned to either the specified intervention algorithm (group 1) or conventional management (group 2) in a 1:1 ratio (**Fig. 1**). Patients in both arms have active monitoring of IEGM data, but AHRE data are made available to treating physicians only for patients in group 1. Patients in group 2 undergo routine device interrogation and physician-directed OAC therapy according to current practice guidelines.[27,28] Patients in both arms undergo device evaluations no less often than every 6 months (±30 days) (see **Fig. 1**), and more frequently as the need arises based on recommendations for management of patients with implanted cardiac arrhythmia devices.[29,30]

Enrolled patients must have a $CHADS_2$ score of at least 1 and implanted Biotronik Lumax HF-T or DR-T device (Biotronik, Incorported, Lake Oswego, Oregon). For those with previously implanted devices, a mean IEGM P-wave amplitude of at least 1.0 mV in sinus rhythm is required. Patients must be eligible to receive OAC therapy if an indication should arise during follow-up, but no prior indication for sustained OAC therapy. Among the exclusion criteria are permanent AF, a history of stroke, TIA or systemic embolism associated and prior AF or AFl, long QT or Brugada syndrome as the sole indication for device implantation, life expectancy less than the anticipated duration of the study, or successful AF ablation with restoration of sinus rhythm within 3 months of entry. The complete rationale, inclusion and exclusion criteria and trial design have been published.[29]

Patients in group 1 are prescribed OAC therapy based on a predefined device-guided protocol (**Fig. 2** and **Table 3**). If the duration of AHRE in a 48-hour period meets the specified criteria, OAC therapy is initiated. The threshold of AHRE warranting initiation of OAC is based on the patient's $CHADS_2$ risk score (**Table 4**); higher stroke risk requires a lower AHRE burden to initiate OAC. The OAC is withdrawn based on freedom from AHRE; termination of therapy requires 30 consecutive days without AHRE in patients with $CHADS_2$ scores 1 or 2 and 90 days without AHRE in patients with $CHADS_2$ scores of 3 or 4. After stopping OAC therapy, detection of recurrent AHRE prompts reinstatement of OAC (**Table 5**), and treatment is stopped again if the criteria for freedom from AHRE are met, as indicated in **Table 6**. For patients with prior ischemic stroke, TIA or systemic embolism, once started because of device-detected AHRE anticoagulation, is

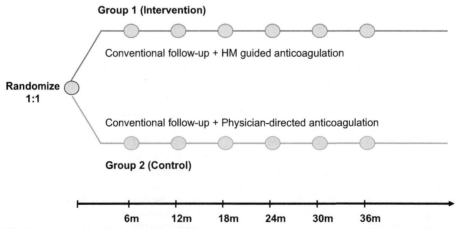

**Fig. 1.** Schedule of patient randomization and follow-up.

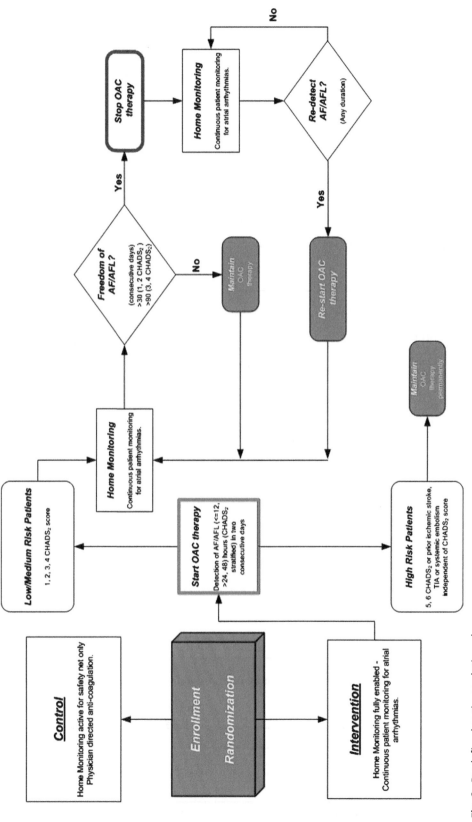

**Fig. 2.** Predefined anticoagulation plan.

**Table 3**
**IMPACT trial: rhythm-guided initiation of anticoagulation in patients with implanted arrhythmia devices**

| CHADS$_2$ Score | AF/AFL Duration to Start Anticoagulation (hours) | Period Free from AF/AFL to Stop Anticoagulation (days) |
|---|---|---|
| 1–2 | 48 | 30 |
| 3–4 | 24 | 60 |
| 5–6 or prior stroke | ≤12 | Maintain anticoagulation |

*Abbreviation:* AF/AFL, Atrial fibrillation/atrial flutter.

**Table 4**
**Duration of atrial fibrillation/atrial flutter to start oral anticoagulation therapy**

| CHADS$_2$ Score | AF/AFL Duration (Over Consecutive 48 h) to Start Anticoagulation |
|---|---|
| 1–2 | 48 h |
| 3–4 | 24 h |
| 5–6 or prior ischemic stroke, TIA or systemic embolism independent of CHADS$_2$ score | ≤12 h |

*Abbreviation:* AF/AFL, Atrial fibrillation/atrial flutter.

**Table 5**
**Duration of atrial fibrillation/atrial flutter to restart oral anticoagulation therapy**

| CHADS$_2$ Score | AF/AFL Duration to Restart Anticoagulation |
|---|---|
| 1–2 | Any |
| 3–4 | Any |
| 5–6 or prior ischemic stroke, transient ischemic attack or systemic embolism independent of CHADS$_2$ score | N/A |

*Abbreviations:* AF/AFL, atrial fibrillation/atrial flutter; NA, not applicable.

**Table 6**
**Duration of freedom from atrial fibrillation/atrial flutter to stop oral anticoagulation therapy**

| CHADS$_2$ Score | Consecutive Days Free from AF/AFL to Stop Anticoagulation |
|---|---|
| 1–2 | 30 |
| 3–4 | 90 |
| 5–6 or prior ischemic stroke, transient ischemic attack or systemic embolism independent of CHADS$_2$ score | Maintain oral anticoagulation |

*Abbreviation:* AF/AFL, Atrial fibrillation/atrial flutter.

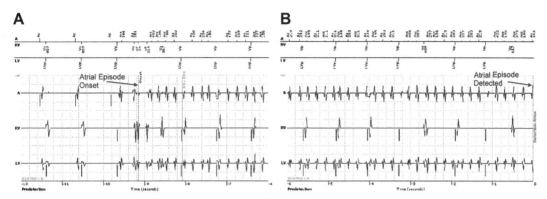

**Fig. 3.** Long atrial episode intracardiac electrogram. (*A*) Onset of atrial episode. (*B*) Atrial episode detected by the device.

continued whether or not atrial tachyarrhythmias continue to occur, because these patients represent a secondary prevention population at high risk of recurrent stroke related to AF. Randomization is stratified by CHADS$_2$ score and device type (ICD or CRT) to ensure balanced distribution of higher and lower risk patients in each arm.

Consistent with recent guideline updates, anticoagulation may be achieved either with a VKA, including warfarin (Coumadin) or phenprocoumon (Markumar) or with dabigatran etexilate (Pradaxa) in conventional doses.[6] For subjects receiving VKA therapy, the intensity of anticoagulation is monitored at least weekly until stable in the therapeutic range (INR 2.0–3.0, target 2.5) and monthly thereafter for the duration of therapy. As they gain regulatory approval for clinical use in this indication, additional novel OAC agents may be acceptable alternatives.

When the intrinsic atrial rate exceeds the preprogrammed device detection rate (eg, 200 beats per minute) for 36 of 48 consecutive heart cycles, the atrial episode IEGM is automatically stored in the implanted device (**Fig. 3**), sent to the physician only for patients assigned to group 1, and sent to a central data repository for all patients in both treatment groups. Information about a device-detected AHRE is transmitted over a wireless connection between the implanted device and a rechargeable external device (**Fig. 4**), which then relays the information to a central monitoring facility using either a built-in cellular telephone module or a wired telephone line using a modem in the base of the unit. Data are transferred to an Internet server that transmits the information to the physician through a secure Web site. Communication from the implanted device to the clinician's email system typically takes less than 5 minutes. Energy consumption for this function during the life of the device is equivalent to that required for delivery of a single 30 J defibrillator shock. The device-based monitoring technology can transmit data every 24 hours at a programmed time or automatically after termination of an AHRE. Both periodic and event-triggered messages follow a schedule of repeated communication

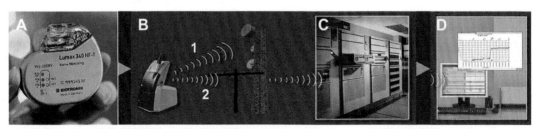

**Fig. 4.** Home monitoring transmission path. (*A, B*) Radiofrequency data transmission (402–405 MHz) from the implantable device to Cardio Messenger II (Lake Oswego, OR, USA). (*B, C*) Transmission from Cardio Messenger II to the Web server; path 1 is wireless (through a GSM cell phone module), and path 2 is a landline with a modem in the charging base. (*C, D*) Transmission from Web server to the physician through a secure Web site. (*Courtesy of* BIOTRONIK, Incorporated, Lake Oswego, OR, USA; with permission.)

attempts. If communication fails, up to 3 additional attempts are made at 60-minute intervals.

The primary outcome measure is the composite rate of stroke, systemic embolism and major bleeding events. The estimated sample size is 2718 patients, based on an estimated primary event rate of 2.8% per year in the group assigned to conventional anticoagulation management and analysis to assess for superiority of the device-guided treatment strategy according to intention to treat.[24]

Early detection and verification of paroxysmal AF may have important implications for prevention of thromboembolism in patients at risk. Initiation, interruption, and restarting of OAC therapy based on a predefined atrial rhythm-guided strategy in conjunction with standard stroke risk stratification could lead to better clinical outcomes compared with conventional clinical care. The IMPACT trial is based on the premise that reducing the risks of both thromboembolism associated with episodes of paroxysmal AF and bleeding during chronic OAC therapy in the absence of AF can improve patient outcomes. Verification of this hypothesis would change the way patients with implanted arrhythmia devices are managed. The results of this study will also determine the clinical utility of remote cardiac rhythm surveillance and define the critical threshold of AHRE burden warranting OAC or antiarrhythmic drug therapy in patients at risk of stroke. Moreover, the findings will help establish whether stroke in patients with AF is directly related to the arrhythmia itself or to other factors that place such patients at ongoing risk.

# REFERENCES

1. Lloyd-Jones DM, Wang TJ, Leip EP, et al. Lifetime risk for development of atrial fibrillation: the Framingham Heart Study. Circulation 2004;110:1042–6.

2. Jessup M, Bronzena S. Heart failure. N Engl J Med 2003;348:2007–18.

3. Benjamin EJ, Levy D, Vaziri SM, et al. Independent risk factors for atrial fibrillation in a population based cohort: the Framingham Heart Study. JAMA 1994; 271:840–4.

4. Cleland JG, Swedberg K, Follath F, et al. The Euro Heart Failure survey programme—a survey on the quality of care among patients with heart failure in Europe. Part 1: patient characteristics and diagnostics. Eur Heart J 2003;24:442–63.

5. Atrial Fibrillation Investigators. Risk factors for stroke and efficacy of antithrombotic therapy in atrial fibrillation. Analysis of pooled data from 5 randomized controlled trials. Arch Intern Med 1994;154:1449–57.

6. SPAF III Writing Committee for the Stroke Prevention in Atrial Fibrillation. Stroke prevention atrial fibrillation III study. JAMA 1998;279:1273–7.

7. Gage BF, van Walraven C, Pearce L, et al. Selecting patients with atrial fibrillation for anticoagulation: stroke risk stratification in patients taking aspirin. Circulation 2004;110:2287–92.

8. Estes NAM III, Halperin JL, Calkins H, et al. ACC/AHA/Physician Consortium 2008 clinical performance measures for adults with nonvalvular atrial fibrillation or atrial flutter: a report of the American College of Cardiology/American Heart Association Task Force on Performance Measures and the Physician Consortium for Performance Improvement (Writing Committee to Develop Clinical Performance Measures for Atrial Fibrillation): developed in collaboration with the Heart Rhythm Society. Circulation 2008;117:1101–20.

9. Albers GW, Dalen JE, Laupacis A, et al. Antithrombotic therapy in atrial fibrillation. Chest 2001;119: 194S–65.

10. Garcia D, Libby E, Crowther MA. The new oral anticoagulants. Blood 2010;115:15–20.

11. Connolly SJ, Ezekowitz MD, Yusuf S, et al. Dabigatran versus Warfarin in patients with atrial fibrillation. N Engl J Med 2009;361:1139–51.

12. ROCKET study investigators. Rivaroxaban-once daily, oral, direct factor Xa inhibition compared with vitamin K antagonism for prevention of stroke and Embolism Trial in Atrial Fibrillation: rationale and design of the ROCKET AF study. Am Heart J 2010; 159:340–7.

13. Lopes RD, Alexander JH, Al-Khatib SM, et al. Apixaban for reduction in stroke and other thromboembolic events in atrial fibrillation (ARISTOTLE) trial: design and rationale. Am Heart J 2010;159:331–9.

14. Ruff CT, Giugliano RP, Elliott M, et al. Evaluation of the novel factor Xa inhibitor edoxaban compared with warfarin in patients with atrial fibrillation: design and rationale for the effective anticoagulation with factor Xa next generation in Atrial Fibrillation–Thrombolysis In Myocardial Infarction study 48 (ENGAGE AF–TIMI 48). Am Heart J 2010;160:635–41.

15. Page RL, Wilkinson WE, Claire WK. Asymptomatic arrhythmias in patients with symptomatic paroxysmal atrial fibrillation. Circulation 1994;89:224–7.

16. Patten M, Maas R, Karim A, et al. Event-recorder monitoring in the diagnosis of atrial fibrillation in symptomatic patients: subanalysis of the SOPAT trial. J Cardiovasc Electrophysiol 2006;17: 1216–20.

17. Strickberger SA, Ip J, Saksena S, et al. Relationship between atrial tachyarrhythmias and symptoms. Heart Rhythm 2005;2:125–31.

18. Spaf I writing committee for the stroke prevention in atrial fibrillation. Stroke prevention in atrial fibrillation study. Circulation 1991;84:933–5.

19. Israel CW, Grönefeld G, Ehrlich JR, et al. Long-term risk of recurrent atrial fibrillation as documented by an implantable monitoring device: implications for optimal patient care. J Am Coll Cardiol 2004;43: 47–52.

20. Schwartzman D, Gold M, Quesada A, et al. Serial evaluation of atrial tachyarrhythmia burden and frequency after implantation of a dual-chamber cardioverter-defibrillator. J Cardiovasc Electrophysiol 2005;16:708–13.

21. Varma N, Epstein AE, Irimpen A, et al. Efficacy and safety of automatic remote monitoring for implantable cardioverter-defibrillator follow-up: the Lumos-T Safely Reduces Routine Office Device Follow-up (TRUST) trial. Circulation 2010;122:325–32.

22. Gillis AM, Morck M. Atrial fibrillation after DDDR pacemaker implantation. J Cardiovasc Electrophysiol 2002;13:542–7.

23. Carlson MD, Ip JH, Messenger J, et al. A new pacemaker algorithm for the treatment of atrial fibrillation. J Am Coll Cardiol 2003;42:627–33.

24. Glotzer TV, Hellkamp AS, Zimmerman J, et al. Atrial high rate episodes detected by pacemaker diagnostics predicts death and stroke: report of the atrial diagnostic ancillary study of the Mode Selection Trial (MOST). Circulation 2003;107:1614–9.

25. Glotzer TV, Daoud EG, Wyse DG, et al. The relationship between daily atrial tachyarrhythmia burden from implantable device diagnostics and stroke risk: the TRENDS study. Circ Arrhythm Electrophysiol 2009;2:474–80.

26. Healy JS, Connolly SJ, Gold MR, et al. The relationship between atrial high-rate episodes and stroke: the Asymptomatic Stroke and Atrial Fibrillation Evaluation in Pacemaker Patients (ASSERT) Trial. Am Heart Association; 2010. Scientific Sessions: abstract 21838.

27. Wann LS, Curtis AB, January CT, et al, writing on behalf of the 2006 ACC/AHA/ESC Guidelines for the Management of Patients With Atrial Fibrillation Writing Committee. 2011 ACCF/AHA/HRS focused update on the management of patients with atrial fibrillation (updating the 2006 guideline): a report of the American College of Cardiology Foundation/ American Heart Association Task Force on Practice Guidelines. Circulation 2011;123:104–23.

28. Wann LS, Curtis AB, Ellenbogen KA, et al, writing on behalf of the 2006 ACC/AHA/ESC Guidelines for the Management of Patients With Atrial Fibrillation Writing Committee. 2011 ACCF/AHA/HRS focused update on the management of patients with atrial fibrillation (update on dabigatran): a report of the American College of Cardiology Foundation/American Heart Association Task Force on Practice Guidelines. J Am Coll Cardiol 2011;57:1330–7.

29. Wilkoff BL, Auricchio A, Brugada J, et al. HRS/EHRA expert consensus on the monitoring of cardiovascular implantable electronic devices (CIEDs): description of techniques, indications, personnel, frequency and ethical considerations. Heart Rhythm 2008;5:907–25.

30. Ip J, Waldo AL, Lip GYH, et al. Multicenter randomized study of anticoagulation guided by remote rhythm monitoring in patients with implantable cardioverter-defibrillator and CRT-D devices: rationale, design, and clinical characteristics of the initially enrolled cohort: the IMPACT study. Am Heart J 2009;158:364–70.

# Implantable Cardioverter-Defibrillators in End-Stage Renal Disease

Mehul B. Patel, MD[a], Swapnil Hiremath, MD, MPH[b],
Tahmeed Contractor, MD[c], Ranjan K. Thakur, MD, MPH, MBA, FHRS[c],*

**KEYWORDS**
- Implantable cardioverter-defibrillator
- End-stage renal disease • Sudden cardiac death
- Randomized controlled trials

The kidney is a multifunctional organ orchestrating numerous hemodynamic and regulatory functions, which are inextricably linked to the cardiovascular system. The incidence of chronic kidney disease (CKD) is rising, and it is estimated that more than 500,000 patients with end-stage renal disease (ESRD) may be dialysis dependent by the year 2020.[1] Patients with ESRD encounter exceptionally high cardiovascular morbidity and mortality, and despite significant advances in pharmacotherapy, dialysis, and other interventions, their 5-year survival rate has improved only marginally from 30% to 33% over the last decade.[1]

The mechanisms of increased cardiovascular mortality in patients with CKD are multifactorial. CKD accelerates the progression of hypertension and diabetes, and aggravates vasculopathy by increasing the obstructive atherosclerotic burden.[1–3] CKD per se is a powerful predictor of cardiovascular death, independent of hypertension, diabetes, ischemic cardiomyopathy, and heart failure.[4] Cardiovascular disease accounts for 41% of all-cause mortality in ESRD patients, with sudden cardiac death (SCD) accounting for two-thirds of this.[1]

Although implantable cardioverter-defibrillators (ICDs) prevent SCD, little is known about their efficacy in ESRD patients because these patients have been selectively excluded from major randomized clinical trials (RCTs) such as MADIT, MADIT-II, and SCDHeFT.[5–7] A post hoc analysis of the MADIT-II trial suggested a significant association between isolated elevated blood urea nitrogen (BUN) and increased mortality in both ICD and control groups.[8] Subsequent analysis showed that the group with BUN of 26 mg/dL to 50 mg/dL had a hazard ratio of 1.56, and the group with BUN greater than 50 mg/dL and creatinine level greater than 2.5 mg/dL derived no benefit from ICD implantation.[9]

These reports suggest that perhaps patients with ESRD may not benefit from primary prevention ICDs. This view can be rationalized based on the fact that patients with renal disease have high mortality rates attributable to SCD as well as competing causes such as sepsis, heart failure, and so forth, and an ICD would not affect mortality from competing causes. Indeed, many small, single-center, uncontrolled, retrospective analyses that have compared ICD efficacy in CKD/ESRD patients with patients with normal renal

---

[a] Department of Clinical Cardiac Electrophysiology, The Bay Pines Veterans Affairs Health Care System, University of South Florida, Tampa, 10000 Bay Pines Boulevard, Bay Pines, FL 33744, USA
[b] Division of Nephrology, The Ottawa Hospital, Riverside Campus, Ottawa, ON K1H 7W9, Canada
[c] Department of Clinical Cardiac Electrophysiology, Thoracic and Cardiovascular Institute, Sparrow Health System, Michigan State University, 405 West Greenlawn, Suite 400, Lansing, MI 48910, USA
* Corresponding author.
*E-mail address:* thakur@msu.edu

Card Electrophysiol Clin 3 (2011) 641–650
doi:10.1016/j.ccep.2011.08.007
1877-9182/11/$ – see front matter © 2011 Elsevier Inc. All rights reserved.

function suggest that ICDs do not appear to prolong life in renal disease patients as much as they do in the population without significant renal disease. On the other hand, because SCD mortality is so high in these patients and because the ICD is an effective tool for decreasing sudden arrhythmic death, its effectiveness in prolonging life also seems plausible. One retrospective analysis using data from two separate registries compared ESRD patients with low ejection fraction (EF) with or without ICD, and found a significant survival advantage in ICD recipients.[10] However, the matter is still far from settled because the efficacy of ICD therapy for primary prevention of SCD in dialysis patients with ischemic or nonischemic cardiomyopathy and depressed EF has not been evaluated in an RCT.

Given these gaps in our understanding of SCD and the clinical equipoise regarding ICD efficacy in dialysis patients, an RCT is the next logical step. The purpose of this article is to discuss the current literature on the role of ICDs in reducing SCD and overall mortality in the dialysis population. After outlining mechanisms responsible for increased incidence of SCD in the setting of renal disease, clinical studies that have evaluated the benefit of ICDs in this population are reviewed.

## EPIDEMIOLOGY OF CHRONIC KIDNEY DISEASE

CKD is defined as either kidney damage (pathologic renal changes or markers of renal damage, such as abnormal blood or urine tests or imaging studies) or glomerular filtration rate (GFR) of less than 60 mL/min/1.73 m$^2$ lasting 3 months or longer. CKD is classified from stage I to V, using the GFR or the estimated GFR values (eGFR) as suggested by the National Kidney Foundation Kidney Disease Outcomes Quality Initiative (KDOQI), using the formula developed by the Modification of Diet in Renal Disease Study Group.[11,12] Stage I represents GFR equal to or greater than 90 mL/min/1.73 m$^2$ with kidney damage; stage II 60 to 89 90 mL/min/1.73 m$^2$ with kidney damage; stage III 30 to 59 90 mL/min/1.73 m$^2$; stage IV 15 to 29 90 mL/min/1.73 m$^2$; and stage V, representing ESRD, with GFR of less than 15 mL/min/1.73 m$^2$ or requiring renal replacement therapy (dialysis or renal transplantation) for survival. Renal replacement therapies consist of hemodialysis, peritoneal dialysis, or renal transplantation. Hemodialysis is the modality of renal replacement therapy that is most readily available for the majority of ESRD patients worldwide.

Over the past 2 decades, the prevalence of CKD has increased dramatically and is expected to continue to increase. By 2030, it is expected that more than 2 million patients in the United States may require renal replacement therapy for stage V CKD. However, the survival of these patients is quite poor, with a 5-year survival of 33% for hemodialysis, which is only marginally better than that for peritoneal dialysis and much worse than that for kidney transplantation (**Fig. 1**).[13]

## SUDDEN CARDIAC DEATH IN ESRD

Cardiovascular causes of death account for 43% of deaths in patients on dialysis, with nearly two-thirds being arrhythmic deaths and, hence, approximately 25% of deaths in these patients being attributable to SCD.[14,15] Furthermore, survival from cardiac arrest in patients with ESRD is roughly half of the survival in the general population.

Many factors predispose dialysis patients to enhanced arrhythmogenicity: volume shifts, endothelial dysfunction, and ventricular repolarization heterogeneity, along with the intense neurohormonal, metabolic, and electrolyte abnormalities associated with kidney failure and dialysis.[16] Ventricular tachycardia degenerating into ventricular fibrillation is the most common cause of SCD in CKD patients. A 24-hour ambulatory electrocardiographic monitoring study on a sizable

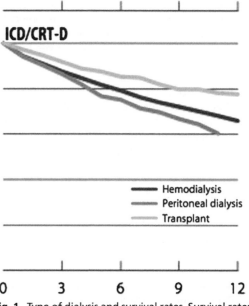

**ICD/CRT-D**

— Hemodialysis
— Peritoneal dialysis
— Transplant

0        3        6        9        12

**Fig. 1.** Type of dialysis and survival rates. Survival rates up to 12 months for the three modes of renal replacement are shown. Survival is shown on the ordinate in increments of 20%. (*From* U.S. Renal Data System, USRDS 2009 Annual Data Report: Atlas of End-Stage Renal Disease in the United States, National Institutes of Health, National Institute of Diabetes and Digestive and Kidney Diseases, Bethesda, MD, 2009.)

number of CKD patients with SCD showed nearly 85% of deaths attributed to ventricular arrhythmias.[17] Dialysis patients with stable myocardial scars may be more prone to ventricular fibrillation as reported in the AVID (Antiarrhythmics vs Implantable Defibrillators) trial, in which a high incidence of SCD occurred even in patients with previously "stable" ventricular tachycardias.[18]

## LEFT VENTRICULAR FUNCTION AND THE RISK OF SUDDEN CARDIAC DEATH IN ESRD

Heart failure is more common in renal disease patients than in the general population, and is an independent predictor of death.[19] Both systolic (left ventricular dysfunction) and diastolic (left ventricular hypertrophy with preserved left ventricular function) heart failure are seen in dialysis patients, and they often coexist.[20,21] Recently, Wang and colleagues[22] described a 5-year prospective study in 230 ESRD patients, aiming to determine the role of echocardiographic parameters and biomarkers in predicting subsequent SCD. SCD accounted for 24% of all-cause mortality in this cohort. Unlike the coronary artery disease population in whom the risk of sudden death begins to increase below an EF of about 30% to 35%, Wang and colleagues found that an EF of 48% or less was the best cutoff threshold for predicting an increased risk of SCD with 80% specificity.[23,24]

## CARDIOPULMONARY RESUSCITATION AND DEFIBRILLATION IN DIALYSIS PATIENTS

The incidence of SCD increases during the peridialysis period, and also as the interdialytic interval lengthens.[25,26] The incidence of ventricular ectopy increases during and immediately after hemodialysis.[2,21] SCD accounts for approximately one-quarter of all deaths in dialysis patients with a 6% to 7% yearly incidence, thus surpassing the SCD incidence even in "high-risk" heart failure patients.[27] With prompt use of defibrillation, more than 60% of the initial rhythm of ventricular tachycardia (VT) or ventricular fibrillation (VF) can be reverted to sinus rhythm.[28] Also, there is observational evidence that automated external fibrillators (AEDs) might prove useful in dialysis centers.[25] However, studies have found varying results regarding the efficacy of cardiopulmonary resuscitation and the use of AEDs in dialysis centers, so it is not surprising that AEDs are still underutilized and their value debated.[29]

## THE ROLE OF IMPLANTABLE CARDIOVERTER-DEFIBRILLATORS

Although none of the clinical trials demonstrating the efficacy of ICDs for primary and secondary prevention included patients with ESRD, clinical guidelines for ICD implantation have not excluded these patients as long as the anticipated long-term survival is not expected to be less than 1 year. The number of patients with ESRD receiving ICDs for primary prevention has risen in recent years, though overall use still remains less in comparison with the general population. Interventional cardiovascular therapies are underused in ESRD patients, and age and gender disparities in the dialysis patients are also quite pronounced.[13] Compared with an ESRD patient aged 45 to 64 years, one 75 years or older is 32% less likely to receive percutaneous coronary intervention, 50% less likely to receive coronary artery bypass surgery, and 36% less likely to receive an ICD or cardiac resynchronization therapy defibrillator (CRT-D). Women with ESRD, for example, are less than half as likely as men to receive an ICD or CRT-D. Even among resuscitated cardiac arrest patients who survived the arrest as well as the subsequent 30 days, only 7.6% received an ICD for secondary prevention. This finding suggests underutilization of ICDs in the dialysis population.[30] Some of this underutilization may be appropriate given that these patients are often quite ill and have multiple medical problems and, in general, that interventional therapies may entail higher risk.

Cardiovascular mortality defined as death because of arrhythmias, cardiomyopathy, cardiac arrest, myocardial infarction, atherosclerotic heart disease, or pulmonary edema in the general population, when compared with ESRD patients treated by dialysis, shows a reduced gap with increasing age.[31] The gap significantly reduces at age 65 years or older (**Fig. 2**). Using a decision analytical model, Amin and colleagues[32] reported that the benefits of ICDs in patients with ESRD might be limited to those younger than 65 years.

Until recently, only one study had been published comparing the survival in dialysis patients with ICDs with those without ICDs for secondary prevention. This survival was evaluated in a retrospective analysis on a select group of Medicare enrolled patients who survived VF/cardiac arrest, were subsequently discharged alive, and survived at least 30 days. ICD implantation was associated with a 42% reduction in risk of mortality in this select group using a propensity-adjusted model (P<.0001), and the 5-year survival was low in both groups as shown in **Fig. 3** (22% in the ICD group vs 12% in the no-ICD group).[33] A recent analysis of the US Renal Data System database of 9528 ESRD patients receiving an ICD in the period 1994 to 2006 (including devices inserted for both primary and secondary prevention)

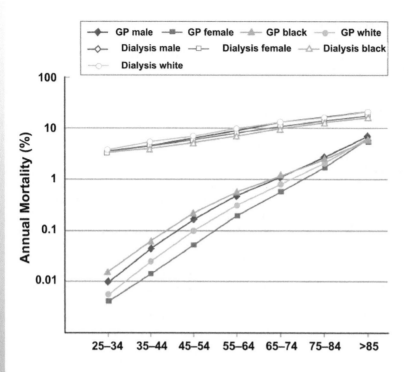

**Fig. 2.** A comparison of all-cause mortality between general population (GP) and end-stage renal disease (ESRD) patients on dialysis. All-cause cardiovascular mortality is defined as death because of arrhythmias, cardiomyopathy, cardiac arrest, myocardial infarction, atherosclerotic heart disease, or pulmonary edema in the GP, compared with ESRD patients treated by dialysis. Data are stratified by age, race, and gender. The reduced gap after the age of 65 years explains the reduced benefit of ICD in dialysis patients. (*From* Foley RN, Pafrey PS, Sarnack MJ. Clinical epidemiology of cardiovascular disease in chronic renal disease. Am J Kidney Dis 1998;32(5 Suppl 3):S112–9; with permission.)

reported a high mortality rate (448/1000 patient-years). Using propensity-matched controls, there was indeed a 14% lower mortality in ICD users after Cox proportional hazards analysis, though the Kaplan-Meier survival curves converged after about 3 years of follow-up.[34]

Several small studies have evaluated the impact of ESRD on outcomes in patients with ICDs. A

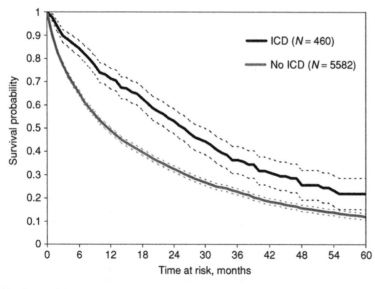

**Fig. 3.** Survival advantage of ICD in dialysis patients. Estimated unadjusted survival of dialysis patients with and without an ICD after cardiac arrest. *P*<.0001 by log-rank test for comparison of patients with ICD with those without ICD. Dashed lines indicate 95% confidence intervals. (*From* Herzog CA, Li S, Weinhandl ED, et al. Survival of dialysis patients after cardiac arrest and the impact of implantable cardioverter defibrillators. Kidney Int 2005;68(2):818–25; with permission.)

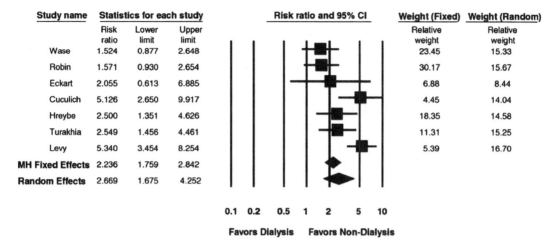

**Fig. 4.** Meta-analysis of mortality in dialysis patients, comparing ICD patients on dialysis with ICD patients not on dialysis. Results from both fixed effects and random effects model are shown, and suggest twofold to threefold better survival in nondialysis patients. (*From* Sakhuja R, Keebler M, Lai TS, et al. Meta-analysis of mortality in dialysis patients with an implantable cardioverter defibrillator. Am J Cardiol 2009;103(5):735–41; with permission.)

meta-analysis of 7 observational studies suggested a 2.7-times higher risk of death in dialysis patients who received an ICD when compared with patients not on dialysis (**Fig. 4**).[35] Data suggest that even though dialysis patients receive appropriate shocks for ventricular arrhythmias, their survival is significantly shorter than nondialysis patients. However, this should not be the point of contention. It seems logical that patients with ESRD may not derive as many "life-years" from a primary-prevention ICD. The main question is, given renal failure with ischemic or nonischemic cardiomyopathy and significant left ventricular dysfunction, would ICDs confer a survival advantage? Only one retrospective study has evaluated these "counterfactual" treatment conditions. Hiremath and colleagues[10] compared the survival of 50 dialysis-dependent ICD patients with 50 dialysis-dependent patients with ischemic or nonischemic cardiomyopathy and EF 35% or less but without ICDs. These investigators reported a significant survival advantage in the ICD group (**Fig. 5**).

As in the general population, there is paucity of data on the utility of available tools for risk stratification in dialysis patients, such as signal-averaged electrocardiograms, QT dispersion, and microvolt T-wave alternans. Biomarkers have not been appropriately tested in ESRD patients, and there are no data on predictive ability of electrophysiology study in this population. Mortality following myocardial infarction in patients with ESRD remains strikingly significant, with a 2-year mortality of more than 70%.[36] It is possible that identification of certain outcome predictors may

help in identifying patients who are most likely to derive benefit from a primary prevention strategy.

The ongoing Implantable Cardioverter Defibrillators in Dialysis Patients (ICD2) trial, a pilot study of 200 patients, will evaluate ICD versus no ICD in dialysis patients 55 to 80 years old, irrespective of left ventricular EF.[37] Until more studies are done to evaluate the benefit of ICDs in ESRD, standard indications for implantation as well as the patient's anticipated survival should guide decisions to implant ICDs. The most recent guidelines consider primary prevention ICD therapy only in those with "a reasonable expectation of survival

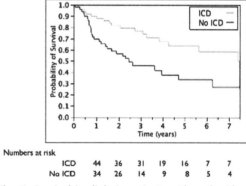

**Fig. 5.** Survival in dialysis patients with and without ICDs. Long-term survival in ESRD patients with ICD compared with patients with ischemic or nonischemic cardiomyopathy (ejection fraction <35%) without ICDs. (*From* Hiremath S, Punnam SR, Brar S, et al. Implantable defibrillators improve survival in end-stage renal disease: results from a multi-center registry. Am J Nephrol 2010;32:305–10; with permission.)

with an acceptable functional status for at least 1 year."[38] With respect to the type of renal replacement therapy and survival, renal transplant fares better than hemodialysis, which fares better than peritoneal dialysis (see **Fig. 1**).

## THE ROLE OF WEARABLE CARDIAC DEFIBRILLATORS

Zareba and colleagues studied the electrocardiographic recordings of wearable cardiac defibrillator (WCD) treatments and asystole events in ESRD patients using the WCD. VT and VF appear to be responsible for the majority of sudden cardiac arrests in dialysis patients, and these events can be successfully resuscitated with the WCD. The survival rate of 69% is far higher than the reported 5% to 10% survival rate of cardiac arrest victims unprotected by a WCD or an ICD.[13] A WCD may represent useful alternative therapy for patients unwilling or unable to receive an ICD or requiring ICD explantation as a result of infection and so forth.[39]

## IMPLANT-RELATED PROCEDURAL COMPLICATIONS IN DIALYSIS PATIENTS

Several studies have suggested that procedural complications may be higher in ESRD patients, thereby detracting from the potential benefits of an ICD. While it is possible that the high complication rates reported in observational studies may be attributable to reporting bias, there are physiologic reasons to explain the observations.

Several factors such as uremia-related immune system dysfunction, coagulopathy, limited venous access, malnutrition, and medical comorbidities associated with ESRD predispose CKD patients to high complication rates during implantation. Overall complication rates range from 2.5% to 6.5%, depending on the type of device implanted and operator experience. In a study by Eberhardt and colleagues,[40] the lead dislodgement rate was approximately 2.0%, pocket hematoma rate was 0.6%, lead insulation defect rate was 0.4%, and pocket or lead infection rate was 0.3% after a mean follow-up of 34 months. Similar complication rates of between 3.5% and 4.8% have been reported in other studies.[41,42] Dasgupta and colleagues,[43] in an observational study, reported hematoma as the most common implant-related complication, which occurred in 12% of patients with ESRD and 2% of patients without ESRD. There was a higher incidence of thrombosis of the dialysis access graft or arteriovenous fistula ipsilateral to pacemaker or ICD implant. The type of hemodialysis access or time on dialysis therapy

before device implantation had no relationship to the complication rate after device implantation. In patients with ESRD, ICD implantation and even generator changes or upgrades offer specific challenges. Uremic coagulopathy, anticoagulant and antiplatelet therapies, and malnutrition increase the risk of bleeding. Delayed wound infection is more common than in the general population: the odds are nearly 5 times higher among those with moderate to severe renal dysfunction.[44] Increased direct bloodstream access for pathogens as well as increased host susceptibility due to the relatively immunocompromised state heightens the risk. Endomyocardial calcification may interfere with lead fixation, and contribute to excess lead trauma and, eventually, lead failure.[45]

Awareness of these issues and attention to detail during the implant procedure may help ameliorate some of these complications. Meticulous hemostasis, avoiding postimplant anticoagulation if possible, placement of intravascular leads on the contralateral side of dialysis access, infection control using an antibiotic envelope, and the use of high-energy devices are often recommended. The liberal use of local hemostatic agents such as topical hemostat, local thrombin injection, and a variety of microfibrillar collagen hemostatic agents have been shown to improve local hemostasis and reduce the incidence of pocket hematoma and its sequelae. The COMMAND study demonstrated the effectiveness of the AIGISRx Antibacterial Envelope (TyRx Pharma, Monmouth Junction, NJ, USA) to significantly reduce infections in patients receiving implantable pacemakers or defibrillators.[46]

Even after ICD implantation, patients continue to have arrhythmic deaths. In part, this may be related to inefficacy of defibrillation. Patients with ESRD have high defibrillation thresholds; one study found that more than 35% of dialysis patients had high defibrillation thresholds compared with less than 10% of patients without renal disease.[47] It is possible that under the right set of metabolic conditions more common in ESRD patients, such as severe hyperkalemia, the ICD may prove ineffective because of failure to terminate VT or VF or recurrent VT/VF.

## CARDIAC RESYNCHRONIZATION THERAPY IN CHRONIC KIDNEY DISEASE

Clinical trials of cardiac resynchronization therapy (CRT) have also excluded patients with advanced renal disease, including patients on dialysis. Therefore, our understanding of the utility of this therapy in patients with ESRD is limited, and its use in this population is based on studies in patients with relatively normal renal function.

Unlike many other interventions such as drug therapy, CRT does not have direct effects on the kidney. Renal function may, however, be affected indirectly by a variety of mechanisms. CRT has been reported to increase cardiac output and improve symptoms, functional status, left ventricular function, morbidity, and mortality. The improvement in ventricular pumping occurs through better temporal coordination of left ventricular activation and contraction, which may result in increased left ventricular pressure generation, mean arterial pressure, cardiac output, and myocardial efficiency, and reduced mitral regurgitation and cardiac filling pressures.[48–50] Increasing aortic pressure and decreasing right-sided pressures may improve renal capillary perfusion pressure and thus improve the GFR.[51] Another possible mechanism for improvement in renal function could be the result of reduced activation of the sympathetic nervous system and reduced cardiac muscle sympathetic nerve traffic.

Fung and colleagues[52] reported 3 months of reverse remodeling of CRT (defined as at least 10% reduction in left ventricular end-systolic volume), with a corresponding increase in eGFR from an average of 51.7 to 54.2 mL/min/1.73 m², in contrast to patients without reverse remodeling who had a decrease from a mean 61.9 to 48.8 mL/min/1.73 m². The major drawback of this study, however, was the absence of a control group. Cowburn and colleagues[53] reported significant improvement in 10 patients with severe decompensated heart failure on inotropic support; CRT enabled weaning from inotropes, improved cardiac output, and reduced serum creatinine. Boerrigter and colleagues[54] reported a randomized placebo-controlled clinical trial demonstrating favorable effects of CRT to improve eGFR and reduce BUN in patients with moderately decreased eGFR at baseline (30–59 mL/min/1.73 m²). Patients with lower eGFR had a lower lean body mass and were more likely to have ischemic heart failure, with lower mean and diastolic blood pressures and therefore reduced renal perfusion pressure.

Impaired cardiovascular hemodynamics and intense neurohumoral activation may play a key role in the impaired renal function that characterizes severe heart failure.[55] A significant reduction in BUN was identified as an important prognostic factor in patients admitted for heart failure.[56] Patients on β-blockers fared well in comparison with those without β-blockers. Subgroup analyses of the Comparison of Medical Therapy, Pacing and Defibrillation in Chronic Heart Failure (COMPANION) and Cardiac Resynchronization-Heart Failure (CARE-HF) trials showed that the respective primary end points were significantly improved with CRT only in patients on β-blockers, further emphasizing the importance of continued β-blockade. Whether changes in eGFR after CRT implantation affects outcome with reduction in hospitalization and mortality requires further study.

Goldenberg and colleagues[57] recently reported a post hoc subgroup analysis on 1803 patients enrolled in the Multicenter Automatic Defibrillator Implantation Trial–Cardiac Resynchronization Therapy (MADIT CRT) trial. Response to CRT-D was assessed by renal function parameter, including serum creatinine (SCr), BUN, and the ratio of BUN to SCr (BUN:SCr), with BUN:SCr dichotomized at median values and into approximate quartiles. Multivariate analysis showed that the benefit of CRT-D was significantly increased with increasing quartiles of BUN:SCr from Q1 to Q4: Q1 (<15): HR = 1.06 ($P$ = .79); Q2 (15–18): HR = 0.64 ($P$ = .04);, Q3 (>18–22): HR = 0.47 ($P$<.001); Q4 (>22): HR = 0.44 ($P$<.001) ($P$ value for trend = .005). These findings suggest CRT-D as a highly effective therapy for mildly symptomatic low-EF patients with prerenal azotemia. The high BUN:SCr quartile showed greater than 50% reduction in the risk of heart failure or death and a pronounced echocardiographic response with CRT-D, whereas among patients with a low BUN:SCr, CRT-D therapy was associated with a significantly lower clinical and echocardiographic response. These findings persisted after multivariate adjustment for medication usage, including diuretic therapy and furosemide dosage. The limitations of post hoc subgroup analysis should be kept in mind before implementing such data in practice.[57]

Lin and colleagues[58] recently reported a retrospective analysis on the impact of CKD on mortality after CRT. Of 482 patients, 342 (71%) had CKD (defined as a GFR of ≤60 mL/min/1.73 m²) at the time of device implantation. After multivariate analysis, patients with normal or mild renal dysfunction showed superior survival compared with patients with CKD (72% vs 57% at 3 years, $P$<.01). The acute hemodynamic benefits failed to confer survival benefit over a mean follow-up period of 36.45 ± 26.55 months. Univariate analysis showed anemia (hemoglobin <12 mg/L), hyponatremia (sodium <135 mmol/L), increased brain natriuretic peptide (>500 ng/dL), male gender, and EF less than 20% were predictive of poor outcomes (death or need for heart transplantation). Nonischemic cardiomyopathy was associated with lower mortality and improved outcomes following CRT. After multivariate analysis, CKD remained a significant predictor of poor outcome, although anemia (hemoglobin <12.0 mg/dL) was the most robust predictor.[58]

## THE WAY FORWARD

Clinical trials that showed the benefit of primary prevention ICDs excluded patients with significant renal disease and dialysis patients. Efficacy of ICD therapy is often extrapolated beyond the strict inclusion criteria used in clinical trials into clinical practice; this is partly why ICD survival benefits in the general population are attenuated in comparison with those seen in clinical trials.[59] However, in the absence of data, and the desire to improve patients' quality of life and to prevent sudden death whenever possible, implantation of ICDs or CRT-D may not be an unreasonable course of action for physicians facing a challenging clinical situations. With respect to patients with advanced renal disease, one can certainly rationalize arguments for implanting or not implanting primary prevention devices, and empirical observations support both these positions. A clinical approach may be reasonable for individual decisions, but public health issues need to be based on solid data.

Given the increasing population of CKD patients requiring dialysis, a clear understanding of the marginal benefit of this therapy in reducing overall mortality is an urgent public health issue. In addition, given the increasing cost of health care, a clear, evidence-based approach is needed to inform public health policy. The ongoing primary prevention pilot study of 200 patients on dialysis (ICD2 Trial) will randomize patients to ICD versus no ICD, irrespective of left ventricular function.[28] Regardless of its findings, this trial will raise many more questions than it will answer. Also needed is a primary prevention trial comparing ICD versus no ICD in cardiomyopathy patients with reduced left ventricular function, as well as a trial to evaluate the marginal benefit of CRT-D therapy in patients with ESRD.

## REFERENCES

1. Herzog CA. Poor long-term survival of dialysis patients after acute myocardial infarction: bad treatment or bad disease? Am J Kidney Dis 2000;35:1217–20.
2. Bleyer AJ, Russell GB, Satko SG. Sudden cardiac death rates in hemodialysis patients. Kidney Int 1999;55(4):1553–9.
3. Parfrey PS, Foley RN, Harnett JD, et al. Outcome and risk factors of ischemic heart disease in chronic uremia. Kidney Int 1996;49:1428–34.
4. Hillege HL, Nitsch D, Pfeffer MA, et al. Renal function as a predictor of outcome in a broad spectrum of patients with heart failure. Circulation 2006;113(5):671–8.
5. Mark DB, Nelson CL, Anstrom KJ, et al. SCD-HeFT Investigators. Cost-effectiveness of defibrillator therapy or amiodarone in chronic stable heart failure: results from the Sudden Cardiac Death in Heart Failure Trial (SCD-HeFT). Circulation 2006;114(2):135–42.
6. Buxton AE, Lee KL, Fisher JD, et al, The Multicenter Unsustained Tachycardia Trial Investigators. A randomized study of the prevention of sudden death in patients with coronary artery disease. N Engl J Med 1999;341:1882–90.
7. Moss AJ, Zareba W, Hall WJ, et al, Multicenter Automatic Defibrillator Implantation Trial II Investigators. Prophylactic implantation of a defibrillator in patients with myocardial infarction and reduced ventricular ejection fraction. N Engl J Med 2002; 346:877–83.
8. Greenberg H, Case RB, Moss AJ, et al. Analysis of mortality events in the Multicenter Automatic Defibrillator Implantation Trial (MADIT-II). J Am Coll Cardiol 2004;43:1459–65.
9. Goldenberg I, Vyas AK, Hall WJ, et al, MADIT-II Investigators. Risk stratification for primary implantation of a cardioverter-defibrillator in patients with ischemic left ventricular dysfunction. J Am Coll Cardiol 2008;51(3):288–96.
10. Hiremath S, Punnam SR, Brar S, et al. Implantable defibrillators improve survival in end-stage renal disease: results from a multi-center registry. Am J Nephrol 2010;32:305–10.
11. National Kidney Foundation. Clinical practice guidelines for chronic kidney disease: evaluation, classification, and stratification. Am J Kidney Dis 2002;2(Suppl 1):S46.
12. Levey AS, Bosch JP, Lewis JB, et al. A more accurate method to estimate glomerular filtration rate from serum creatinine: a new prediction equation. Modification of Diet in Renal Disease Study Group. Ann Intern Med 1999;130(6):461–70.
13. Bhatt DL, Roe MT, Peterson ED, et al. Utilization of early invasive management strategies for high-risk patients with non-ST segment elevation acute coronary syndromes: results from the CRUSADE Quality Improvement Initiative. JAMA 2004;292:2096–104.
14. Herzog CA. Cardiac arrest in dialysis patients: approaches to alter an abysmal outcome. Kidney Int Suppl 2003;84:S197–200.
15. Port FK. Morbidity and mortality in dialysis patients. Kidney Int 1994;46:1728–37.
16. Morris ST, Galiatsou E, Stewart GA, et al. QT dispersion before and after hemodialysis. J Am Soc Nephrol 1999;10:160–3.
17. Bayes de Luna A, Coumel P, Leclercq JF. Ambulatory sudden cardiac death: mechanisms of production of fatal arrhythmia on the basis of data from 157 cases. Am Heart J 1989;117(1):151–9.

18. The Antiarrhythmic versus Implantable Defibrillators (AVID) Investigators. A comparison of antiarrhythmic-drug therapy with implantable defibrillators in patients resuscitated from near-fatal ventricular arrhythmias. N Engl J Med 1997;337:1576–83.

19. Harnett JD, Foley RN, Kent GM, et al. Congestive heart failure in dialysis patients: prevalence, incidence, prognosis and risk factors. Kidney Int 1995;47:884–90.

20. Foley RN, Parfrey PS, Harnett JD, et al. Clinical and echocardiographic disease in patients starting end-stage renal disease therapy: prevalence, associations and prognosis. Kidney Int 1995;47:186–92.

21. Hutting J, Kramer W, Schutterle G, et al. Analysis of left ventricular changes associated with chronic hemodialysis: a non-invasive follow-up study. Nephron 1988;49:284–90.

22. Wang AY, Lam CW, Chan IH, et al. Sudden cardiac death in end-stage renal disease patients: a 5-year prospective analysis. Circulation 2010;56:210–6.

23. Bigger JT, Fleiss JL, Kleiger R, et al. The relationship among ventricular arrhythmias, left ventricular dysfunction, and mortality in the 2 years after myocardial infarction. Circulation 1984;69:250–8.

24. Mukharji J, Rude RE, Poole WK, et al. Risk factors for sudden death after acute myocardial infarction: two-years follow-up. Am J Cardiol 1984;54:31–6.

25. Davis TR, Young BA, Eisenberg MS, et al. Outcome of cardiac arrests attended by emergency medical services staff at community outpatient dialysis centers. Kidney Int 2008;73(8):933–9.

26. Bleyer AJ, Hartman J, Brannon PC, et al. Characteristics of sudden death in hemodialysis patients. Kidney Int 2006;69(12):2268–73.

27. US Renal Data System. USRDS 2010 Annual Data Report: Atlas of chronic kidney disease and end-stage renal disease in the United States. Bethesda (MD): National Institutes of Health, National Institute of Diabetes and Digestive and Kidney Diseases; 2010.

28. Becker L, Eisenberg M, Fahrenbruch C, et al. Cardiac arrest in medical and dental practices: implications for automated external defibrillators. Arch Intern Med 2001;161(12):1509–12, 23.

29. Lafrance JP, Nolin L, Senécal L, et al. Predictors and outcome of cardiopulmonary resuscitation (CPR) calls in a large haemodialysis unit over a seven-year period. Nephrol Dial Transplant 2006;21(4):1006–12.

30. United States Renal Data System. USRDS 2009. Annual data report. Available at: http://www.usrds. org/. Accessed July 16, 2011.

31. Foley RN, Parfey PS, Sarnak MJ. Clinical epidemiology of cardiovascular disease in chronic renal disease. Am J Kidney Dis 1998;32(5 Suppl 3):S112–9.

32. Amin MS, Fox AD, Kalahasty G, et al. Benefit of primary prevention implantable cardioverter-defibrillators in the setting of chronic kidney disease: a decision model analysis. J Cardiovasc Electrophysiol 2008;19:1275–80.

33. Herzog CA, Li S, Weinhandl ED, et al. Survival of dialysis patients after cardiac arrest and the impact of implantable cardioverter defibrillators. Kidney Int 2005;68(2):818–25.

34. Charytan DM, Patrick AR, Liu J, et al. Trends in the use and outcomes of implantable cardioverter-defibrillators in patients undergoing dialysis in the United States. Am J Kidney Dis 2011;58(3):409–17. [Epub ahead of print].

35. Sakhuja R, Keebler M, Lai TS, et al. Meta-analysis of mortality in dialysis patients with an implantable cardioverter defibrillator. Am J Cardiol 2009;103(5): 1515, 735–41.

36. Chertow GM, Normand SL, Silva LR, et al. Survival after acute myocardial infarction in patients with end-stage renal disease: results from the cooperative cardiovascular project. Am J Kidney Dis 2000;35:1044–51.

37. De Bie MK, Lekkerkerker JC, van Dam B, et al. Prevention of sudden cardiac death: rationale and design of the Implantable Cardioverter Defibrillators in Dialysis patients (ICD2) Trial—a prospective pilot study. Curr Med Res Opin 2008;24(8):2151–7. [Epub 2008 Jun 17].

38. Epstein AE, DiMarco JP, Ellenbogen KA, et al. ACC/AHA/HRS 2008 Guidelines for Device-Based Therapy of Cardiac Rhythm Abnormalities: a report of the American College of Cardiology/American Heart Association Task Force on Practice Guidelines (Writing Committee to Revise the ACC/AHA/NASPE 2002 Guideline Update for Implantation of Cardiac Pacemakers and Antiarrhythmia Devices) developed in collaboration with the American Association for Thoracic Surgery and Society of Thoracic Surgeons. American College of Cardiology/American Heart Association Task Force on Practice Guidelines (Writing Committee to Revise the ACC/AHA/NASPE 2002 Guideline Update for Implantation of Cardiac Pacemakers and Antiarrhythmia Devices); American Association for Thoracic Surgery; Society of Thoracic Surgeons [Erratum appears in J Am Coll Cardiol 2009;53(16):1473. J Am Coll Cardiol 2009; 53(1):147]. J Am Coll Cardiol 2008;51(21):e1–62, No abstract available.

39. Zareba W, Bianco N, Szymkiewicz S. Abstract 2845: Sudden cardiac arrest in end-stage renal disease: successful resuscitation with wearable cardiac defibrillator. Circulation 2009;120:S701–2.

40. Eberhardt F, Bode F, Bonnemeier H, et al. Long term complications in single and dual chamber pacing are influenced by surgical experience and patient morbidity. Heart 2005;91:500–6.

41. Lamas GA, Lee KL, Sweeney MO, et al. Ventricular pacing or dual-chamber pacing for sinus-node dysfunction. N Engl J Med 2002;346:1854–62.

42. Moller M, Arnsbo P, Asklund M, et al. Quality assessment of pacemaker implantation in Denmark. Europace 2002;4:107–12.

43. Dasgupta A, Montalvo J, Medendorp S, et al. Increased complication rates of cardiac rhythm management devices in ESRD patients. Am J Kidney Dis 2007;49(5):656–63.

44. Bloom H, Heeke B, Leon A, et al. Renal insufficiency and the risk of infection from pacemaker or defibrillator surgery. Pacing Clin Electrophysiol 2006;29(2): 142–5.

45. Rostand SG, Sanders C, Kirk KA, et al. Myocardial calcification and cardiac dysfunction in chronic renal failure. Am J Med 1988;85:651–7.

46. Hansen LK, Brown M, Johnson D, et al. In vivo model of human pathogen infection and demonstration of efficacy by an antimicrobial pouch for pacing devices. Pacing Clin Electrophysiol 2009; 32(7):898–907.

47. Wase A, Basit A, Nazir R, et al. Impact of chronic kidney disease upon survival among implantable cardioverter-defibrillator recipients. J Interv Card Electrophysiol 2004;11(3):199–204.

48. Sutton MG, Plappert T, Abraham WT, et al. Effect of cardiac resynchronization therapy on left ventricular size and function in chronic heart failure. Circulation 2003;107:1985, e90.

49. Bristow MR, Saxon LA, Boehmer J, et al. Cardiac-resynchronization therapy with or without an implantable defibrillator in advanced chronic heart failure. N Engl J Med 2004;350:2140, e50.

50. Cleland JG, Daubert JC, Erdmann E, et al. The effect of cardiac resynchronization on morbidity and mortality in heart failure. N Engl J Med 2005;352:1539. e49.

51. Burnett JC Jr, Knox FG. Renal interstitial pressure and sodium excretion during renal vein constriction. Am J Physiol 1980;238:F279, e82.

52. Fung JW, Szeto CC, Chan JY, et al. Prognostic value of renal function in patients with cardiac resynchronization therapy. Int J Cardiol 2007;122:10–6.

53. Cowburn PJ, Patel H, Jolliffe RE, et al. Cardiac resynchronization therapy: an option for inotrope-supported patients with end-stage heart failure? Eur J Heart Fail 2005;7:215–7.

54. Boerrigter G, Costello-Boerrigter LC, Abraham WT, et al. Cardiac resynchronization therapy improves renal function in human heart failure with reduced glomerular filtration rate. J Card Fail 2008;14(7):539–46.

55. Hillege HL, Girbes AR, de Kam PJ, et al. Renal function, neurohormonal activation, and survival in patients with chronic heart failure. Circulation 2000;102:203, e10.

56. Fonarow GC, Adams KF Jr, Abraham WT, et al. Risk stratification for in-hospital mortality in acutely decompensated heart failure: classification and regression tree analysis. JAMA 2005; 293:572, e80.

57. Goldenberg I, Moss AJ, McNitt S, et al, Multicenter Automatic Defibrillator Implantation Trial-Cardiac Resynchronization Therapy Investigators. Relation between renal function and response to cardiac resynchronization therapy in Multicenter Automatic Defibrillator Implantation Trial—Cardiac Resynchronization Therapy (MADIT-CRT). Heart Rhythm 2010;7(12):1777–82.

58. Lin G, Gersh BJ, Greene EL, et al. Renal function and mortality following cardiac resynchronization therapy. Eur Heart J 2011;32(2):184–90.

59. Lee DS, Tu JV, Austin PC, et al. Effect of cardiac and non-cardiac conditions on survival after defibrillator implantation. J Am Coll Cardiol 2007;49: 2408–15.

# Antiarrhythmic Drug Therapy for New-Onset Ventricular Arrhythmia (VT/VF) in ICD Patients

Girish M. Nair, MBBS, FRCPC[a],*,
Jeffrey S. Healey, MD, MSc, FRCPC[a],
Syamkumar M. Divakaramenon, MBBS, MD, DM[b],
Stuart J. Connolly, MD, FRCPC[a],
Carlos A. Morillo, MD, FRCPC[c]

**KEYWORDS**

- Implantable cardioverter-defibrillator
- Ventricular arrhythmia • Antiarrhythmic drug therapy

Implantable cardioverter-defibrillators (ICD) have been firmly established as the most effective treatment for primary and secondary prevention of sudden cardiac death (SCD) in a variety of conditions such as ischemic cardiomyopathy, nonischemic dilated cardiomyopathy, and other inherited genetic conditions affecting the heart (arrhythmogenic right ventricular cardiomyopathy, hypertrophic cardiomyopathy, the ion channelopathies, and so forth).[1–4] The use of ICD for prevention of SCD has increased exponentially over the past decade, and this has resulted in a large population of patients living with ICDs.[5–7] ICD patients and physicians treating them have to contend with the prospect of recurrent ventricular arrhythmia (ventricular tachycardia [VT] and ventricular fibrillation [VF]) resulting in therapy, including both shocks and antitachycardia pacing (ATP). Multiple randomized controlled trials (RCTs) have shown that about 20% of patients receiving ICDs will need adjunctive antiarrhythmic therapy to prevent ventricular arrhythmia and resultant ICD therapy.[8–14] There is growing evidence to suggest that ventricular arrhythmia resulting in ICD therapy is associated with a higher risk of morbidity and mortality.[15–17] Patients with symptomatic ventricular arrhythmia and ICD shocks may have restrictions imposed on them (eg, driving restrictions, inability to operate heavy machinery) that may result in loss of employment. In addition, frequent ICD therapy results in increased use of health care resources.[18–21] The purpose of this review is to understand the role of antiarrhythmic therapy in management of ICD patients with new-onset ventricular arrhythmia.

Financial Disclosures: Drs Nair, Healey, Connolly and Morillo have received grants and honoraria from St Jude Medical and Boston Scientific Corporation Inc.

[a] Division of Cardiology, Department of Medicine, Population Health Research Institute and Hamilton Health Sciences, McMaster University, C3-204, David Braley Research Institute Building, 237 Barton Street East, Hamilton, Ontario L8L 2X2, Canada

[b] Division of Cardiology, Department of Medicine, McMaster University and Hamilton Health Sciences, Room# 502, 5th Floor McMaster Clinic Building, 237 Barton Street East, Hamilton, Ontario L8L 2X2, Canada

[c] Division of Cardiology, Department of Medicine, Population Health Research Institute and Hamilton Health Sciences, McMaster University, C3-120, David Braley Research Institute Building, 237 Barton Street East, Hamilton, Ontario L8L 2X2, Canada

* Corresponding author.

*E-mail address:* Girish.Nair@phri.ca

## INCIDENCE OF VENTRICULAR ARRHYTHMIA IN PATIENTS WITH ICD AND PROGNOSTIC SIGNIFICANCE

Data from large, randomized ICD trials have shown that by 4 years after implantation of an ICD 30% to 35% patients have experienced at least one shock. Further analysis revealed that two-thirds (16%–20%) of the shocks resulted from ventricular arrhythmia and one-third resulted from supraventricular arrhythmia, inappropriate sensing, or patient-related and device-related issues. This result translates to a 6% to 10% annual incidence of ventricular arrhythmia in ICD patients.[13–15,22] Data from trials incorporating ICD programming strategies to reduce shocks have shown that 85% of ventricular arrhythmias occurring in ICD patients were secondary to monomorphic VT (rates ranging from 188 to 250 beats/min) with VF accounting for the remaining 15%.[23–25]

Long-term follow-up data from large ICD trials, including the Multicenter Automatic Defibrillator Implantation Trial-II (MADIT-II) and the Sudden Cardiac Death in Heart Failure Trial (SCD-HeFT), have shown that new-onset ventricular arrhythmia in ICD patients conferred a threefold increase in the risk of death. The most common cause of death in these patients was progressive heart failure and nonsudden cardiac death. Recent trials evaluating optimal programming of ICD antitachycardia therapy parameters have shown that both appropriate and inappropriate shocks resulted in increased risk of death. Patients without any ventricular arrhythmia and patients treated with ATP alone fared better than patients receiving shocks (survival rates at 1 year were 5% lower).[11–14] Another interesting observation was that patients receiving ICD shocks were likely to have a high rate of recurrent ventricular arrhythmia, and in about 10% to 20% of cases the initial presentation was in the form of an electrical storm (ES; ≥3 episodes of VT separated by >5 minutes during a 24-h period, each resulting in an appropriate shock by the ICD). Electrical storms were associated with a very poor prognosis and resulted in a twofold to threefold increase in all-cause and cardiac mortality.[26–28] Lastly, in 8% to 10% of patients supraventricular arrhythmias, especially atrial fibrillation (AF), may be responsible for triggering ventricular arrhythmia, resulting in ICD shocks.[29] Multivariate analyses of pooled data from primary and secondary prevention ICD trials have identified risk factors for ventricular arrhythmia and ICD shocks (summarized in **Box 1**).[12,15]

Patients receiving frequent ICD shocks have poor health-related quality of life and psychological distress ranging from posttraumatic stress disorder to depression. Such patients require

---

**Box 1**
**Clinical predictors of recurrent ventricular arrhythmia and ICD therapy**

Secondary prevention indication and/or appropriate therapy after ICD implantation

Congestive heart failure

Severe left ventricular systolic dysfunction (left ventricular ejection fraction <25%)

Associated acute coronary syndrome

Associated supraventricular tachycardia (especially atrial fibrillation)

---

frequent emergency department and hospital visits, and may have accelerated battery depletion resulting in increased use of health care resources.[18–20,30]

The trials quoted have exclusively included patients with ischemic or nonischemic dilated cardiomyopathy. Patients receiving ICD for other indications such as arrhythmogenic right ventricular cardiomyopathy, hypertrophic cardiomyopathy, cardiac valve disease, and ion channelopathies are underrepresented in these studies. Information regarding incidence of ventricular arrhythmia and ICD shocks in these patients is based on anecdotal reports and small cohort studies. A French cohort study including more than 2000 patients reported that the incidence of ventricular arrhythmia in the group of ICD patients, without ischemic or nonischemic dilated cardiomyopathy, was similar to that observed in the large, randomized ICD trials quoted previously. However, the incidence of appropriate ICD shocks was noted to be lower in this cohort of patients.[31]

It is clear that most patients will develop ventricular arrhythmia at some point in time after ICD implantation and that this is a poor prognostic indicator, contributing to morbidity and mortality. Therefore, there is growing interest in prevention of ventricular arrhythmia and ICD shocks in these patients. However, it is as yet not clear if ventricular arrhythmia in this situation is causative of death or simply a marker for poor prognosis resulting from progressive ventricular systolic dysfunction and other comorbid conditions. The available data seem to suggest that both factors may be responsible for the poor prognosis noted in ICD patients developing ventricular arrhythmia. The final question that is yet to be answered is: will prevention and treatment of ventricular arrhythmia translate to improved survival in ICD patients?

## STRATEGIES FOR MANAGEMENT OF VENTRICULAR ARRHYTHMIA AND ICD SHOCK PREVENTION

Antiarrhythmic drugs (AAD), optimal ICD programming, and catheter ablation are the most commonly used approaches to treat ventricular arrhythmia and prevent shocks in the ICD population. AAD were used to treat ventricular arrhythmia and prevent SCD in high-risk patients before the invention of the ICD.[32-38] Therefore it was logical to use AAD to treat ventricular arrhythmia in ICD patients. The initial ICD trials used the device as a "shock-box," restricting therapy to shocks for most ventricular arrhythmia. However, it was observed that a significant proportion of ventricular arrhythmia in these patients could have been safely terminated with ATP, reducing the need for shocks. Subsequent randomized trials, evaluating optimal ICD programming, demonstrated that introducing ATP as the first step in ICD-tachycardia treatment algorithms resulted in significant reduction of shocks without compromising efficacy or safety. Reducing shocks in patients with ICD clearly has a significant role to play in improving the quality of life. However, it is not clear whether this will improve patient outcomes such as death and other major adverse cardiac events.[23-25] Recent trials have demonstrated the safety and efficacy of catheter ablation in reducing ventricular arrhythmia and ICD shocks.[39-42] The scope of this review is restricted to the role of AAD in the management of ventricular arrhythmia in ICD patients.

## ANTIARRHYTHMIC DRUG THERAPY FOR PREVENTION OF VENTRICULAR ARRHYTHMIA AND SHOCKS IN ICD PATIENTS

The use of AAD therapy has not been completely eliminated from the treatment of SCD patients even though the ICD has become the primary treatment modality in recent years. The ICD is capable of treating ventricular arrhythmia and preventing SCD. However, it cannot prevent or reduce the incidence of ventricular arrhythmia in patients at risk of SCD. Therefore, AAD therapy is being increasingly used as an adjunctive therapy in patients with ICD shocks. To understand the role of AAD in the treatment of ventricular arrhythmia, trials evaluating these medications in SCD prevention prior to the routine use of ICD are reviewed. In this article the authors use the Vaughan-Williams classification of AAD, which refers to the type of ion channel blocked and the effect of AAD on the electrophysiologic properties of cardiac tissue.[43]

A survey done in ICD patients over the span of a decade (1989–1997) showed a decreasing trend in AAD use. This finding was thought to be related to the advent of the ICD and the expectation that most ventricular arrhythmia could be treated by ATP. The survey noted a significant decrease in the use of class I AAD, probably related to the results of the Cardiac Arrhythmia Suppression Trial (CAST).[32] However, during the second half of the study period an increase in the use of AAD was noted, with 40% to 50% of ICD patients receiving concomitant therapy. During the second half of the study, class III AAD were used more commonly, with one-half of all treated patients receiving amiodarone. This increase was probably related to the promising results of SCD prevention trials evaluating sotalol and amiodarone.[32-38,44]

### Class I AAD (Encainide, Flecainide, Moricizine, Mexiletine)

Clinical trials evaluating class I AAD (encainide, flecainide, mexiletine, and moricizine) for the prevention of SCD in the "pre-ICD" era were terminated early, due to the increased mortality in the AAD treatment arm. The proarrhythmic effects (QT prolongation and torsade de pointe [TDP]) of the class I AAD were thought to be responsible for the increase in mortality noted in these trials.[32-34] These agents are very seldom used to treat ventricular arrhythmia in ICD patients. In a trial evaluating catheter ablation for drug refractory ES, only 6% of patients received class I AAD therapy.[42] Amiodarone and sotalol have been shown to be more effective than class I AAD in the prevention of recurrent ventricular events.[35-38] No randomized trials using class I AAD for the treatment of ventricular arrhythmia in the ICD population have been conducted. Their role as adjunctive therapy in ICD patients with ventricular arrhythmia refractory to AAD (amiodarone/sotalol) and patients undergoing catheter ablation has not yet been evaluated. At present there is no evidence to suggest that this class of medications is safe or effective for the treatment of ICD patients with ventricular arrhythmia and shocks. Quinidine has been reported to suppress VF in patients with Brugada syndrome by depressing the $I_{to}$ current, which plays an important role in the arrhythmogenesis of this disease. Quinidine and isoproterenol have also been used to treat ES in ICD patients with Brugada syndrome.[45,46]

### Class II AAD (β-Blockers)

There is very strong evidence to suggest that β-blockers are effective in reducing mortality in post-myocardial infarction patients and in patients with congestive heart failure (CHF). The beneficial effects of β-blockers seem to be due to a greater relative reduction in SCD.[47,48] However, β-blockers have not been formally evaluated for the treatment of ventricular arrhythmia in ICD patients. In the OPTIC (Optimal Pharmacologic Therapy in Cardioverter Defibrillator) trial comparing amiodarone along with β-blockers, sotalol, and β-blockers alone for prevention of ICD shocks, the β-blocker–alone arm had a 38.5% shock rate at 1 year.[49] Therefore, β-blockers alone may not offer adequate therapy for reduction of ventricular arrhythmia in ICD patients. All ICD patients with CHF and a previous myocardial infarction should be on maximally tolerated doses of β-blockers. β-Blockers also have a special role in patients with the congenital long-QT syndrome type I and catecholaminergic polymorphic VT.

### Class III AAD (Sotalol, Amiodarone, Azimilide, Dofetilide)

Sotalol was the first class III AAD to be evaluated for prevention of recurrent shocks in ICD patients. Sotalol is a β-blocker and in addition has antiarrhythmic actions, the latter effect predominating at higher doses. A placebo-controlled randomized trial evaluated sotalol (160–320 mg) in ICD patients who had received at least one appropriate shock during the 6 months preceding enrollment. The primary end point of the trial was death from any cause or the delivery of a first shock for any reason (except those resulting from electrophysiologic testing). At the end of the follow-up period of 12 months there was a significant reduction of the primary end point in the sotalol treatment arm, with a relative risk reduction (RRR) of 48% (P<.001). The beneficial effect of sotalol in preventing recurrent ICD shocks was equally effective in patients with normal and depressed left ventricular ejection fraction. An added benefit of sotalol was to reduce inappropriate ICD shocks resulting from supraventricular arrhythmia. There was no significant difference in the incidence of TDP between the sotalol arm and the placebo arm.[50]

Azimilide, a potassium-channel blocker selective for the $I_{Ks}$ and $I_{Kr}$ currents, was the next AAD evaluated in this clinical situation. The Shock Inhibition Evaluation with Azimilide (SHIELD) trial, a placebo-controlled randomized trial, evaluated the efficacy of azimilide in preventing recurrent ICD shocks. Patients with poor left ventricular systolic function (ejection fraction <40%) with a prophylactic ICD for secondary prevention of SCD or with new-onset ventricular arrhythmia were included. The primary end points of the trial

were all-cause shocks plus symptomatic VT terminated by ATP and all-cause shocks. This trial was also a dose-finding study, and used 75 mg or 125 mg azimilide for prevention of recurrent ventricular arrhythmia resulting in ICD shocks. A significant reduction in the composite primary end point of all-cause shocks plus symptomatic VT terminated by ATP was noted in the azimilide arm, with RRR of 57% (hazard ratio [HR] = 0.43, 95% confidence interval [CI] 0.26–0.69, P = .0006) and 47% (HR = 0.53, 95% CI 0.34–0.83, P = .0053) at 75-mg and 125-mg doses, respectively. However, the risk reduction in the second primary outcome of all-cause shocks did not reach statistical significance. Five patients in the azimilide arm developed TDP, all of whom were successfully treated by the ICD.[51] A subgroup analysis of the SHIELD trial using 125 mg/d showed a significant reduction in the risk of recurrent ES, with an RRR of 55% (HR = 0.45, 95% CI 0.23–0.87, P = .018) compared with placebo.[52] Azimilide is an investigational agent, and has not yet been approved by the Food and Drug Administration for use in this clinical situation.

The Optimal Pharmacologic Therapy in Cardioverter Defibrillator Patients (OPTIC) trial was designed to compare amiodarone (administered with a β-blocker) and sotalol with standard β-blocker therapy for prevention of ICD shocks in patients with spontaneous or inducible ventricular arrhythmia (VT or VF), receiving an ICD. Eligible patients were randomized to receive amiodarone (with β-blockers), sotalol, or β-blockers in a blinded fashion (1:1:1 concealed allocation). The average doses of medications used were 285 mg for amiodarone and 180 mg for sotalol. All patients had their ICD programmed in a standardized fashion to maximize ATP and avoid shocks during ventricular arrhythmia. The primary outcome of the study was the time to first recurrence of any shock delivered by the ICD. A reduction in the risk of shock was observed with use of amiodarone plus β-blocker or sotalol versus β-blocker alone (HR = 0.44, 95% CI 0.28–0.68; P<.001). Amiodarone plus β-blocker also reduced the risk of shock compared with β-blocker alone (HR = 0.27, 95% CI 0.14–0.52; P<0,001) and sotalol (HR = 0.43; 95% CI 0.22–0.85; P = .02). There was a trend for sotalol to reduce shocks compared with β-blocker alone (HR = 0.61; 95% CI 0.37–1.01; P = .055). The rates of AAD discontinuation at 1 year were 18.2% for amiodarone, 23.5% for sotalol, and 5.3% for β-blockers.[49] This trial demonstrated the efficacy of amiodarone in preventing recurrent ventricular arrhythmia in ICD patients. However, amiodarone therapy is associated with pulmonary, thyroid, hepatic, and dermatologic side effects, resulting in poor patient compliance and eventual discontinuation in most patients.[53]

Dofetilide, a potassium-channel blocker ($I_{Kr}$ current), is another class III AAD that has been compared with sotalol for prevention of ventricular arrhythmia in patients with ischemic cardiomyopathy. This randomized trial was conducted before ICDs were routinely used for SCD prevention in this population. The study evaluated the efficacy of the AAD in suppressing ventricular arrhythmia during programmed electrical stimulation during electrophysiologic testing. Dofetilide and sotalol were found to be equally effective in reducing the primary end point (35.9% responders in the dofetilide group vs 33.6% in the sotalol; $P$ not significant). In patients responding to the AAD during electrophysiologic testing there was no difference in the incidence of recurrent ventricular arrhythmia in either group, during long-term follow-up.[54] Dofetilide has not been evaluated in ICD patients for prevention of recurrent ventricular arrhythmia (**Table 1**).

## Novel Antiarrhythmic Drugs

Dronedarone and celivarone are AAD similar to amiodarone in their pharmacologic actions. A randomized trial evaluating the efficacy of dronedarone in improving cardiovascular outcomes in patients with moderate to severe CHF was prematurely terminated because of increased mortality in the dronedarone arm. Dronedarone has not been evaluated for prevention or treatment of ventricular arrhythmia in ICD patients. Celivarone is being evaluated for its efficacy in preventing ventricular arrhythmia and shocks in ICD patients with left ventricular ejection fraction of less than 40%.[55–57]

## Combination AAD Therapy

Combinations of AAD have been used to manage ICD patients with drug-refractory (amiodarone and sotalol) ventricular arrhythmia, especially in the setting of ES.[41] This strategy has not been systematically evaluated, and is potentially associated with enhanced proarrhythmia and risk of CHF secondary to adverse drug interactions.

## Beneficial Effects of AAD in the ICD Patient with Shocks: Beneficial Drug-Device Interactions

AAD therapy in ICD patients with ventricular arrhythmia and shocks is primarily intended to eliminate or at least reduce recurrence. An additional benefit of AAD therapy is the potential to reduce the burden of concomitant supraventricular arrhythmia, which may be responsible for ICD shocks in a proportion of patients. AAD drug therapy may slow the rate of ventricular arrhythmia, making it more hemodynamically tolerable and amenable to termination by ATP before a shock is delivered. Certain AAD (sotalol and dofetilide) also reduce the defibrillation threshold (DFT) and may help in easier termination of ventricular arrhythmia.[58–61]

## Adverse Effects of AAD in the ICD Patient with Shocks: Adverse Drug-Device Interactions

AAD therapy may cause slowing of ventricular arrhythmia and, if the rate is slower than the programmed ICD detection rate, may result in failure to deliver therapy. This failure can have potentially lethal outcomes in ICD patients, many of whom have severely impaired systolic ventricular function. Class I and III agents have the most pronounced effect on ventricular arrhythmia cycle length, and may cause the tachycardia to slow by as much as 80 milliseconds. The slowing of ventricular arrhythmia cycle length may result in overlap with sinus and supraventricular tachycardia rates, making discrimination from VT difficult. This situation may result in inappropriate shocks during exercise or AF. The pacing threshold may rise with concomitant AAD therapy, and this may cause failure to capture during rapid ATP. To prevent this it may be required to test pacing thresholds during rapid ATP to obtain a safety margin of at least 4 to 5 times.[62,63] AAD therapy is also known to result in small increments in DFT (class I and III agents). However, most ICDs in use currently have the ability to deliver 31 to 41 J of energy during defibrillation, and this provides an adequate safety margin to account for the increase in DFT. ICD patients on adjunctive AAD therapy may develop suppression of sinus node function and atrioventricular node conduction, leading to dependence on the ICD for bradycardia pacing; this may result in fatigue or CHF, especially if the rate response feature has not been activated, and reduction in battery life. Finally, the proarrhythmic actions of AAD may result in ventricular arrhythmia and ICD shocks.[64,65]

These "drug-device" interactions are summarized in **Table 2**.

## Catheter Ablation of Ventricular Arrhythmia

Two recent trials have evaluated the role of prophylactic catheter ablation for prevention of recurrent ventricular arrhythmia and shock in ICD patients. In both trials there was significant reduction in recurrent ventricular arrhythmia and ICD shocks in the catheter ablation arm.[40,42] Two ongoing trials are comparing the efficacy of prophylactic catheter ablation with AAD therapy

**Table 1**
Randomized trials comparing AAD therapy for prevention of ventricular arrhythmia and shocks in patients with an ICD

| Trial | Study Design | Study Population | Primary Outcome | Treatment Arm | Control Arm | Results |
|---|---|---|---|---|---|---|
| Pacifico et al,[50] 1999 | RCT; Placebo controlled | ICD implanted for secondary prevention of SCD | Risk of death from any cause or the delivery of a first shock for any reason | Sotalol 160–320 mg/d | Placebo | Treatment with sotalol was associated with a lower incidence of the primary end point (reduction in risk, 48%; P<.001 by the log-rank test) |
| Dorian et al,[51] 2004 SHIELD Trial | RCT; Placebo controlled | ICD implanted for secondary or primary prevention of SCD with an ICD shock for spontaneous VT/VF | All-cause shocks plus symptomatic tachyarrhythmia terminated by ATP, and all-cause shocks | Azimilide; 75 or 125 mg/d | Placebo | Treatment with azimilide significantly reduced the composite primary end point, with relative risk reductions of 57% (HR 0.43, 95% CI 0.26–0.69, P = .0006) and 47% (HR 0.53, 95% CI 0.34–0.83, P = .0053) at 75-mg and 125-mg doses, respectively The reduction in all-cause shocks did not reach statistical significance |
| Connolly et al,[49] 2006 OPTIC Trial | RCT | ICD implanted for secondary prevention of SCD with spontaneous VT/VF or inducible VT/VF on electrophysiologic study | First occurrence of any shock delivered by the ICD at 1 year | Amiodarone + β-blockers; sotalol | β-Blockers | Amiodarone + β-blockers significantly reduced the primary end point at 1 year compared with sotalol and β-blockers alone (HR 0.27 [P<.001] and 0.43 [P = .02], respectively) |

*Abbreviations:* AAD, antiarrhythmic drugs; ATP, antitachycardia pacing; HR, hazard ratio; ICD, implantable cardioverter-defibrillator; RCT, randomized controlled trial; VF, ventricular fibrillation; VT, ventricular tachycardia.

**Table 2**
**Beneficial and adverse "drug-device" interactions**

| Beneficial Drug-Device Interactions | Adverse Drug-Device Interactions |
|---|---|
| Slowing the rate of VT making the arrhythmia hemodynamically better tolerated | Slowing the rate of VT below the programmed ICD detection rate |
| Slower VT may be terminated by ATP, thereby avoiding shocks | Overlap of slower VT with sinus tachycardia and SVT resulting in inappropriate ICD therapy |
| Reduction in SVT burden prevents inappropriate ICD shocks | Amiodarone increases DFT |
| Sotalol and dofetilide lower DFT | Sinus node dysfunction and AV conduction block resulting in forced ventricular pacing |
|  | Proarrhythmic effects of AAD may lead to ICD therapy |

*Abbreviations:* AAD, antiarrhythmic drugs; ATP, antitachycardia pacing; AV, atrioventricular; DFT, defibrillation threshold; ICD, implantable cardioverter-defibrillator; SVT, supraventricular tachycardia; VT, ventricular tachycardia.

in preventing recurrent ventricular arrhythmia and shocks in ICD patients.[66,67] A detailed evaluation of the role of catheter ablation in shock prevention in ICD patients is beyond the scope of this review.

### Approach to AAD Therapy in Patients with ICD and Recurrent Ventricular Arrhythmia

The most difficult issues facing physicians who are treating patients with ventricular arrhythmia and ICD shocks are when to start AAD therapy and which AAD to select as first-line therapy (**Fig. 1**). The evidence presented herein suggests that patients with ICD for secondary prevention of SCD and those with ICD for primary prevention indications and at least one appropriate ICD therapy (shock or symptomatic VT terminated by ATP) are most likely to benefit from AAD therapy. Amiodarone is the most effective antiarrhythmic available for prevention of recurrent ventricular arrhythmia and shocks in these patients. However, amiodarone is associated with significant side

effects that limit its use in the long term. Sotalol is the next best alternative in patients who cannot tolerate amiodarone or refuse to take it. Sotalol at doses necessary to manifest its class III antiarrhythmic actions is often associated with troublesome side effects such as fatigue and depression.

All patients with poor systolic function and structural heart disease (ischemic/nonischemic dilated cardiomyopathy) should be started on maximally tolerated doses of β-blockers. In addition, any reversible causes responsible for precipitating ventricular arrhythmia (eg, thyrotoxicosis) should be managed. The ICD should be programmed optimally to maximize ATP and prevent unnecessary shocks.

In patients tolerating and responding to amiodarone therapy, the lowest effective dose (usually 200 mg/d) should be continued. Patients not having recurrences can be cautiously taken off AAD therapy after a reasonable period of follow-up (12–18 months), In case of recurrences the dose of amiodarone can be increased to 300 or 400 mg/d. Patients having recurrent ventricular arrhythmia and shocks while on adequate doses of amiodarone may need additional therapy with class I or substitution by other class III (dofetilide/azimilide) AAD. It should be noted that this approach has not been validated in clinical trials. Sotalol is a less effective alternative in patients intolerant to amiodarone.

Clinical trials have shown that catheter ablation is an effective first-line and adjunctive treatment for ventricular arrhythmia and prevention of ICD shocks.[39–42] However, these trials have not compared catheter ablation with AAD therapy directly. Randomized clinical trials are under way to evaluate the role of catheter ablation as first-line treatment instead of AAD therapy, and as an adjunct to AAD therapy in refractory cases.[66,67]

This approach is not applicable to special situations such as patients with ion channelopathies, for whom treatment should be individualized.

## UNRESOLVED ISSUES AND LIMITATIONS

Clinical trials evaluating the efficacy of AAD therapy in preventing ventricular arrhythmia and shocks in ICD patients have mainly included patients with structural heart disease and left ventricular systolic dysfunction (ischemic or nonischemic cardiomyopathy). Therefore, the information and recommendations provided in this review should be used only in this patient population. Prevention of recurrent ventricular arrhythmia is very important to the patient with symptoms and poor quality of life resulting from ICD therapy. However, as yet it is not clear

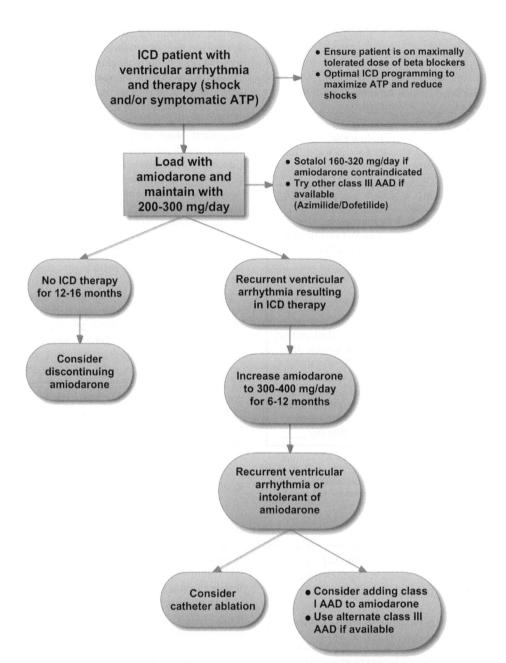

**Fig. 1.** Approach to management of the ICD patient with ventricular arrhythmia and frequent shocks. AAD, antiarrhythmic drugs; ATP, antitachycardia pacing; ICD, implantable cardioverter-defibrillator.

whether preventing ventricular arrhythmia and shocks in ICD patients can prevent the increased risk of mortality associated with this condition. The optimal treatment strategy for managing ICD patients with ventricular arrhythmia has not yet been defined clearly. Ongoing trials comparing AAD with catheter ablation and "hybrid" treatment (AAD with catheter ablation) will, it is hoped, clarify this issue.[66,67]

## SUMMARY

ICDs have been firmly established as the treatment of choice in patients at high risk of SCD. However, a majority of patients will invariably develop recurrent ventricular arrhythmia and receive shocks at some point after ICD implantation. Ventricular arrhythmia and ICD therapy are poor prognostic markers in such patients, and are associated with an increased risk of mortality and morbidity. AAD therapy should be initiated in patients with ventricular arrhythmia and ICD shocks. Amiodarone is the most effective AAD available, with sotalol being the next best alternative. Side effects associated with commonly used AAD therapy are responsible for discontinuation of medications in a significant proportion of patients. The clinician also needs to be aware of interactions between AAD and the ICD that may potentially harm the patient. There are very few pharmacologic alternatives to amiodarone and sotalol in this clinical situation, making it difficult to manage the patient refractory to or intolerant of these two AAD. Catheter ablation has emerged as a new management strategy in ICD patients with ventricular arrhythmia and shocks. Clinical trials comparing AAD therapy with catheter ablation or as adjunctive therapy are required to test the efficacy of these two management strategies.

## REFERENCES

1. The Antiarrhythmics Versus Implantable Defibrillators (AVID) investigators. A comparison of antiarrhythmic-drug therapy with implantable defibrillators in patients resuscitated from near-fatal ventricular arrhythmias. N Engl J Med 1997;337:1576–83.
2. Connolly SJ, Gent M, Roberts R, et al. Canadian implantable defibrillator study (CIDS): a randomized trial of the implantable cardioverter defibrillator against amiodarone. Circulation 2000;101:1297–302.
3. Moss AJ, Zareba W, Hall WJ, et al. Prophylactic implantation of a defibrillator in patients with myocardial infarction and reduced ejection fraction. N Engl J Med 2002;346:877–83.
4. Bardy GH, Lee KL, Mark DB, et al. Amiodarone or an implantable cardioverter-defibrillator for congestive heart failure. N Engl J Med 2005;352:225–37.
5. Birnie DH, Sambell C, Johansen H, et al. Use of implantable cardioverter defibrillators in Canadian and US survivors of out-of-hospital cardiac arrest. CMAJ 2007;177:41–6.
6. Mond HG, Irwin M, Ector H, et al. The world survey of cardiac pacing and cardioverter-defibrillators: calendar year 2005. An international cardiac pacing and electrophysiology society (ICPES) project. Pacing Clin Electrophysiol 2008;31:1202–12.
7. Goldberger Z, Lampert R. Implantable cardioverter-defibrillators—expanding indications and technologies. JAMA 2006;295:809–18.
8. Grimm W, Flores BT, Marchlinski FE, et al. Implantable cardioverter-defibrillator: shock occurrence and survival in 241 patients with implantable cardioverter-defibrillator therapy. Circulation 1993;87(6):1880–8.
9. Villacastin J, Almendral J, Arenal A, et al. Incidence and clinical significance of multiple consecutive, appropriate, high-energy discharges in patients with implanted cardioverter-defibrillators. Circulation 1996;93:753–62.
10. Saxon LA, Bristow MR, Boehmer J, et al. Predictors of sudden cardiac death and appropriate shock in the comparison of medical therapy, pacing, and defibrillation in heart failure (COMPANION) trial. Circulation 2006;114:2766–72.
11. Poole JE, Johnson GW, Hellkamp AS, et al. Prognostic importance of defibrillator shocks in patients with heart failure. N Engl J Med 2008;359:1009–17.
12. Daubert JP, Zareba W, Cannom DS, et al. Inappropriate implantable cardioverter-defibrillator shocks in MADIT II: frequency, mechanisms, predictors, and survival impact. J Am Coll Cardiol 2008;51:1357–65.
13. Gradaus R, Block M, Brachmann J, et al. Mortality, morbidity and complications in 3344 patients with implantable cardioverter defibrillators: result from the Germany ICD registry EURID. Pacing Clin Electrophysiol 2003;26:1511–8.
14. Moss AJ, Greenberg H, Case RB, et al. Long-term clinical course of patients after termination of ventricular tachyarrhythmia by an implanted defibrillator. Circulation 2004;110:3760–5.
15. Al-Khatib SM, Hellkamp AS, Lee KL, et al. Implantable cardioverter defibrillator therapy in patients with prior coronary revascularization in the Sudden Cardiac Death in Heart Failure Trial (SCD-HeFT). J Cardiovasc Electrophysiol 2008;19:1059–65.
16. Sweeney MO, Sherfesee L, DeGroot PJ, et al. Differences in effects of electrical therapy type for ventricular arrhythmias on mortality in implantable cardioverter-defibrillator patients. Heart Rhythm 2010;7:353–60.
17. VanRees JB, Borleffs JW, de Bie MK, et al. Inappropriate implantable cardioverter-defibrillator shocks—incidence, predictors, and impact on mortality. J Am Coll Cardiol 2011;57:556–62.
18. Irvine J, Dorian P, Baker B, et al. Quality of life in the Canadian Implantable Defibrillator Study (CIDS). Am Heart J 2002;144:282–9.
19. Schron EB, Exner DV, Yao Q, et al. Quality of life in the antiarrhythmics versus implantable defibrillators trial. Impact of therapy and influence of adverse symptoms and defibrillator shocks. Circulation 2002;105:589–94.
20. Mark DB, Anstrom KJ, Sun JL, et al. Quality of life with defibrillator therapy or amiodarone in heart failure. N Engl J Med 2008;359:999–1008.
21. Namerow PB, Firth BR, Heywood GM, et al. Quality-of-life six months after CABG surgery in patients randomized to ICD versus no ICD therapy: Findings from the CABG patch trial. Pacing Clin Electrophysiol 1999;22:1305–13.
22. Freedberg NA, Hill JN, Fogel RI, et al. Recurrence of symptomatic ventricular arrhythmias in patients with implantable cardioverter defibrillator after the first device therapy. J Am Coll Cardiol 2001;37:1910–5.

23. Wathen MS, Sweeney MO, DeGroot PJ, et al. Shock reduction using antitachycardia pacing for spontaneous rapid ventricular tachycardia in patients with coronary artery disease. Circulation 2001;104: 796–801.

24. Wathen MS, DeGroot PJ, Sweeney MO, et al. Prospective randomized multicenter trial of empirical antitachycardia pacing versus shocks for spontaneous rapid ventricular tachycardia in patients with implantable cardioverter-defibrillators: Pacing Fast Ventricular Tachycardia Reduces Shock Therapies (Pain FREE Rx II) trial results. Circulation 2004; 110:2591–6.

25. Wilkoff BL, Williamson BD, Stern RS, et al. Strategic programming of detection and therapy parameters in implantable cardioverter-defibrillators reduces shocks in primary prevention patients: results from the PREPARE (Primary Prevention Parameters Evaluation) study. J Am Coll Cardiol 2008;52:541–50.

26. Verma A, Kilicaslan F, Marrouche NF, et al. Prevalence, predictors, and mortality significance of the causative arrhythmia in patients with electrical storm. J Cardiovasc Electrophysiol 2004;15:1265–70.

27. Exner DV, Pinski SL, Wyse DG, et al. Electrical storm presages nonsudden death: The antiarrhythmics versus implantable defibrillators (AVID) trial. Circulation 2001;103:2066–71.

28. Gatzoulis KA, Andrikopoulos GK, Apostolopoulos T, et al. Electrical storm is an independent predictor of adverse long-term outcome in the era of implantable defibrillator therapy. Europace 2005;7:184–92.

29. Stein KM, Euler DE, Mehra R, et al. Do atrial tachyarrhythmias beget ventricular tachyarrhythmias in defibrillator recipients? J Am Coll Cardiol 2002;40:335–40.

30. Dorian P, Al-Khalidi HR, Hohnloser SH, et al. Azimilide reduces emergency department visits and hospitalizations in patients with an implantable cardioverter-defibrillator in a placebo-controlled clinical trial. J Am Coll Cardiol 2008;52:1076–83.

31. Otmani A, Trinquart L, Marijon E, et al. Rates and predictors of appropriate implantable cardioverter-defibrillator therapy delivery: results from the EVA-DEF cohort study. Am Heart J 2009;158:230–7.

32. CAST Investigators. Preliminary report: effect of encainide and flecainide on mortality in a randomized trial of arrhythmia suppression after myocardial infarction. N Engl J Med 1989;321:406–12.

33. IMPACT Research Group. International Mexiletine and Placebo Antiarrhythmic Coronary Trial: I. Report on arrhythmia and other findings. J Am Coll Cardiol 1984;4:1148–63.

34. The Cardiac Arrhythmia Suppression Trial II (CAST) Investigators. Effect of the antiarrhythmic agent moricizine on survival after myocardial infarction. N Engl J Med 1992;327:227–33.

35. Waldo AL, Camm AJ, de Ruyter H, et al. The SWORD Investigators. Effect of d-sotalol on mortality in patients with left ventricular dysfunction after myocardial infarction. Lancet 1996;348:7–12.

36. Dorian P, Cass D, Shwartz B, et al. Amiodarone as compared with lidocaine for shock resistant ventricular fibrillation. N Engl J Med 2002;346(12):884–90.

37. Cairns JA, Connolly SJ, Roberts R, et al. Randomised trial of outcome after myocardial infarction in patients with frequent or repetitive ventricular premature depolarisations: CAMIAT. Canadian Amiodarone Myocardial Infarction Arrhythmia Trial Investigators. Lancet 1997;349(9053):675–82.

38. Julian DG, Camm AJ, Frangin G, et al. European Myocardial Infarct Amiodarone Trial Investigators. Randomised trial of effect of amiodarone on mortality in patients with left ventricular dysfunction after recent myocardial infarction: EMIAT. Lancet 1997;349:667–74.

39. Della Bella P, De Ponti R, Uriarte JA, et al. Catheter ablation and antiarrhythmic drugs for haemodynamically tolerated post-infarction ventricular tachycardia; long-term outcome in relation to acute electrophysiologic findings. Eur Heart J 2002;23: 414–24.

40. Reddy VY, Reynolds MR, Neuzil P, et al. Prophylactic catheter ablation for the prevention of defibrillator therapy. N Engl J Med 2007;357:2657–65.

41. Carbucicchio C, Santamaria M, Trevisi N, et al. Catheter ablation for the treatment of electrical storm in patients with implantable cardioverter-defibrillators: short- and long-term outcomes in a prospective single-center study. Circulation 2008;117:462–9.

42. Kuck KH, Schaumann A, Eckardt L, et al. Catheter ablation of stable ventricular tachycardia before defibrillator implantation in patients with coronary heart disease (VTACH): a multicentre randomised controlled trial. Lancet 2010;375:31–40.

43. Nattel S, Singh BN. Evolution, mechanisms, and classification of antiarrhythmic drugs: focus on class III actions. Am J Cardiol 1999;84:11R–9R.

44. Marchlinski FE, Zado ES, Deely MP, et al. Concomitant device and drug therapy: current trends, potential benefits, and adverse interactions. Am J Cardiol 1999;84:69R–75R.

45. Belhassen B, Glick A, Viskin S. Efficacy of quinidine in high-risk patients with Brugada syndrome. Circulation 2004;110:1731–7.

46. Jongman JK, Jepkes-Bruin N, Ramdat Misier AR, et al. Electrical storms in Brugada syndrome successfully treated with isoproterenol infusion and quinidine orally. Neth Heart J 2007;15:151–4.

47. Yusuf S, Peto R, Lewis J, et al. Beta blockade during and after myocardial infarction: an overview of the randomized trials. Prog Cardiovasc Dis 1985;27: 335–71.

48. CIBIS-II Investigators and Committees. The Cardiac Insufficiency Bisoprolol Study II (CIBIS-II): a randomised trial. Lancet 1999;353:9–13.

49. Connolly SJ, Dorian P, Roberts RS, et al. Comparison of beta-blockers, amiodarone plus beta-blockers, or sotalol for prevention of shocks from implantable cardioverter defibrillators: the OPTIC Study: a randomized trial. JAMA 2006;295:165–71.

50. Pacifico A, Hohnloser SH, Williams JH, et al. Prevention of implantable-defibrillator shocks by treatment with sotalol. d,l-Sotalol Implantable Cardioverter-Defibrillator Study Group. N Engl J Med 1999;340:1855–62.

51. Dorian P, Borggrefe M, Al-Khalidi HR, et al. SHock Inhibition Evaluation with azimilide (SHIELD) investigators. Placebo-controlled, randomized clinical trial of azimilide for prevention of ventricular tachyarrhythmias in patients with an implantable cardioverter defibrillator. Circulation 2004;110:3646–54.

52. Hohnloser S, Dorian P, Al-Khalidi H, et al. Electrical storms in patients with implantable defibrillators: results from Shock Inhibition Evaluation with Azimilide (SHIELD) trial [abstract 2361]. Circulation 2005;112(Suppl II):II-492.

53. Bokhari F, Newman D, Greene M, et al. Long-term comparison of the implantable cardioverter defibrillator versus amiodarone: eleven year follow-up of a subset of patients in the Canadian Implantable Defibrillator Study (CIDS). Circulation 2004;110:112–6.

54. Boriani G, Lubinski A, Capucci A, et al. A multicentre, double blind randomized crossover comparative study on the efficacy and safety of dofetilide vs sotalol in patients with inducible sustained ventricular tachycardia and ischaemic heart disease. Eur Heart J 2001;22:2180–91.

55. Hohnloser SH, Crijns HJ, van Eickels M, et al. Effect of dronedarone on cardiovascular events in atrial fibrillation. N Engl J Med 2009;360:668–78.

56. Kober L, Torp-Pedersen C, McMurray JJ, et al. Increased mortality after dronedarone therapy for severe heart failure. N Engl J Med 2008;358:2678–87.

57. Gautier P, Serre M, Cosnier-Pucheu S, et al. In vivo and in vitro antiarrhythmic effects of SSR149744C in animal models of atrial fibrillation and ventricular arrhythmias. J Cardiovasc Pharmacol 2005;45:125–35.

58. Dorian P, Newman D. Effect of sotalol on ventricular fibrillation and defibrillation in humans. Am J Cardiol 1993;72(Suppl):72A–9A.

59. Beatch GN, Dickenson DR, Tang ASL. Dofetilide: relationship between refractory period extension and defibrillation threshold [abstract]. Pacing Clin Electrophysiol 1995;18:820.

60. Naccarelli GV, Zipes DP, Rahilly T, et al. Influence of tachycardia cycle length and antiarrhythmic drugs on pacing termination and acceleration of ventricular tachycardia. Am Heart J 1983;105:1–5.

61. Roy D, Waxman HL, Buxton AE, et al. Termination of ventricular tachycardia: role of tachycardia cycle length. Am J Cardiol 1982;50:1346–50.

62. Marchlinski FE, Buxton AE, Kindwall KE, et al. Comparison of individual and combined effects of procainamide and amiodarone in patients with sustained ventricular tachyarrhythmias. Circulation 1988;78:583–91.

63. Hook BG, Perlman RL, Callans DJ, et al. Acute and chronic cycle length dependent increase in ventricular pacing threshold. Pacing Clin Electrophysiol 1992;15:1437–44.

64. Brode SE, Schwartzman D, Callans DJ, et al. ICD-antiarrhythmic drug and ICD-pacemaker interactions. J Cardiovasc Electrophysiol 1997;8:830–42.

65. Johnson N, Marchlinski FE. The need to enhance diagnostic specificity to avoid device response to supraventricular rhythms and the risk of induced ventricular arrhythmias. J Am Coll Cardiol 1991;18:1418–22.

66. Ventricular Tachycardia (VT) Ablation Versus Enhanced Drug Therapy (VANISH). Available at: http://clinicaltrials.gov/ct2/show/NCT00905853?term=VANISH&rank=1. Accessed February 16, 2011.

67. Catheter Ablation Versus Amiodarone for Shock Prophylaxis in Defibrillator Patients With Ventricular Tachycardia (CEASE-VT). Available at: http://clinicaltrials.gov/ct2/show/study/NCT01097330. Accessed February 16, 2011.

# Should Every Broken Lead Be Extracted?

Melanie Maytin, MD*, Laurence M. Epstein, MD

## KEYWORDS

- Lead extraction • Lead management
- Implantable cardioverter-defibrillator • Pacemaker

With expanded indications for device therapy, the use of cardiovascular implantable electronic devices (CIEDs) has greatly increased over the past decade.[1–3] In fact, it estimated that there are more than 4.5 million active devices with more than 1 million new leads implanted annually.[4,5] Coincident with the increase in CIED use, there has been a similar increase in device complications.[6–12] As a result of longer patient life expectancies and the occurrence of more frequent device system revisions for complications[7] and/or lead malfunction,[6,8–11] clinicians increasingly are faced with the challenging choice of extraction or abandonment of sterile, superfluous leads. The decision is difficult and highly controversial,[5,13–21] with limited rigorous evidence on either side.

As with any intervention, the decision to proceed with lead extraction for the management of lead malfunctions mandates a comparison of the risks of extraction with the risks of lead abandonment (**Fig. 1**). In this article the authors present available data that can help clinicians with this complex issue.

## LEAD ABANDONMENT

In evaluating the best management strategy of superfluous leads, rigorous evidence from large-scale randomized trials is lacking and the available reported observational and cohort studies of lead abandonment are often underpowered, generating more confusion than answers (**Table 1**). Objective risk evaluation for lead abandonment, as for any procedure, includes an assessment of the procedural risks as well as the potential future risks.

### Procedural Risk

The REPLACE registry provides current, real-world experience regarding the short-term periprocedural risks associated with lead abandonment. Poole and colleagues[22] compared the major complication rates between patients undergoing generator replacement with lead addition for replacement or upgrade and patients undergoing generator replacement alone. The 6-month major complication rates for lead revision in comparison with generator change alone were astonishingly high (15.3% vs 4%) with a 1.8% procedural complication rate (0.7% cardiac perforation, 0.8% pneumothorax or hemithorax and 0.3% cardiac arrest) and the majority of late complications resulting from lead dislodgement or malfunction. Although typically thought of as having little to no associated procedural risks, lead abandonment in the REPLACE registry was associated with procedural complication rates in excess of those reported for lead extraction.[16,17,23,24]

### Future Risk: Venous Access

The controversy surrounding the management of superfluous leads often focuses on the argument of maintaining venous patency. As life expectancies and the number of younger individuals receiving CIEDs increase, the device-years per person increases along with the attendant potential risks of infection, lead malfunction, and the need for system upgrade, escalating the chance of the eventual need for implantation via the contralateral venous system. Thus, the primary

Dr Maytin has no disclosures. Dr Epstein has received research grants from and is a consultant for Boston Scientific, Medtronic, Spectranetics and St Jude Medical; and has equity in and served as a board member for Carrot Medical.

Division of Cardiovascular Medicine, Brigham and Women's Hospital, 75 Francis Street, Boston, MA 02215, USA
* Corresponding author.
*E-mail address:* mmaytin@partners.org

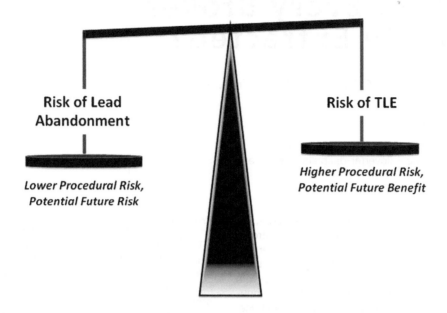

## Risk vs. Risk

**Fig. 1.** Risk versus risk. The decision regarding lead extraction or abandonment requires comparison of the current risks of lead extraction with the future risks of both lead abandonment and potential lead extraction. TLE, transvenous lead extraction.

benefit of removing rather than replacing a lead is preserving venous access, ie, the continued use of the implant vein to preserve contralateral or alternative venous access for future use. Consequently, implanting physicians are required to evaluate and implement the best lead-management strategy for each individual for both the immediate procedure and future procedures—hence the imperative to preserve venous access and not venous patency.

In fact, venous patency is likely not maintained with either lead revision or extraction. Within 4 to 5 days of implant, extensive thrombosis and near complete encapsulation of intravascular pacing leads with a fibrin sheath have been observed.[25,26] In addition, younger patients develop more vigorous fibrotic responses and frequently develop progressive calcification of the areas of fibrosis.[27] Several clinical studies have demonstrated frequent occurrence of asymptomatic venous stenoses and occlusion after endovascular pacing and defibrillator lead placement.[28–30] Similarly, asymptomatic venous thrombosis is commonly observed in patients with abandoned leads, again with little clinical significance.[31–34] By contrast, little is known about the effects of lead extraction on venous patency, and attempts to study this have been confounded by ipsilateral reimplantation, making it impossible to isolate the effects of extraction.[35]

CIED lead revision can be and has been accomplished despite venous occlusion. The solution frequently involves venoplasty,[36] unconventional ipsilateral venous entry,[37–40] or contralateral venous access with tunneling or complete abandonment of the original system. Each approach has its limitations. Tunneled leads can be painful both at implant and chronically, and can be apt to erode.[41] Contralateral implantation fails to preserve venous access, and should not be considered responsible lead management (**Fig. 2**) or a reasonable alternative to lead extraction. Although venoplasty and unconventional ipsilateral venous access avoid the unnecessary use of the contralateral venous system, both result in increased lead burden, have uncertain effects on lead survival, and carry potential present and future risks. Furthermore, in some cases venoplasty of the occluded vein may not be possible.

### Future Risk: Infection

With the surge in CIED use, there has been a disproportionate increase in CIED infection (0.8%–19.9% CIED patients).[42–44] The number of CIED implants increased by 12% between 2003 and 2006, while the number of CIED infections rose by an alarming 57%.[44] The presence of more than 2 pacing leads[45] has been identified as a risk factor for CIED infection (**Fig. 3**). Despite this, data regarding the risk of CIED infection in patients with abandoned leads have failed to demonstrate an increased risk of device-related infection, likely attributable to small sample size and abbreviated follow-up periods.[33,46–49] For example, among young patients with abandoned leads, Silvetti and Drago[33] observed a startling 11% incidence of CIED infection compared with a 2% incidence in all pacemaker patients, although the trial was underpowered to reach statistical significance. All patients with CIED infection required definitive treatment with lead removal. Similarly, Suga and colleagues[34] noted a significant increase in infection and asymptomatic venous occlusion in patients with multiple leads, although the end point was driven largely by venous pathology. As with the experience of Silvetti and colleagues, all patients with CIED infection underwent complete device system removal. Moreover, 44% of patients with asymptomatic venous occlusion required transvenous lead extraction (TLE) for ipsilateral venous access while the remaining 56% underwent contralateral implantation for lead revision, demonstrating that a significant percentage of patients with abandoned leads may eventually require extraction.

Mortality in device-related infection is reduced from 66% to 18% in patients treated with extraction and antibiotics. Eradication of CIED infection requires complete removal of the entire system.[50–52] The occurrence of device-related infection in the setting of previously abandoned leads increases both the difficulty and risk of the extraction procedure, due to the longer implant duration and lead-lead binding. While rigorous data regarding CIED infection risk and lead abandonment are lacking, the risk of device-related infection with increasing lead burden and the associated mortality with incomplete treatment require careful consideration of an individual's future risk in the management decision regarding superfluous leads.

### Future Risk: Lead-Lead Interaction

Lead-lead interaction between superfluous and active leads can result in the oversensing of specious signals and inappropriate inhibition of pacing, with potential serious sequelae (**Fig. 4**).[53–55] Although most implanters believe that lead-lead interaction can be avoided by eliminating contact between the active and abandoned lead, in fact physical lead-lead interaction is only one mechanism of spurious signal generation. False signals can be created by the production of galvanic current between two electrodes of different composition without physical contact

between the active and abandoned electrodes.[53,54] Observational studies of patients with abandoned leads have failed to demonstrate a significant occurrence of lead-lead interaction.[32,49,56] The lack of supportive data is a reflection of underpowered studies unable to detect a significant difference. For example, Wollmann and colleagues[56] observed a twofold increase in oversensing with inappropriate shocks in patients with an added as compared with replaced high-voltage lead. Moreover, in a prior observational study of added pace-sense leads, Wollmann and colleagues[49] found a 28.5% failure rate of the new pace-sense lead with half of the failures attributed to oversensing. As neither study clearly delineated the mechanism of oversensing (ie, lead fracture, T/P wave oversensing, or lead-lead interaction), the exact incidence of lead-lead interaction is not known.

### Future Risk: Central Venous System Stenosis and Thrombosis

Endovascular lead-induced venous stenosis and thrombosis is not limited to the implant veins. Multiple reports of superior vena cava (SVC) syndrome exist in the literature (**Fig. 5**).[57–64] Identified risk factors for the development of SVC syndrome include device infection, polyurethane leads, thrombophilia, and multiple leads.[60,61,64] Symptomatic SVC syndrome requires an invasive approach with surgical or percutaneous venoplasty frequently in association with lead extraction.[62] As a result, the 2009 Heart Rhythm Society Expert Consensus on Lead Extraction[20] has deemed any CIED procedure that would result in more than 4 leads on one side or 5 leads through the SVC a class IIa indication for lead extraction.

### Future Risk: Tricuspid Valve

Fibrous adhesion of electrodes to the tricuspid valve[25,26] and regurgitant valve disease of varying clinical significance are observed commonly following endovascular lead placement.[65,66] The incremental risk of lead burden on tricuspid regurgitation has not been defined, although small observational series of patients with abandoned leads have not demonstrated an increased risk of clinically significant regurgitant disease.[31,33] More recently, isolated cases of severe tricuspid stenosis from excessive lead burden have been reported in patients with 4 and 5 endovascular pacing leads.[67,68]

### Risk of Future Lead Extraction

Perhaps the most important risk of lead abandonment is the potential need for future lead extraction. As emphasized previously, the increasing

**Table 1**
Risks of lead abandonment

| Study | Study Type | Groups Studied | No. of Patients | No. of Leads | Follow-up (Years) | Primary End Point | Abandon Versus Remove | Comments |
|---|---|---|---|---|---|---|---|---|
| Wollmann et al[56] | RC | Add HV (A) vs Replace HV (R) | 33 A vs 53 R[a] | 2.6 ± 0.8 vs 1.4 ± 0.7[b] | 9.3 ± 2.7 vs 6.7 ± 3.8[b] | Event-free survival | ⇆ | Add HV decision due to failed TLE attempt in 70% |
| Wollmann et al[49] | PO | Add P/S | 151 | 2.3 | 3.6 ± 2.3 | Event-free survival | N/A | 28.5% failure rate of new P/S requiring repeat procedure |
| Suga et al[34] | RO | Patients with ≥1 abandoned lead | 433 | 2.8 | 3.1 ± 2.7 | Event-free survival | N/A | No. of abandoned leads higher in those with complications[b] |
| Furman et al[46] | RO | Patients with ≥1 abandoned lead | 152 | na | 4 | Event-free survival | N/A | One fatal case of DRE |
| Rettig et al[48] | RO | Patients with ≥1 abandoned lead | 25 | na | 1.8 | Event-free survival | N/A | Fatal embolization of cut lead |
| Silvetti and Drago[33] | RO | Young patients with abandoned leads | 18 | 1.1 ± 0.3 (abandoned) | 4 | Event-free survival | N/A | 11% DRE and 28% new contralateral implant |

| Study | | | Abandoned HV or P/S | | | Event-free survival | N/A | No sensing malfunction, VO, or change in DFT |
|---|---|---|---|---|---|---|---|---|
| Glikson et al[32] | RO | Abandoned HV or P/S | 78 | 1.5 (abandoned) | 3.1 ± 2.0 | Event-free survival | N/A | No sensing malfunction, VO, or change in DFT |
| de Cock et al[31] | PO | Patients with ≥3 leads vs age-matched dual chamber controls | 48 | 3.2 vs 2.0 | 7.4 ± 2.0 | Clinical VO, RHF, hospitalizations, AF & mortality | N/A | |
| Bohm et al[79] | RO | Patients with ≥1 abandoned lead (epi-/endocardial) | 60 | 1.0 (abandoned) | na | Event-free survival | N/A | 20% event rate driven by migration of cut leads |
| Sweeney et al[80] | PO | Device upgrades: Add vs Replace | 58 | na | 1.1 ± 1.1 | Event-free survival | ⇆ | |
| Parry et al[47] | RO | Patients with ≥1 abandoned lead (infectious vs noninfectious) | 119 | na | na | Event-free survival | N/A | 42% vs 3% rate of major complications infectious vs noninfectious |

*Abbreviations:* AF, atrial fibrillation; DFT, defibrillation threshold; DRE, device-related endocarditis; HV, high-voltage defibrillation lead; na, not available; N/A, not applicable—refers to studies in which comparative analysis is not possible; No., number; PO, prospective observational; P/S, pace-sense lead; RC, retrospective cohort; RHF, right heart failure; RO, retrospective observational; TLE, transvenous lead extraction; VO, venous occlusion.

[a] Mean lead implant duration 7.4 ± 2.9 years in the add HV group versus 4.1 ± 3.4 years in the replace group (*P*<.05).

[b] *P*<.05.

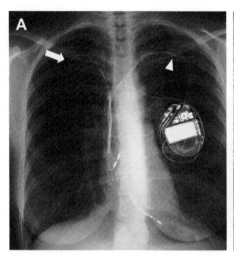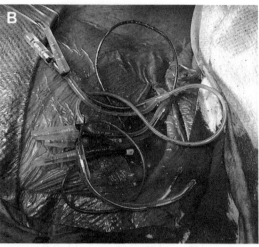

**Fig. 2.** (*A, B*) Excessive lead burden in the setting of repeated lead malfunction. (*A*) Posteroanterior chest radiography of a 37-year-old woman with long QT syndrome and bradycardia-dependent torsades des pointes, status post left pectoral dual-chamber pacemaker in 1993. She developed atrial lead failure in 1999. Attempted removal of the failed atrial lead was unsuccessful; new atrial lead was placed and failed, so lead was cut and abandoned (*arrowhead*). In 2003 she was upgraded to an ICD system. At the time of upgrade, the left subclavian vein was found to be occluded. The ventricular pace-sense lead was abandoned and a high-voltage lead was placed via the right subclavian vein and tunneled to the left pectoral pocket (*arrow*). She then presented with a nonfunctional atrial lead and was referred for extraction. The extraction procedure was complicated by lead burden, the need for bilateral lead removal, cut and abandoned leads, and long implant duration of the abandoned pacing leads. (*B*) Opened ICD pocket demonstrating tremendous lead burden in a 53-year-old man with ischemic cardiomyopathy, status post single-chamber ICD implant complicated by repeated high-voltage lead fracture with lead replacement and abandonment. The extraction procedure was made challenging by the intense lead-lead binding, particularly at the level of the superior vena cava coil.

incidence of CIED complications and longer patient life expectancies significantly increase the incremental likelihood of TLE over an individual lifetime. Moreover, lead extraction failure and complications are directly related to both lead implant duration and lead burden.[4,20,69–73] Byrd and colleagues[70] observed a twofold increase in the risk of extraction failure with every 3 years of implant duration in a prospective registry of more than 3500 leads extracted at 266 centers. Roux and colleagues[72] noted a similar association between unsuccessful TLE and lead implant duration as well as a higher complication rate among patients requiring bilateral extraction. More recently, 212 consecutive patients undergoing TLE were noted to have a 3.5-fold increase in TLE complications per additional right ventricular lead extracted, and a 50% increase in the need for powered sheath assistance per year increase in implant duration of the oldest lead.[4] These data are consistent with the authors' own observations that lead-to-lead binding, particularly in the setting of multiple endovascular leads, is frequently more technically challenging than vessel-to-lead fibrosis. Although quantification of this potential risk is difficult, it cannot be ignored.

## LEAD EXTRACTION

With the introduction of locking stylets and successful intravascular countertraction techniques, transvenous lead extraction has grown from a rare specialty reserved for life-threatening conditions to an increasingly practiced and often used tool with continually expanding indications.[20] The estimated demand for TLE has reached an annual extraction rate of 10,000 to 15,000 leads worldwide.[74] This growth is a result of both expanding device indications and the use and development of new tools and techniques, with higher success rates and lower morbidity and mortality.[16,17,23,24] The creation of the locking stylet and telescoping sheath represented a significant advance in transvenous lead extraction, allowing for critical opposing forces of traction and countertraction and yielding a higher degree of success and safety. Moreover, the introduction of the laser sheath further improved extraction success rates from 64% with traditional extraction techniques to 94% with laser-assisted extraction.[75]

Complication rates with TLE directly parallel operator experience. With an increase in operator experience from 20 to 120 cases to greater than 300 cases performed, major and minor complications are

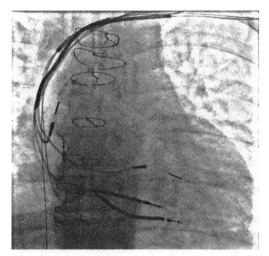

**Fig. 3.** High lead burden and pocket infection. Anteroposterior fluoroscopy of a 42-year-old man with ischemic heart disease and sinus node dysfunction, status post left pectoral dual-chamber pacemaker in 1998. Device system was upgraded to a left pectoral dual-chamber implantable cardioverter-defibrillator (ICD) in 2006 with abandonment of the atrial and ventricular pacemaker leads. ICD lead fracture occurred in September 2008 with addition of a new high-voltage lead and abandonment of the fractured lead. He presented 1 month later with pocket infection. Transvenous lead extraction proved technically challenging because of lead burden, lead-lead binding, and long implant duration of abandoned pacing leads.

reduced by half.[70] Large-scale multicenter randomized trials have confirmed the effect of experience on outcomes.[24,70,73,75,76] In addition, observational registries of experienced, high-volume extractionists have consistently demonstrated high success rates

(>99%) with exceedingly low major complication (<1.0%) and mortality rates (<0.3%).[16,17,23]

Similar outcomes have been reported with TLE for lead revision.[77,78] The safety and efficacy of lead extraction using mechanical dilation in the setting of subclavian vein thrombosis was first reported by Le Franc and colleagues,[78] who described 2 patients with defibrillator systems and thrombosis of the implant vein who required the implantation of new pacing and defibrillator electrodes. Recanalization of the implant vein was achieved without complication through the use of locking stylets and telescoping sheaths. Bracke and colleagues[77] presented a case series of 3 patients with subclavian vein stenosis and need for lead replacement who underwent successful laser-assisted extraction of a nonfunctional lead to gain access to the venous circulation. Venous dilation and/or stenting were not needed following recanalization of the implant vein with the laser sheath.

## RISK VERSUS RISK

The risks of TLE are concrete, with success and complication rates defined by large-scale randomized trials and registries, although this risk must be individualized on a case-by-case basis. The consideration of patient and lead characteristics and, perhaps most importantly, operator experience must be factored into the risk assessment of extraction (**Box 1**). Specific attention to the number of leads, implant duration, defibrillator versus pacing electrodes, and patient age must enter into the risk assessment process. By contrast, the risks of lead abandonment and, by extension, the potential risk of future TLE, are difficult to quantify. The majority of studies of

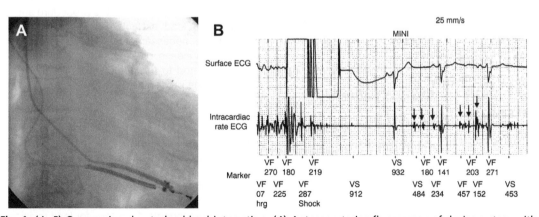

**Fig. 4.** (*A, B*) Oversensing due to lead-lead interaction. (*A*) Anteroposterior fluoroscopy of device system with abandoned ICD lead. (*B*) Intracardiac electrocardiogram (ECG) of a single-chamber ICD demonstrating noise with oversensing, resulting in inappropriate arrhythmia detection (*arrows*). Device interrogation demonstrated normal lead parameters.

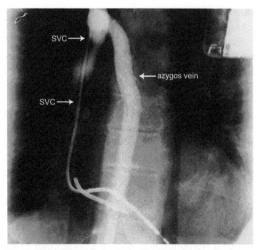

**Fig. 5.** Superior vena cava (SVC) stenosis. Contrast venography demonstrating complete occlusion of the SVC with a patent and dilated azygos vein in a patient with a left-sided ICD with a high-voltage lead and additional pace-sense lead.

abandoned leads are small registries or observational reports with a finite period of follow-up. In fact, most of these studies have follow-up times of less than 5 years. By contrast, in many of the extraction studies the average implant duration was 6 to 7 years with leads as old as 32 years. Observed complications, not surprisingly, often do not reach statistical significance, due to the short duration of follow-up and the small number of events that are frequently ascribed away or deemed unimportant. Moreover, most extraction experts would agree that the irrefutable risks of lead abandonment are related to the potential need for future extraction—a risk that is essentially ignored despite the frequent need for transvenous or surgical extraction in patients with complications of abandoned leads (29%–100% of abandoned leads with complications).[33,34,47,49,79] The potential need for future extraction is compounded

by the increased risk of extraction following lead abandonment given the increase in lead burden, lead-lead binding, and increase in implant duration in the time following the initial lead replacement. Thus, lead decisions at the time of device system revision must weigh the present risks of extraction with the future risks of both lead abandonment and potential future lead extraction.

The risk-risk analysis must also incorporate the indication for extraction. Device system revision in the setting of bilateral subclavian vein thrombosis, SVC occlusion, or ipsilateral venous occlusion preventing ipsilateral implantation with contraindications to contralateral implant (eg, arteriovenous fistula, vascular access port, mastectomy, and so forth) are class I indications for TLE.[20] Class IIa indications include need for lead implantation, with ipsilateral venous occlusion preventing ipsilateral implantation without contraindications to contralateral implant or lead implantation that would result in more than 4 leads in the implant vein or more than 5 leads through the SVC. Despite the compelling nature of these TLE indications, careful consideration of patient and lead characteristics as well as operator experience is integral to risk evaluation and the decision process. Superfluous leads with the potential for CIED interference and abandoned or redundant leads represent a class IIb indication for extraction, and are more controversial, requiring even more scrutiny of the potential complications.

Decisions regarding lead extraction must be made on an individual case-by-case basis, integrating various patient and lead characteristics and operator-related variables. TLE has the potential for significant morbidity and mortality, and may not be warranted in patients with a poor prognosis or for whom the risks of intervention clearly outweigh the risks of lead abandonment. In addition, those inexperienced in the procedure should not perform lead extractions, nor should those without the necessary tools available to attain complete success or in a setting not prepared and committed to the complete and safe performance of the procedure.[20]

## SUMMARY

The authors contend that while decisions regarding extraction of sterile, superfluous leads must be made on a case-by-case basis considering multiple patient-related and physician-related variables, lead extraction should be the preferred management strategy for lead revisions. Randomized controlled trials of extraction versus abandonment are lacking, but the available evidence from observational, cohort, and registry

---

**Box 1**
**Risk analysis in lead abandonment versus extraction**

Operator experience

TLE indication

Patient age, comorbidities, and life expectancy

Patient's wishes

Lead implant duration

Number of leads

Lead type (ie, pace-sense vs defibrillator lead)

studies support the contention that the potential future benefit of lead extraction outweighs the risks of lead abandonment, and that lead abandonment should be viewed as a "palliative procedure" that "just postpone[s] the inevitable future lead extraction."[33]

## REFERENCES

1. DeFrances CJ, Lucas CA, Buie VC, et al. 2006 National hospital discharge survey. Natl Health Stat Report 2008;(5):1.
2. Hammill SC, Kremers MS, Kadish AH, et al. Review of the ICD registry's third year, expansion to include lead data and pediatric ICD procedures, and role for measuring performance. Heart Rhythm 2009;6: 1397.
3. Maisel WH, Moynahan M, Zuckerman BD, et al. Pacemaker and ICD generator malfunctions: analysis of Food and Drug Administration annual reports. JAMA 2006;295:1901.
4. Agarwal SK, Kamireddy S, Nemec J, et al. Predictors of complications of endovascular chronic lead extractions from pacemakers and defibrillators: a single-operator experience. J Cardiovasc Electrophysiol 2009;20:171.
5. Borek PP, Wilkoff BL. Pacemaker and ICD leads: strategies for long-term management. J Interv Card Electrophysiol 2008;23:59.
6. Dorwarth U, Frey B, Dugas M, et al. Transvenous defibrillation leads: high incidence of failure during long-term follow-up. J Cardiovasc Electrophysiol 2003;14:38.
7. Eckstein J, Koller MT, Zabel M, et al. Necessity for surgical revision of defibrillator leads implanted long-term: causes and management. Circulation 2008;117:2727.
8. Ellenbogen KA, Wood MA, Shepard RK, et al. Detection and management of an implantable cardioverter defibrillator lead failure: incidence and clinical implications. J Am Coll Cardiol 2003;41:73.
9. Haqqani HM, Mond HG. The implantable cardioverter-defibrillator lead: principles, progress, and promises. Pacing Clin Electrophysiol 2009;32:1336.
10. Kleemann T, Becker T, Doenges K, et al. Annual rate of transvenous defibrillation lead defects in implantable cardioverter-defibrillators over a period of >10 years. Circulation 2007;115:2474.
11. Luria D, Glikson M, Brady PA, et al. Predictors and mode of detection of transvenous lead malfunction in implantable defibrillators. Am J Cardiol 2001;87:901.
12. Pakarinen S, Oikarinen L, Toivonen L. Short-term implantation-related complications of cardiac rhythm management device therapy: a retrospective single-centre 1-year survey. Europace 2010;12:103.
13. Bracke F, Meijer A, van Gelder B. Complications due to abandoned noninfected pacemaker leads. Pacing Clin Electrophysiol 2002;25:1533 [author reply: 1533].
14. Bracke FA. Yes we can! But should we? Lead extraction for superfluous pacemaker and implanted cardioverter-defibrillator leads. Europace 2009;11:546.
15. Bracke FA, Meijer A, Van Gelder LM. Malfunction of endocardial defibrillator leads and lead extraction: where do they meet? Europace 2002;4:19.
16. Jones SO, Eckart RE, Albert CM, et al. Large, single-center, single-operator experience with transvenous lead extraction: outcomes and changing indications. Heart Rhythm 2008;5:520.
17. Kennergren C, Bjurman C, Wiklund R, et al. A single-centre experience of over one thousand lead extractions. Europace 2009;11:612.
18. Levine PA. Should lead explantation be the practice standard when a lead needs to be replaced? Pacing Clin Electrophysiol 2000;23:421.
19. Venkataraman G, Hayes DL, Strickberger SA. Does the risk-benefit analysis favor the extraction of failed, sterile pacemaker and defibrillator leads? J Cardiovasc Electrophysiol 2009;20:1413.
20. Wilkoff BL, Love CJ, Byrd CL, et al. Transvenous lead extraction: heart rhythm society expert consensus on facilities, training, indications, and patient management: this document was endorsed by the American Heart Association (AHA). Heart Rhythm 2009;6:1085.
21. Xu W, Moore HJ, Karasik PE, et al. Management strategies when implanted cardioverter defibrillator leads fail: survey findings. Pacing Clin Electrophysiol 2009;32:1130.
22. Poole JE, Gleva MJ, Mela T, et al. Complication rates associated with pacemaker or implantable cardioverter-defibrillator generator replacements and upgrade procedures: results from the REPLACE registry. Circulation 2010;122:1553.
23. Bongiorni MG, Soldati E, Zucchelli G, et al. Transvenous removal of pacing and implantable cardiac defibrillating leads using single sheath mechanical dilatation and multiple venous approaches: high success rate and safety in more than 2000 leads. Eur Heart J 2008;29:2886.
24. Wazni O, Epstein LM, Carrillo RG, et al. Lead extraction in the contemporary setting: the LExICon study an observational retrospective study of consecutive laser lead extractions. J Am Coll Cardiol 2010;55:579.
25. Huang TY, Baba N. Cardiac pathology of transvenous pacemakers. Am Heart J 1972;83:469.
26. Robboy SJ, Harthorne JW, Leinbach RC, et al. Autopsy findings with permanent pervenous pacemakers. Circulation 1969;39:495.
27. Smith MC, Love CJ. Extraction of transvenous pacing and ICD leads. Pacing Clin Electrophysiol 2008;31:736.

28. Da Costa SS, Scalabrini Neto A, Costa R, et al. Incidence and risk factors of upper extremity deep vein lesions after permanent transvenous pacemaker implant: a 6-month follow-up prospective study. Pacing Clin Electrophysiol 2002;25:1301.

29. Haghjoo M, Nikoo MH, Fazelifar AF, et al. Predictors of venous obstruction following pacemaker or implantable cardioverter-defibrillator implantation: a contrast venographic study on 100 patients admitted for generator change, lead revision, or device upgrade. Europace 2007;9:328.

30. Korkeila P, Ylitalo A, Koistinen J, et al. Progression of venous pathology after pacemaker and cardioverter-defibrillator implantation: a prospective serial venographic study. Ann Med 2009;41:216.

31. de Cock CC, Vinkers M, Van Campe LC, et al. Long-term outcome of patients with multiple (>or = 3) noninfected transvenous leads: a clinical and echocardiographic study. Pacing Clin Electrophysiol 2000;23:423.

32. Glikson M, Suleiman M, Luria DM, et al. Do abandoned leads pose risk to implantable cardioverter-defibrillator patients? Heart Rhythm 2009;6:65.

33. Silvetti MS, Drago F. Outcome of young patients with abandoned, nonfunctional endocardial leads. Pacing Clin Electrophysiol 2008;31:473.

34. Suga C, Hayes DL, Hyberger LK, et al. Is there an adverse outcome from abandoned pacing leads? J Interv Card Electrophysiol 2000;4:493.

35. Bracke FA, Meijer A, Van Gelder LM. Symptomatic occlusion of the access vein after pacemaker or ICD lead extraction. Heart 2003;89:1348.

36. Worley SJ. Implant venoplasty: dilation of subclavian and coronary veins to facilitate device implantation: indications, frequency, methods, and complications. J Cardiovasc Electrophysiol 2008;19:1004.

37. Aleksic I, Kottenberg-Assenmacher E, Kienbaum P, et al. The innominate vein as alternative venous access for complicated implantable cardioverter defibrillator revisions. Pacing Clin Electrophysiol 2007;30:957.

38. Antonelli D, Freedberg NA, Turgeman Y. Supraclavicular vein approach for upgrading an implantable cardioverter defibrillator to a biventricular device. Pacing Clin Electrophysiol 2010;33:634.

39. Bhakta M, Obioha CC, Sorajja D, et al. Nontraditional implantable cardioverter defibrillator placement in adult patients with limited venous access: a case series. Pacing Clin Electrophysiol 2010;33:217.

40. Ranjan R, Henrikson CA. ICD implantation after crossing a totally occluded subclavian vein via collaterals from the superior vena cava. Pacing Clin Electrophysiol 2010;33:e14.

41. Gula LJ, Ames A, Woodburn A, et al. Central venous occlusion is not an obstacle to device upgrade with the assistance of laser extraction. Pacing Clin Electrophysiol 2005;28:661.

42. Bluhm G. Pacemaker infections. A clinical study with special reference to prophylactic use of some isoxazolyl penicillins. Acta Med Scand Suppl 1985;699:1.

43. Cabell CH, Heidenreich PA, Chu VH, et al. Increasing rates of cardiac device infections among Medicare beneficiaries: 1990-1999. Am Heart J 2004;147:582.

44. Voigt A, Shalaby A, Saba S. Continued rise in rates of cardiovascular implantable electronic device infections in the united states: temporal trends and causative insights. Pacing Clin Electrophysiol 2010;33:414.

45. Sohail MR, Uslan DZ, Khan AH, et al. Risk factor analysis of permanent pacemaker infection. Clin Infect Dis 2007;45:166.

46. Furman S, Behrens M, Andrews C, et al. Retained pacemaker leads. J Thorac Cardiovasc Surg 1987; 94:770.

47. Parry G, Goudevenos J, Jameson S, et al. Complications associated with retained pacemaker leads. Pacing Clin Electrophysiol 1991;14:1251.

48. Rettig G, Doenecke P, Sen S, et al. Complications with retained transvenous pacemaker electrodes. Am Heart J 1979;98:587.

49. Wollmann CG, Bocker D, Loher A, et al. Incidence of complications in patients with implantable cardioverter/defibrillator who receive additional transvenous pace/sense leads. Pacing Clin Electrophysiol 2005;28:795.

50. Baddour LM, Bettmann MA, Bolger AF, et al. Nonvalvular cardiovascular device-related infections. Circulation 2003;108:2015.

51. Chua JD, Wilkoff BL, Lee I, et al. Diagnosis and management of infections involving implantable electrophysiologic cardiac devices. Ann Intern Med 2000;133:604.

52. Samuels LE, Samuels FL, Kaufman MS, et al. Management of infected implantable cardiac defibrillators. Ann Thorac Surg 1997;64:1702.

53. Tyers GF, Larrieu AJ, Nishimura A, et al. Suppression of a demand pacemaker in the presence of redundant transvenous right ventricular leads. Pacing Clin Electrophysiol 1980;3:84.

54. Waxman HL, Lazzara R, El-Sherif N. Apparent malfunction of demand pacemakers due to spurious potentials generated by contact between two endocardial electrodes. Pacing Clin Electrophysiol 1978; 1:531.

55. Widmann WD, Mangiola S, Lubow LA, et al. Suppression of demand pacemakers by inactive pacemaker electrodes. Circulation 1972;45:319.

56. Wollmann CG, Bocker D, Loher A, et al. Two different therapeutic strategies in ICD lead defects: additional combined lead versus replacement of the lead. J Cardiovasc Electrophysiol 2007;18:1172.

57. Gilard M, Perennes A, Mansourati J, et al. Stent implantation for the treatment of superior vena

cava syndrome related to pacemaker leads. Europace 2002;4:155.

58. Goudevenos JA, Reid PG, Adams PC, et al. Pacemaker-induced superior vena cava syndrome: report of four cases and review of the literature. Pacing Clin Electrophysiol 1989;12:1890.

59. Matthews DM, Forfar JC. Superior vena caval stenosis: a complication of transvenous endocardial pacing. Thorax 1979;34:412.

60. Mazzetti H, Dussaut A, Tentori C, et al. Superior vena cava occlusion and/or syndrome related to pacemaker leads. Am Heart J 1993;125:831.

61. Melzer C, Lembcke A, Ziemer S, et al. Pacemaker-induced superior vena cava syndrome: clinical evaluation of long-term follow-up. Pacing Clin Electrophysiol 2006;29:1346.

62. Riley RF, Petersen SE, Ferguson JD, et al. Managing superior vena cava syndrome as a complication of pacemaker implantation: a pooled analysis of clinical practice. Pacing Clin Electrophysiol 2010; 33(4):420–5.

63. Rossi A, Baravelli M, Cattaneo P, et al. Acute superior vena cava syndrome after insertion of implantable cardioverter defibrillator. J Interv Card Electrophysiol 2008;23:247.

64. van Rooden CJ, Molhoek SG, Rosendaal FR, et al. Incidence and risk factors of early venous thrombosis associated with permanent pacemaker leads. J Cardiovasc Electrophysiol 2004;15:1258.

65. Kim JB, Spevack DM, Tunick PA, et al. The effect of transvenous pacemaker and implantable cardioverter defibrillator lead placement on tricuspid valve function: an observational study. J Am Soc Echocardiogr 2008;21:284.

66. Klutstein M, Balkin J, Butnaru A, et al. Tricuspid incompetence following permanent pacemaker implantation. Pacing Clin Electrophysiol 2009; 32(Suppl 1):S135.

67. Krishnan A, Moulick A, Sinha P, et al. Severe tricuspid valve stenosis secondary to pacemaker leads presenting as ascites and liver dysfunction: a complex problem requiring a multidisciplinary therapeutic approach. J Interv Card Electrophysiol 2009;24:71.

68. Rosenberg Y, Myatt JP, Feldman M, et al. Down to the wire: tricuspid stenosis in the setting of multiple pacing leads. Pacing Clin Electrophysiol 2010;33:e49.

69. Byrd CL, Wilkoff BL, Love CJ, et al. Clinical study of the laser sheath for lead extraction: the total experience in the United States. Pacing Clin Electrophysiol 2002;25:804.

70. Byrd CL, Wilkoff BL, Love CJ, et al. Intravascular extraction of problematic or infected permanent pacemaker leads: 1994-1996. U.S. Extraction Database, MED Institute. Pacing Clin Electrophysiol 1999;22:1348.

71. Kay GN, Brinker JA, Kawanishi DT, et al. Risks of spontaneous injury and extraction of an active fixation pacemaker lead: report of the Accufix Multicenter Clinical Study and Worldwide Registry. Circulation 1999;100:2344.

72. Roux JF, Pagé P, Dubuc M, et al. Laser lead extraction: predictors of success and complications. Pacing Clin Electrophysiol 2007;30:214.

73. Smith HJ, Fearnot NE, Byrd CL, et al. Five-years experience with intravascular lead extraction. U.S. lead extraction database. Pacing Clin Electrophysiol 1994;17:2016.

74. Hauser RG, Katsiyiannis WT, Gornick CC, et al. Deaths and cardiovascular injuries due to device-assisted implantable cardioverter-defibrillator and pacemaker lead extraction. Europace 2010;12:395.

75. Wilkoff BL, Byrd CL, Love CJ, et al. Pacemaker lead extraction with the laser sheath: results of the Pacing Lead Extraction with the Excimer Sheath (PLEXES) trial. J Am Coll Cardiol 1999; 33:1671.

76. Epstein LM, Byrd CL, Wilkoff BL, et al. Initial experience with larger laser sheaths for the removal of transvenous pacemaker and implantable defibrillator leads. Circulation 1999;100:516.

77. Bracke FA, van Gelder LM, Sreeram N, et al. Exchange of pacing or defibrillator leads following laser sheath extraction of non-functional leads in patients with ipsilateral obstructed venous access. Heart 2000;83:E12.

78. Le Franc P, Klug D, Jarwe M, et al. Extraction and re-implantation of defibrillation leads through a thrombotic subclavian vein. Pacing Clin Electrophysiol 1999;22:977.

79. Bohm A, Pinter A, Duray G, et al. Complications due to abandoned noninfected pacemaker leads. Pacing Clin Electrophysiol 2001;24:1721.

80. Sweeney MO, Shea JB, Ellison KE. Upgrade of permanent pacemakers and single chamber implantable cardioverter defibrillators to pectoral dual chamber implantable cardioverter defibrillators: indications, surgical approach, and long-term clinical results. Pacing Clin Electrophysiol 2002;25:1715.

# Primary Ablation for Ventricular Tachycardia: When and How?

Pasquale Santangeli, MD[a], Luigi Di Biase, MD, PhD, FHRS[a,b,c],
Amin Al-Ahmad, MD, FHRS[d], Henry Hsia, MD, FACC, FHRS[d],
J. David Burkhardt, MD, FHRS[a], Javier Sanchez, MD[a],
Rong Bai, MD[a], Michela Casella, MD, PhD[e],
Antonio Dello Russo, MD, PhD[e], Claudio Tondo, MD, PhD[e],
Andrea Natale, MD, FACC, FHRS[a,b,d,f,g,h,*]

## KEYWORDS

• Ventricular tachycardia • Catheter ablation • Cardiac arrest

Sudden cardiac arrest accounts for more than 450,000 deaths in United States each year, with ventricular tachycardia (VT) being the most common arrhythmia leading to sudden death.[1,2] Overall, event rates in Europe are similar to those in the United States. Coronary artery disease is the most frequent substrate underlying sudden cardiac arrest,[1,2] and scar-related reentry is the mechanism leading to sustained VT in most of these patients.[3] Multiple randomized trials have demonstrated the effectiveness of implantable cardioverter-defibrillators (ICD) in reducing mortality in patients at high risk of sudden cardiac death; namely, those who already experienced a sudden cardiac arrest (secondary prevention), and those with severe left ventricular dysfunction who have not yet experienced major arrhythmic events (primary prevention).[4]

However, ICDs do not prevent the occurrence of VT, and many of these patients receive multiple and painful ICD shocks, resulting in decreased quality of life[5] and, even, increased risk of nonarrhythmic mortality.[6-8] Approximately 30% of patients who were implanted with a primary prevention indication receive an ICD shock for rapid sustained VT within 3 years after ICD implantation,[8,9] and this event rate rises to 45% at 1 year in patients receiving an ICD for the secondary prevention of sudden cardiac death.[10] A well-represented subset of patients develop VT storm, defined as three or more appropriate ICD therapies within a 24-hour period for VT. The reported incidence of VT storm in primary prevention ICD recipients is 4%[11] and reaches 20% in patients who received an ICD for the secondary prevention of sudden cardiac death.[12]

[a] Texas Cardiac Arrhythmia Institute, St. David's Medical Center, 3000 North I-35, Suite 720, Austin, TX 78705, USA
[b] Department of Biomedical Engineering, The University of Texas at Austin, 1 University Station, C0800 Austin, TX 78712, USA
[c] Department of Cardiology, University of Foggia, Viale Pinto 1, 71100 Foggia, Italy
[d] Division of Cardiology, Stanford University, Cardiovascular Medicine Clinic, 300 Pasteur Drive, MC 5319 A260 Stanford, CA 94305, USA
[e] Cardiac Arrhythmia Research Centre, Centro Cardiologico Monzino IRCCS, Via Parea 4, 20138 Milano, Italy
[f] Case Western Reserve University, 450 Sears Building, 2083 Martin Luther King Jr Drive, Cleveland, OH, USA
[g] Interventional Electrophysiology, Scripps Clinic, 9888 Genesee Avenue La Jolla, San Diego, CA 92037, USA
[h] EP Services, California Pacific Medical Center, 2333 Buchanan Street, San Francisco, CA 94115, USA
* Corresponding author. Texas Cardiac Arrhythmia Institute, St. David's Medical Center, 3000 North I-35, Suite 720, Austin, TX 78705.
E-mail address: dr.natale@gmail.com

Card Electrophysiol Clin 3 (2011) 675–688
doi:10.1016/j.ccep.2011.08.014

Importantly, few treatment strategies have been demonstrated to reduce the occurrence of VT these patients. In this regard, the clinical experience with antiarrhythmic drugs has led to disappointing results; although some compounds such as sotalol, azimilide, and amiodarone have proven to significantly reduce the number of ICD-treated ventricular arrhythmias.[13–15] Multiple, properly designed, randomized trials have clearly shown a neutral or harmful effect of antiarrhythmic drug therapy on survival in patients at risk of tachyarrhythmic sudden cardiac death.[2]

Radiofrequency catheter ablation is an established treatment of drug-refractory recurrent VT, providing quite satisfactory results even without the use of antiarrhythmic drug therapy.[11,16–26] In the setting of VT storm, catheter ablation can be life-saving.[3,26,27] Over the years, significant advances in techniques and technologies for VT ablation, such as improvements in mapping systems,[3] the introduction of percutaneous epicardial approaches for epicardial ablation,[28] and open-irrigation ablation platforms,[26] have further advanced VT ablation and increased the number of patients referred for ablative treatment, with improved outcomes. Available data on catheter ablation are largely limited to patients experiencing multiple episodes of VT refractory to antiarrhythmic drug therapy (ie, secondary VT ablation).[3,16,19,24,26,29] Thus far, only three studies have evaluated the role of catheter ablation early in the treatment of VT.[17,18,20] Such "primary VT

ablation" strategy has been essentially implemented in patients undergoing secondary prevention ICD implantation,[17,18,20] with scant data on patients who were implanted with a primary prevention indication and had a subsequent appropriate ICD therapy for sustained VT.[17] This article summarizes the available evidence on primary VT ablation and discusses its clinical indications and outcomes compared with standard catheter ablation of drug-refractory recurrent VT.

## PRIMARY ABLATION FOR VT: WHEN?

Three randomized trials (published as two full-text articles and one abstract) have evaluated the benefit of primary VT ablation compared with standard medical therapy.[17,18,20] These studies enrolled only patients with ischemic cardiomyopathy.

In a small, pilot, randomized trial, Schreieck and colleagues[20] reported the results of early intervention with VT ablation with ICD implantation versus ICD alone in a sample of 39 patients (19 randomized to ablation) undergoing secondary prevention ICD placement for postinfarct, sustained VT. After a mean follow-up of 11.3 plus or minus 8.9 months, 47% of the ablated patients and 60% of controls had VT recurrence, resulting in a nonsignificant benefit of VT ablation (Fig. 1).[20] The small sample size of this trial coupled with the absence of detailed results in the abstract do not allow

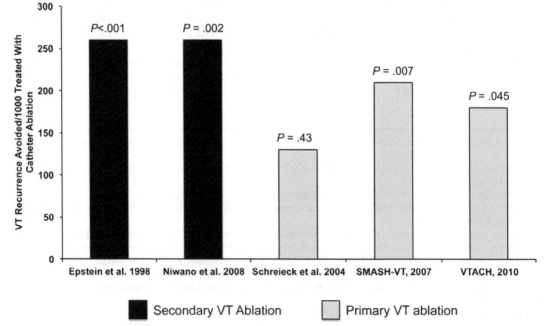

Fig. 1. Benefit of catheter ablation of VT in preventing arrhythmia recurrence compared with medical therapy.

any definite conclusions on the role of primary VT ablation on the VT recurrence rate.

The Substrate Mapping and Ablation in Sinus Rhythm to Halt Ventricular Tachycardia (SMASH-VT) trial was a physician-initiated and self-sponsored multicenter, prospective, unblinded, randomized trial that tested the hypothesis that catheter ablation would reduce the recurrence of sustained ventricular arrhythmias in patients undergoing ICD implantation for the secondary prevention of sudden cardiac death.[18] The investigators referred to such an ablation strategy as "prophylactic catheter ablation," although this definition may be semantically misleading given that enrolled patients had already experienced an episode of life-threatening, sustained, ventricular arrhythmia. Initially, only patients undergoing secondary prevention ICD implantation (within a 6-month period from study enrollment) were eligible for randomization. Among these, no distinction was made with regard to the index arrhythmia responsible for secondary prevention ICD implantation, and the investigators recruited patients with a history of ventricular fibrillation, hemodynamically unstable VT, or syncope with inducible VT during invasive electrophysiological testing. Subsequently, enrollment criteria were extended to patients who had received an ICD for primary prophylaxis and had an appropriate ICD therapy for a single event (**Table 1**). These figures introduce substantial clinical heterogeneity because the prognosis of patients with ventricular fibrillation may not be the same as that of patients with spontaneous VT, or only inducible VT. Of note, patients were excluded if they were being treated with antiarrhythmic drugs (class I or class III), and if they were experiencing VT storm. Patients were randomized in a 1:1 ratio to catheter ablation (see later discussion) or medical therapy (no antiarrhythmic drugs). The primary study endpoint was survival free from any appropriate ICD therapy, defined as ICD shock or antitachycardia pacing. Freedom from any appropriate ICD shock, overall mortality, and VT storm were among the secondary endpoints analyzed. Importantly, the investigators did not report details on the ICDs programming, which may account for a degree of reporting bias in case of different ICD programming between the groups.

One hundred and twenty eight patients (64 in each group) underwent randomization. The baseline clinical characteristics were similar in the two groups, with the notable exception of patients with severe left ventricular dysfunction (left ventricular ejection fraction $\leq$ 20%) who were more represented in the catheter ablation group (25% vs 11%, $P$ = .06). After completing a 2-year follow-up, 12% of patients in the ablation group and 33% of those in the control group received an appropriate ICD intervention (hazard ratio [HR] = 0.35, 95% CI 0.15 to 0.78, $P$ = .007), which was driven by a significant decrease of ICD shocks (9% vs 31%, HR = 0.27, 95% CI 0.11 to 0.67, $P$ = .003). Translating such figures into treatment effects, the number of patients that need to be ablated (ie, number needed to treat [NNT]) to avoid one appropriate ICD intervention is five, resulting in 200 appropriated ICD interventions prevented every 1000 patients treated with catheter ablation (see **Fig. 1**). It bears emphasis that absence of an active control group with antiarrhythmic drug therapy (eg, amiodarone) may have skewed the results toward an increased benefit of catheter ablation. Further, whether such striking reduction of recurrent ventricular arrhythmias is mirrored by a reduction of mortality remains obscure. The sample size of the SMASH-VT was inadequate to address this issue; notwithstanding, the investigators reported a trend toward improved survival in the catheter ablation group (HR = 0.59, 95% CI 0.22 to 1.59, $P$ = .29).

In a subsequent paper, the investigators reported a retrospective analysis aimed at assessing the predictors of appropriate ICD intervention in the catheter ablation group.[30] The procedural variables entered in the Cox proportional hazards model included location of scar, number of induced VT morphologies, tachycardia cycle lengths, use of open-irrigation catheters, total procedural duration, and VT inducibility after ablation. Among the clinical variables tested in the model were age, index arrhythmia, New York Heart Association (NYHA) functional class, ejection fraction, history of prior revascularization, and baseline medications. The only variable associated with occurrence of appropriate ICD intervention at follow-up was the number of VT induced in the baseline electrophysiological study (mean number of induced VTs = 3.9 $\pm$ 2.1 vs 1.9 $\pm$ 1.8, $P$ = .05; HR for each additional VT induced = 1.51, 95% CI 1.07 to 2.13, $P$ = .02), whereas inducibility after ablation did not influence long-term clinical success.[30]

The multicenter Catheter Ablation of Stable Ventricular Tachycardia Before Defibrillator Implantation in Patients With Coronary Artery Disease (VTACH) trial was a physician-initiated and industry-sponsored (St Jude Medical, St Paul, MD, USA) prospective, unblinded, randomized controlled trial testing the hypothesis that early intervention with catheter ablation in patients with previous myocardial infarction, reduced left ventricular ejection fraction (ie, $\leq$50%), and documented first episode of hemodynamically tolerated, sustained VT undergoing secondary prevention ICD

**Table 1**
**Characteristics of studies comparing catheter ablation of VT with medical therapy**

| Study Characteristic | Epstein et al[19] | Schreieck et al[20] | SMASH-VT[18] | Niwano et al[21] | VTACH[17] |
|---|---|---|---|---|---|
| Year | 1998 | 2004 | 2007 | 2008 | 2010 |
| Design | Randomized controlled | Randomized controlled | Randomized controlled | Observational controlled | Randomized controlled |
| Primary VT Ablation | — | X | X | — | X |
| Inclusion Criteria | Structural heart disease; ≥2 sustained VT episodes; hemodynamically stable spontaneous VT; failure of ≥2 AADs | First episode of postinfarct sustained VT; pts undergoing secondary prevention ICD implantation | First episode of postinfarct sustained VT[a] | Congestive heart failure; spontaneous recurrent VT refractory to multiple AADs | Stable postinfarct sustained VT; left ventricular ejection fraction ≤50%; pts undergoing secondary prevention ICD implantation |
| Primary Endpoint | VT recurrence | VT recurrence | VT recurrence | VT recurrence | VT recurrence |
| Endpoint Assessment | Not reported | ICD interrogation | ICD interrogation | ICD interrogation or rate of sudden cardiac death | ICD interrogation |
| Number of Patients | 105 | 39 | 128 | 78 | 107 |
| Catheter Ablation, n (%) | 73 (70) | 19 (49) | 64 (50) | 58 (74) | 52 (49) |
| Medical Therapy, n (%) | 32 (30%) | 20 (51) | 64 (50) | 20 (26) | 55 (51) |
| Mean Follow-up, Months | 6 | 12 | 23 | 31 | 23 |

*Abbreviations:* AADs, antiarrhythmic drugs; n, size of subsample; pts, patients.

[a] Patients with resuscitated sudden cardiac arrest, patients with syncope and inducible sustained VT, or patients who received an ICD for the primary prevention of sudden cardiac death and subsequently had an appropriated ICD intervention.

implantation, would reduce the rate of recurrent VT or ventricular fibrillation compared with standard medical therapy plus ICD implantation (see **Table 1**).[17] In this study, antiarrhythmic drug therapy was allowed, although only 35% of patients in both groups were treated with amiodarone at baseline and no data were reported on the use of antiarrhythmic drugs at follow-up. Patients with VT storm were excluded also from this trial. The primary endpoint was the time from ICD implantation to recurrence of any sustained VT or ventricular fibrillation; the rates of total mortality, syncope, hospitalization for cardiovascular causes, VT storm, and number of appropriate ICD intervention at follow-up were among the secondary endpoints analyzed. Unlike the SMASH-VT trial, detailed information on ICDs programming modes were clearly reported in the VTACH, and consisted of a ventricular fibrillation zone with a cut-off rate of 200 to 220 beats per minute and a VT zone with a cut-off cycle length of 60 milliseconds more than the slowest clinically documented VT, with antitachycardia pacing followed by ICD shock.

One hundred and seven patients were randomized in a 1:1 ratio to catheter ablation with ICD implantation or ICD implantation only, and patients were followed-up for at least 1 year. After a mean follow-up of 22.5 plus or minus 9 months, patients allocated to catheter ablation had significantly longer time to arrhythmia recurrence compared with those randomized to ICD only (median 18.6 months vs 5.9 months), and lower 2-year arrhythmia recurrence rates (53% vs 71%, HR = 0.61, 95% CI 0.37 to 0.99, $P$ = .045). The number needed to treat with catheter ablation to prevent one episode of recurrent ventricular arrhythmia was six, which accounted for 180 malignant ventricular arrhythmias prevented every 1000 patients treated (see **Fig. 1**). It is important to underline that underreported differences in antiarrhythmic drug use in the two groups at follow-up might have introduced bias and affected the quality of the results.

Also in the VTACH, the overall mortality rates were not different between the two groups (8.5% vs 8.6%, $P$ = .68). Of note, the mortality rate in the ICD-only group was extraordinarily low. For instance, the 2-year mortality rate in the ICD-only group of the Antiarrhythmics Versus Implantable Defibrillators (AVID) trial was of 18.4%[10]; that is, more than double than that reported in the ICD-only group of the VTACH. Therefore, the power to disclose a significant mortality reduction with catheter ablation was very poor. On the other side, VTACH-like patients with hemodynamically stable VT have been excluded from secondary prevention ICD trials,[7,10,31] and data about the real clinical outcome of such patients are lacking. In this regard, several early studies suggest a relatively good arrhythmic prognosis of postinfarct, hemodynamically tolerated VT, with an average annual rate of sudden cardiac death of about 2% when treated with antiarrhythmic drug therapy or surgery.[32,33] Unfortunately, the long-term rate of sudden cardiac death in patients presenting with hemodynamically tolerated postinfarct VT and treated with catheter ablation is unknown and is likely to remain unknown because it is nowadays accepted that all of these patients should receive an ICD.[17] On the other side, more than half of the patients allocated to catheter ablation in the VTACH experienced ventricular arrhythmia recurrence at 2 years, which does not support the use of ablation as a stand-alone procedure in these patients.

In conclusion, there is adequate evidence to support the early use of catheter ablation of VT (ie, primary VT ablation) with ICD therapy to decrease arrhythmia recurrence in patients with history of malignant ventricular arrhythmias. Available data do not allow full evaluation the impact of primary VT ablation on mortality (see later discussion) and further studies with larger sample sizes are warranted.

## PRIMARY ABLATION FOR VT: HOW?

Primary VT ablation has been performed through a substrate-based approach in most of the patients included in the studies referenced above (**Table 2**).[17,18,20] Schreieck and colleagues[20] reported a stepwise approach beginning with programmed ventricular stimulation to test inducibility of VTs. Therefore, the exit points of all documented or inducible VTs were defined by pace mapping in sinus rhythm, and radiofrequency applications using cooled-tip or large-tip ablation catheters were delivered to target VT exit points along the scar-border zone guided by electroanatomical voltage mapping (CARTO, Biosense-Webster, Diamond Bar, CA, USA) or noncontact mapping (ENSITE, St Jude Medical, St Paul, MD, USA).

In the SMASH-VT, all the ablation procedures were performed with a substrate-based approach after programmed ventricular stimulation to induce VTs and obtain 12-lead ECGs.[18] A three-dimensional voltage mapping of the left ventricle was obtained during sinus rhythm (CARTO), and pace-mapping maneuvers were performed to reproduce the 12-lead ECG morphology of the inducible VT. Once putative VT exit sites were identified by pace mapping maneuvers, two ablation lines were performed: one from the VT exit site (site of optimal pace mapping) toward the center of the scar and the other perpendicular to the

**Table 2**
Clinical and procedural characteristics of studies comparing catheter ablation of VT with medical therapy

| Study Characteristic | Age | | Male Sex, n (%) | | LVEF, % | | Mapping Technique | Procedural Characteristics | |
| | Abl. | Med. | Abl. | Med. | Abl. | Med. | | Abl. Approach | Abl. Catheter |
| --- | --- | --- | --- | --- | --- | --- | --- | --- | --- |
| Epstein et al[19] | 63 ± 20 | 67 ± 20 | 67 (92) | 27 (84) | 31 ± 13 | 29 ± 12 | NR | NR | CIC |
| Schreieck et al[20] | -ª | -ª | NR | NR | -ª | -ª | CARTO (n = 11), ENSITE (n = 8) | PES for VT induction; exit sites determined by PM | OIC or NIC |
| SMASH-VT[18] | 67 ± 9 | 66 ± 10 | 59 (92) | 52 (81) | 31 ± 10 | 33 ± 9 | CARTO | PES for VT induction; exit sites determined by PM; 2 perpendicular abl. lines; entrainment for stable VT | OIC or NIC |
| Niwano et al[21] | 65 ± 8 | 62 ± 10 | 35 (60) | 13 (65) | 36 ± 6 | 35 ± 9 | CARTO | PES for VT induction; exit sites determined by PM | NR |
| VTACH[17] | 68 ± 8 | 64 ± 8 | 50 (96) | 50 (91) | 34 ± 10 | 34 ± 9 | CARTO (n = 32), ENSITE (n = 11), Conventional (n = 2) | PES for VT induction; activation and entrainment for stable VT; exit sites determined by PM for unstable VT | NR |

Data are reported as mean ± standard deviation, or n (%).

*Abbreviations:* Abl., ablation; CIC, internally cooled radiofrequency catheter; LVEF, left ventricular ejection fraction; Med., medical therapy; n, size of subsample; NIC, nonirrigated radiofrequency catheter; NR, not reported; OIC, open-irrigated radiofrequency catheter; PES, programmed ventricular stimulation; PM, pace mapping.

ª Data sorted per group not reported. Age of the overall population = 65 ± 9 years; LVEF = 33 ± 14%.

first line along the border zone of the scar. In patients with severe left ventricular dysfunction, a second strategy targeting late and fractionated potentials within the scar was used. Entrainment mapping was done only in case hemodynamically stable VT (the number of patients was not reported). Radiofrequency lesions were delivered primarily with an open-irrigated ablation catheter, and no patient underwent epicardial mapping and ablation. In this regard, no appreciable endocardial scar was reported in the 5% of patients in whom an epicardial procedure might have been warranted.

As mentioned above, the only independent predictor of arrhythmia recurrence was the number of VT induced at electrophysiological study, which suggests the presence of multiple VT circuits within the scar.[30] Contemporary cohorts of patients with postinfarct VT often present complex arrhythmogenic substrates, which may be linked to the widespread use of pharmacologic or mechanical reperfusion therapies for acute myocardial infarction.[34] Animal studies have shown that the duration of coronary occlusion influences the size, transmurality, and geometry of postinfarct scar.[35–37] Kumar and colleagues[38] recently reported a significant association in humans between the timing of coronary reperfusion with primary percutaneous coronary intervention and the 2-year rate of spontaneous ventricular arrhythmias, with an incidence ranging from 0% to 14% according to different timings of coronary reperfusion. Although in the SMASH-VT no correlation was found between persistence of VT inducibility after ablation and long-term outcome, the predictive value of the number of induced VTs supports the appropriateness of an extensive substrate-based ablation approach targeting all the putative VT circuits within the scar. Accordingly, at the authors' institution, postinfarct VTs are currently managed with an extensive, endoepicardial, substrate-based ablation approach targeting all the potential circuits within the scar. Preliminary data suggest that such an extensive ablation approach may increase the success rate compared with limited endocardial substrate ablation (**Fig. 2**).[39]

In the VTACH, the three-dimensional electroanatomical reconstruction of the left ventricle was done either with a contact mapping system (CARTO) or with a noncontact system (ENSITE).[17] Activation and entrainment mapping were performed in case of stable VT, whereas a substrate-based approach similar to the SMASH-VT approach was implemented in case of noninducible or unstable VT. No information was provided with regard to the type of ablation catheters used. As mentioned above, all patients enrolled in the VTACH had history of hemodynamically stable

VT and those with hemodynamically unstable VTs were excluded. Accordingly, a monomorphic-stable VT was induced in 94 out of 107 (88%) patients and matched the documented clinical VT in 83% of cases. Notably, even though an acute procedural failure (ie, inducibility of VT after the procedure) was reported in only 13% of cases, more than half of the patients randomized to catheter ablation had ventricular arrhythmia recurrence after 2 years of follow-up. Although a more extensive use of entrainment mapping in addition to substrate modification might have improved the overall long-term outcome this trial, the limited long-term success rate further supports the concept that extensive endo-epicardial substrate based approaches targeting all the potential VT circuits within the scar are important to increase the procedural success in contemporary patients with infarct-related VT (see later discussion).

## PRIMARY VT ABLATION VERSUS SECONDARY VT ABLATION
### Introduction and Methods

The actual benefit of primary VT ablation compared with secondary VT ablation (ie, ablation of drug-refractory recurrent VT) merits an adequate prospective evaluation in properly designed studies. Because, thus far, both ablation approaches have been extensively evaluated against medical therapy, an indirect comparison analysis can be performed to summarize the available evidence. The authors reviewed all randomized controlled trials and nonrandomized studies evaluating the role of radiofrequency catheter ablation of VT compared with medical therapy through a systematic literature search in multiple electronic databases (MEDLINE, PubMed, EMBASE, CENTRAL, Scopus, and ISI Web of Science) using the terms: ventricular tachycardia, tachycardia, catheter ablation, radiofrequency, ischemic cardiomyopathy, implantable cardioverter-defibrillators, and defibrillator* (where * denotes a wildcard). No language or publication-type restrictions were used. Proceedings from the annual American Heart Association (AHA), American College of Cardiology (ACC), European Society of Cardiology (ESC), Heart Rhythm, and Europace meetings for the past 10 years were also manually searched. Web sites of ACC, AHA, and ESC were also screened for oral presentations and/or expert slide presentations. Two independent reviewers performed study selection. Citations initially selected by systematic search were first retrieved as a title and/or abstract and preliminarily screened. Potentially relevant reports were then retrieved as complete manuscripts (when

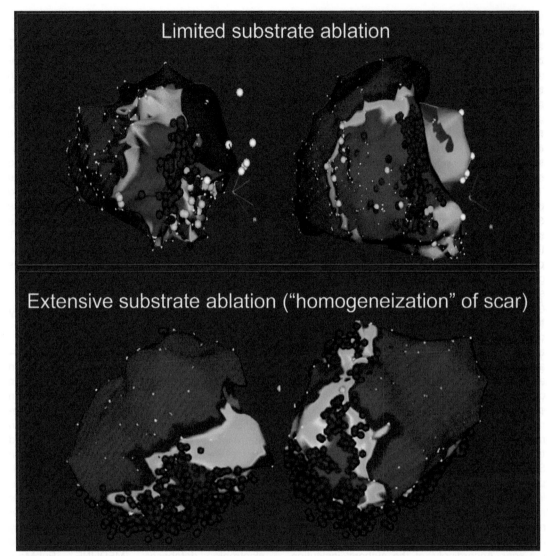

**Fig. 2.** Different approaches for substrate-based ablation of VT. A limited substrate ablation approach based on VTs induction, and targeting only the VTs exit sites (identified with entrainment or activation mapping and/or pace mapping) has been the approach adopted in all clinical trials evaluating the role of primary VT ablation. A more extensive endoepicardial, substrate-based ablation approach, targeting all the potential circuits within the scar (irrespective of the exit sites of clinical or induced VTs) and presenting delayed and fragmented potentials (homogeneization of scar) may improve the outcome. On the left are endocardial maps of the left ventricle, whereas on the right are epicardial maps. Red areas represent scar (bipolar voltage amplitude <0.5 mV), with normal myocardium depicted in purple (bipolar voltage amplitude >1.5 mV). Intermediate colors represent scar-border zone (bipolar voltage amplitude between 0.5 and 1.5 mV).

possible) and assessed for compliance to inclusion criteria. Reviewers evaluated the studies for inclusion in the analysis and extracted the data regarding inclusion criteria, the total number of patients included, the number of patients receiving VT catheter ablation or only medical therapy, the techniques used for VT ablation, the duration of follow-up, the definition of VT recurrence within the studies, the number of patients experiencing VT recurrence at follow-up and, separately, the number of VT storms and the number of deaths and of procedure-related complications. Data are expressed as odds ratio (OR) with its 95% CI. Relative-risk estimates from individual studies were analyzed according to the Mantel-Haenszel model to compute individual ORs with pertinent 95% CI, and the pooled summary-effect estimate was calculated by means of a random-effect model.[40] To appraise the impact on VT recurrence of primary VT ablation (ie, early intervention with catheter ablation) compared with secondary VT ablation (ie, late intervention after multiple antiarrhythmic drug therapy failures), an indirect comparison meta-analysis was performed applying a direct test of statistical significance between the pooled results of primary VT ablation studies[17,18,20] and that of studies on secondary VT ablation.[19,21] To this aim, the authors used the test for interaction by Altman and Bland,[41] which calculates zeta equals the ratio of the difference between the treatment effect estimates of two subgroups to the standard error of this difference. The zeta value, when referred to a table of normal distribution, gives the corresponding P value. Statistical level of significance was defined at a P<.05 [two tailed]. Analyses were performed using the STATA 11.1 software package (Stata Corporation, College Station, TX, USA).

## Results

Five studies (four randomized and one nonrandomized) were selected and included in the analysis.[17–21] As mentioned, three studies (one abstract)[20] tested primary VT ablation against medical therapy[17,18,20]; the remaining two studies (one abstract)[19] compared adjunctive catheter ablation of drug-refractory recurrent VT (secondary VT

ablation) to medical therapy alone.[19,21] All studies reported a long-term follow-up of at least 6 months. Overall, 457 patients were included in the analysis, of whom 266 (58%) were treated with catheter ablation. Primary VT ablation studies enrolled only patients with ischemic cardiomyopathy,[17,18,20] whereas secondary VT ablation studies included patients with both ischemic and nonischemic cardiomyopathy.[19,21] Characteristics of included studies are summarized in **Tables 1** and **2**.

During follow-up ranging from 6 to 22.5 months, a total of 93 (35%) patients in the catheter ablation group experienced VT recurrence, compared with 105 (51%) patients in the medical therapy group (OR = 0.37, 95% CI 0.24 to 0.57, P<.001). The number needed to treat with catheter ablation to avoid one episode of VT recurrence was five, accounting for 200 sustained VT episodes prevented for every 1000 patients ablated.

In studies evaluating a primary VT ablation approach,[17,18,20] the VT recurrence rate at follow-up was 32%, and was significantly lower compared with that occurring in the medical therapy group (51%, OR = 0.41, 95% CI 0.24 to 0.70, P = .001). These figures account for 192 sustained VT episodes prevented for every 1000 patients treated with primary VT ablation (**Fig. 3**). The same degree of benefit was

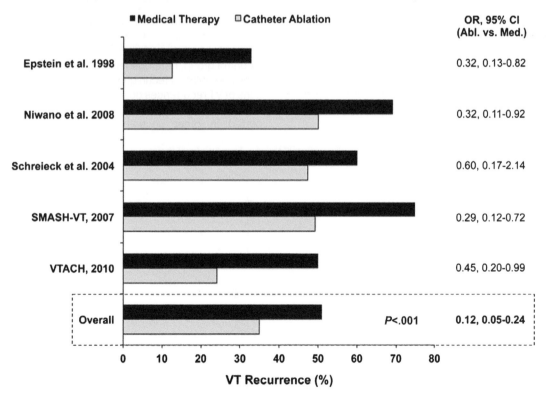

**Fig. 3.** Individual and pooled event rates and ORs with 95% CI of VT recurrence comparing catheter ablation (Abl.) with medical therapy (Med.).

observed in the studies testing secondary VT ablation against medical therapy.[19,21] Indeed, the VT recurrence rate at follow-up in the ablation group was of 38% compared with a rate of 65% in patients treated with medical therapy (OR = 0.32, 95% CI 0.16 to 0.65, P = .001). The number of VT episodes prevented every 1000 patients ablated was higher than that found in primary VT ablation studies; that is, 272 versus 192 (see **Fig. 3**). This could be explained by a higher VT recurrence rate in the medical therapy group of secondary VT ablation studies compared with that reported in primary VT ablation trials (ie, 65% vs 51%). Indirect comparison analysis failed to disclose a difference in long-term success rates between the two ablation strategies (primary VT ablation vs secondary VT ablation), with an OR of 1.28 (95% CI 0.53 to 3.09, P = .58) (**Fig. 4**). It should be also emphasized that only limited ablations were deployed for the primary VT ablation studies, and the ablation approaches for the secondary VT ablation were likely to be more extensive due to the inclusion of patients with larger numbers of arrhythmia events/VT storm pre-procedure. As previously mentioned, limited ablations may be insufficient for long-term arrhythmia control, and more extensive lesions with "homogenization" of the scar may be required to improve the long-term VT control.

Data on the incidence of VT storm at follow-up were reported in only two studies, both testing a primary VT ablation strategy (SMASH-VT and VTACH).[17,18] Pooled analysis of these two studies showed a trend toward a significant reduction of VT storm with catheter ablation (OR = 0.53, 95% CI 0.27 to 1.04, P = .07).

Data on long-term mortality were available in three studies (two primary VT ablation studies).[17,18,21] Mortality occurred in 20 out of 174 (11%) patients of the VT ablation group compared with 14 out of 139 (10%) patients of the medical therapy group (OR = 0.73, 95% CI 0.36 to 1.46, P = .37), without significant interaction between primary and secondary VT ablation strategies (ratio of OR = 0.97, 95% CI 0.21 to 4.53, P = .97) (see **Fig. 4**). As outlined above, none of the included trials had an adequate statistical power to evaluate the effect of catheter ablation on mortality and further studies with larger sample sizes are necessary.

Data on procedure-related complications were retrievable from three studies (**Table 3**).[17–19] Pooled complication rate associated with catheter ablation was 6.3%, including death (1%), cardiac tamponade (1%), and periprocedural thromboembolism (1%).

In conclusion, analysis of the available evidence supports a significant benefit of catheter ablation of VT over medical therapy in preventing VT recurrence. Early intervention with catheter ablation (ie, primary VT ablation strategy) does not seem to improve the outcome.

### Primary VT Ablation Versus Uncontrolled Studies on Secondary VT Ablation

Most of the published studies on VT catheter ablation consist of large case series without a control group (**Table 4**).[16,22,24–26,29,42–49] The absence of a control group, heterogeneities in patient populations and ablation techniques, and different definitions of VT recurrences do not allow comparison of the outcome of primary VT ablation with that reported in other uncontrolled case series on

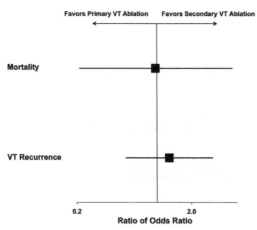

**Fig. 4.** Indirect comparison of the benefit of primary versus secondary VT ablation compared with medical therapy. Based on the available evidence, primary VT ablation does not seem to confer increased benefit. The main implication is that the timing of intervention is not important to improve the long-term outcome and that future research should focus on improving the VT ablation approaches.

**Table 3**
**Catheter ablation-related complications reported in studies included in the analysis**

| Study | Complications |
|---|---|
| Epstein et al[19] | 2 deaths, 1 stroke, 1 cardiac tamponade, 3 third-degree atrioventricular block |
| Schreieck et al[20] | Not reported |
| SMASH-VT[18] | 1 pericardial effusion, 1 worsening heart failure, 1 deep venous thrombosis |
| Niwano et al[21] | Not reported |
| VTACH[17] | 1 transient ST-segment elevation, 1 transient ischemic attack |

secondary VT ablation without introducing significant bias. Notwithstanding these limitations, an exploratory pooled analysis discloses similar long-term VT recurrence rates when comparing studies testing primary VT ablation with those evaluating secondary VT ablation (32% vs 37%, respectively) (see **Table 4**). These findings are in line with those found in the indirect comparison analysis and support the concept that the timing of intervention with VT ablation (early ablation vs delayed ablation after multiple failed antiarrhythmic drugs) is not a major determinant of outcome.

As a corollary, future research on VT ablation should focus on improving the techniques and technologies of ablation to increase the long-term success rate, rather than testing current ablation techniques in broader patient populations. As mentioned above, extensive substrate-based approaches that target all the arrhythmogenic areas within the scar (homogeneization of scar) (see **Fig. 2**) have shown promising results in preliminary studies.[39]

**Table 4**
**Comparison of long-term VT recurrence rates between primary VT ablation studies and uncontrolled clinical studies on catheter ablation of postmyocardial infarction VT**

| | Year | Number of Patients | LVEF, % | Follow-Up, mo | VT Recurrence, % |
|---|---|---|---|---|---|
| Secondary VT Ablation | | | | | |
| Morady et al[29] | 1993 | 15 | 27 | 9 | 13 |
| Kim et al[45] | 1994 | 21 | 32 | 13 | 45 |
| Rothman et al[22] | 1997 | 35 | 24 | 14 | 31 |
| Stevenson et al[24] | 1998 | 52 | 33 | 18 | 31 |
| Ortiz et al[48] | 1999 | 34 | 31 | 26 | 38 |
| El-Shalakany et al[44] | 1999 | 15 | 26 | 15 | 27 |
| Calkins et al[16] | 2000 | 119 | 31 | 8 | 46 |
| O'Callaghan et al[46,*] | 2001 | 55 | 32 | 39 | NR |
| Borger et al[42] | 2002 | 89 | 29 | 34 | 23 |
| Della Bella et al[43] | 2002 | 124 | 34 | 41 | 28 |
| O'Donnell et al[47] | 2002 | 109 | NR | 61 | 23 |
| Segal et al[49] | 2005 | 40 | 36 | 36 | 57 |
| Verma et al[51] | 2005 | 46 | NR | 16 | 37 |
| Stevenson et al[26] | 2008 | 231 | 25 | 6 | 47 |
| Tanner et al[50] | 2010 | 63 | 30 | 12 | 49 |
| Summary | — | 993 | — | — | 37 |
| Primary VT Ablation | | | | | |
| Schreieck et al[20] | 2004 | 39 | 33 | 12 | 47 |
| SMASH-VT[18] | 2007 | 128 | 32 | 23 | 12 |
| VTACH[17] | 2010 | 107 | 34 | 23 | 53 |
| Summary | — | 274 | — | — | 32 |

*Abbreviations:* LVEF, left ventricular ejection fraction; NR, not reported.
* Not included in the summary.

## SUMMARY

Primary VT ablation through a substrate-based approach reduces the VT recurrence rate compared with medical therapy (no antiarrhythmic drugs) in patients with ischemic cardiomyopathy undergoing secondary prevention ICD implantation. Whether such benefit translates into a mortality reduction or whether it may also be extended to patients with nonischemic substrates is unclear. According to current evidence, early intervention with VT ablation does not seem to improve the long-term success rate compared with a secondary VT ablation (ie, ablation of recurrent VT after multiple failed attempts at controlling the arrhythmia with antiarrhythmic drugs). In fact, more than one-third of patients experience VT recurrence after ablation at long-term follow-up independently of the timing of intervention (ie, primary vs secondary VT ablation). Therefore, the main objective of future research should be to improve the overall success rate of current ablation procedures through the development of new techniques and technologies for VT ablation, rather than testing current approaches in broader patient populations.

## REFERENCES

1. Huikuri HV, Castellanos A, Myerburg RJ. Sudden death due to cardiac arrhythmias. N Engl J Med 2001;345(20):1473–82.
2. Zipes DP, Camm AJ, Borggrefe M, et al. ACC/AHA/ESC 2006 guidelines for management of patients with ventricular arrhythmias and the prevention of sudden cardiac death: a report of the American College of Cardiology/American Heart Association Task Force and the European Society of Cardiology Committee for Practice Guidelines (Writing Committee to Develop Guidelines for Management of Patients with Ventricular Arrhythmias and the Prevention of Sudden Cardiac Death): developed in collaboration with the European Heart Rhythm Association and the Heart Rhythm Society. Circulation 2006;114(10):e385–484.
3. Natale A, Raviele A, Al-Ahmad A, et al. Venice Chart International Consensus document on ventricular tachycardia/ventricular fibrillation ablation. J Cardiovasc Electrophysiol 2010;21(3):339–79.
4. Epstein AE, DiMarco JP, Ellenbogen KA, et al. ACC/AHA/HRS 2008 guidelines for device-based therapy of cardiac rhythm abnormalities: a report of the American College of Cardiology/American Heart Association Task Force on Practice Guidelines (Writing Committee to Revise the ACC/AHA/NASPE 2002 Guideline Update for Implantation of Cardiac Pacemakers and Antiarrhythmia Devices) developed in collaboration with the American Association for Thoracic Surgery and Society of Thoracic Surgeons. J Am Coll Cardiol 2008;51(21):e1–62.
5. Kamphuis HC, de Leeuw JR, Derksen R, et al. Implantable cardioverter defibrillator recipients: quality of life in recipients with and without ICD shock delivery: a prospective study. Europace 2003;5(4):381–9.
6. Goldenberg I, Moss AJ, Hall WJ, et al. Causes and consequences of heart failure after prophylactic implantation of a defibrillator in the multicenter automatic defibrillator implantation trial II. Circulation 2006;113(24):2810–7.
7. Kuck KH, Cappato R, Siebels J, et al. Randomized comparison of antiarrhythmic drug therapy with implantable defibrillators in patients resuscitated from cardiac arrest: the Cardiac Arrest Study Hamburg (CASH). Circulation 2000;102(7):748–54.
8. Poole JE, Johnson GW, Hellkamp AS, et al. Prognostic importance of defibrillator shocks in patients with heart failure. N Engl J Med 2008;359(10):1009–17.
9. Moss AJ, Greenberg H, Case RB, et al. Long-term clinical course of patients after termination of ventricular tachyarrhythmia by an implanted defibrillator. Circulation 2004;110(25):3760–5.
10. A comparison of antiarrhythmic-drug therapy with implantable defibrillators in patients resuscitated from near-fatal ventricular arrhythmias. The Antiarrhythmics versus Implantable Defibrillators (AVID) Investigators. N Engl J Med 1997;337(22):1576–83.
11. Sesselberg HW, Moss AJ, McNitt S, et al. Ventricular arrhythmia storms in postinfarction patients with implantable defibrillators for primary prevention indications: a MADIT-II substudy. Heart Rhythm 2007;4(11):1395–402.
12. Exner DV, Pinski SL, Wyse DG, et al. Electrical storm presages nonsudden death: the antiarrhythmics versus implantable defibrillators (AVID) trial. Circulation 2001;103(16):2066–71.
13. Pacifico A, Hohnloser SH, Williams JH, et al. Prevention of implantable-defibrillator shocks by treatment with sotalol. d,l-Sotalol Implantable Cardioverter-Defibrillator Study Group. N Engl J Med 1999;340(24):1855–62.
14. Dorian P, Borggrefe M, Al-Khalidi HR, et al. Placebo-controlled, randomized clinical trial of azimilide for prevention of ventricular tachyarrhythmias in patients with an implantable cardioverter defibrillator. Circulation 2004;110(24):3646–54.
15. Connolly SJ, Dorian P, Roberts RS, et al. Comparison of beta-blockers, amiodarone plus beta-blockers, or sotalol for prevention of shocks from implantable cardioverter defibrillators: the OPTIC Study: a randomized trial. JAMA 2006;295(2):165–71.
16. Calkins H, Epstein A, Packer D, et al. Catheter ablation of ventricular tachycardia in patients with

structural heart disease using cooled radiofrequency energy: results of a prospective multicenter study. Cooled RF Multi Center Investigators Group. J Am Coll Cardiol 2000;35(7):1905–14.

17. Kuck KH, Schaumann A, Eckardt L, et al. Catheter ablation of stable ventricular tachycardia before defibrillator implantation in patients with coronary heart disease (VTACH): a multicentre randomised controlled trial. Lancet 2010;375(9708):31–40.

18. Reddy VY, Reynolds MR, Neuzil P, et al. Prophylactic catheter ablation for the prevention of defibrillator therapy. N Engl J Med 2007;357(26):2657–65.

19. Epstein AE, Wilber D, Calkins H, et al. Randomized controlled trial of ventricular tachycardia treatment by cooled tip catheter ablation vs drug therapy. J Am Coll Cardiol 1998;31(2 Suppl A): 118A.

20. Schreieck J, Schneider MAE, Röhling M, et al. Preventive ablation of post infarction ventricular tachycardias: Results of a prospective randomized study. Heart Rhythm 2004;1(Suppl):S35–7.

21. Niwano S, Fukaya H, Yuge M, et al. Role of electrophysiologic study (EPS)-guided preventive therapy for the management of ventricular tachyarrhythmias in patients with heart failure. Circ J 2008; 72(2):268–73.

22. Rothman SA, Hsia HH, Cossu SF, et al. Radiofrequency catheter ablation of postinfarction ventricular tachycardia: long-term success and the significance of inducible nonclinical arrhythmias. Circulation 1997;96(10):3499–508.

23. Sacher F, Tedrow UB, Field ME, et al. Ventricular tachycardia ablation: evolution of patients and procedures over 8 years. Circ Arrhythm Electrophysiol 2008;1(3):153–61.

24. Stevenson WG, Friedman PL, Kocovic D, et al. Radiofrequency catheter ablation of ventricular tachycardia after myocardial infarction. Circulation 1998; 98(4):308–14.

25. Strickberger SA, Man KC, Daoud EG, et al. A prospective evaluation of catheter ablation of ventricular tachycardia as adjuvant therapy in patients with coronary artery disease and an implantable cardioverter-defibrillator. Circulation 1997;96(5):1525–31.

26. Stevenson WG, Wilber DJ, Natale A, et al. Irrigated radiofrequency catheter ablation guided by electroanatomic mapping for recurrent ventricular tachycardia after myocardial infarction: the multicenter thermocool ventricular tachycardia ablation trial. Circulation 2008;118(25):2773–82.

27. Carbucicchio C, Santamaria M, Trevisi N, et al. Catheter ablation for the treatment of electrical storm in patients with implantable cardioverter-defibrillators: short- and long-term outcomes in a prospective single-center study. Circulation 2008;117(4):462–9.

28. Sosa E, Scanavacca M, d'Avila A, et al. A new technique to perform epicardial mapping in the electrophysiology laboratory. J Cardiovasc Electrophysiol 1996;7(6):531–6.

29. Morady F, Harvey M, Kalbfleisch SJ, et al. Radiofrequency catheter ablation of ventricular tachycardia in patients with coronary artery disease. Circulation 1993;87(2):363–72.

30. Tung R, Josephson ME, Reddy V, et al. Influence of clinical and procedural predictors on ventricular tachycardia ablation outcomes: an analysis from the substrate mapping and ablation in Sinus Rhythm to Halt Ventricular Tachycardia Trial (SMASH-VT). J Cardiovasc Electrophysiol 2010;21(7):799–803.

31. Connolly SJ, Gent M, Roberts RS, et al. Canadian implantable defibrillator study (CIDS): a randomized trial of the implantable cardioverter defibrillator against amiodarone. Circulation 2000;101(11): 1297–302.

32. Sarter BH, Finkle JK, Gerszten RE, et al. What is the risk of sudden cardiac death in patients presenting with hemodynamically stable sustained ventricular tachycardia after myocardial infarction? J Am Coll Cardiol 1996;28(1):122–9.

33. Brugada P, Talajic M, Smeets J, et al. The value of the clinical history to assess prognosis of patients with ventricular tachycardia or ventricular fibrillation after myocardial infarction. Eur Heart J 1989;10(8): 747–52.

34. Santangeli P, Di Biase L, Burkhardt JD, et al. Lesion recovery, epicardial substrate, or new circuit? exploring the dark side of recurrent VT after endocardial ablation. Heart Rhythm Jul 5 2011. [Epub ahead of print].

35. Arnold JM, Antman EM, Przyklenk K, et al. Differential effects of reperfusion on incidence of ventricular arrhythmias and recovery of ventricular function at 4 days following coronary occlusion. Am Heart J 1987; 113(5):1055–65.

36. Miyazaki S, Fujiwara H, Onodera T, et al. Quantitative analysis of contraction band and coagulation necrosis after ischemia and reperfusion in the porcine heart. Circulation 1987;75(5):1074–82.

37. Sager PT, Perlmutter RA, Rosenfeld LE, et al. Electrophysiologic effects of thrombolytic therapy in patients with a transmural anterior myocardial infarction complicated by left ventricular aneurysm formation. J Am Coll Cardiol 1988;12(1):19–24.

38. Kumar S, Sivagangabalan G, Thiagalingam A, et al. Effect of reperfusion time on inducible ventricular tachycardia early and spontaneous ventricular arrhythmias late after ST elevation myocardial infarction treated with primary percutaneous coronary intervention. Heart Rhythm 2011;8(4):493–9.

39. Di Biase L, Burkhardt JD, Sanchez J, et al. Endoepicardial homogenization of the scar versus limited endocardial substrate ablation for the treatment of electrical storms in patients with ischemic cardiomyopathy. Circulation 2010;122:A17371.

40. Cochrane Handbook for systematic reviews of interventions, Version 5.0.1. Updated September 2008. The Cochrane Collaboration, 7.7.7.2. Available at: http://www.cochrane-handbook.org/. Accessed March, 2010.

41. Altman DG, Bland JM. Interaction revisited: the difference between two estimates. BMJ 2003; 326(7382):219.

42. Borger van der Burg AE, de Groot NM, van Erven L, et al. Long-term follow-up after radiofrequency catheter ablation of ventricular tachycardia: a successful approach? J Cardiovasc Electrophysiol 2002;13(5): 417–23.

43. Della Bella P, De Ponti R, Uriarte JA, et al. Catheter ablation and antiarrhythmic drugs for haemodynamically tolerated post-infarction ventricular tachycardia; long-term outcome in relation to acute electrophysiological findings. Eur Heart J 2002;23(5):414–24.

44. El-Shalakany A, Hadjis T, Papageorgiou P, et al. Entrainment/mapping criteria for the prediction of termination of ventricular tachycardia by single radiofrequency lesion in patients with coronary artery disease. Circulation 1999;99(17):2283–9.

45. Kim YH, Sosa-Suarez G, Trouton TG, et al. Treatment of ventricular tachycardia by transcatheter radiofrequency ablation in patients with ischemic heart disease. Circulation 1994;89(3):1094–102.

46. O'Callaghan PA, Poloniecki J, Sosa-Suarez G, et al. Long-term clinical outcome of patients with prior myocardial infarction after palliative radiofrequency catheter ablation for frequent ventricular tachycardia. Am J Cardiol 2001;87(8):975–9, A974.

47. O'Donnell D, Bourke JP, Anilkumar R, et al. Radiofrequency ablation for post infarction ventricular tachycardia. Report of a single centre experience of 112 cases. Eur Heart J 2002;23(21):1699–705.

48. Ortiz M, Almendral J, Villacastin J, et al. [Radiofrequency ablation of ventricular tachycardia in patients with ischemic cardiopathy]. Rev Esp Cardiol 1999;52(3):159–68 [in Spanish].

49. Segal OR, Chow AW, Markides V, et al. Long-term results after ablation of infarct-related ventricular tachycardia. Heart Rhythm 2005;2(5):474–82.

50. Tanner H, Hindricks G, Volkmer M, et al. Catheter ablation of recurrent scar-related ventricular tachycardia using electroanatomical mapping and irrigated ablation technology: results of the prospective multicenter Euro-VT-study. J Cardiovasc Electrophysiol 2010;21(1):47–53.

51. Verma A, Marrouche NF, Schweikert RA, et al. Relationship between successful ablation sites and the scar border zone defined by substrate mapping for ventricular tachycardia post-myocardial infarction. J Cardiovasc Electrophysiol 2005;16(5):465–71.

# Catheter Ablation of Ventricular Fibrillation Storms: Will this Replace Defibrillators?

Ashok J. Shah, MD, Shinsuke Miyazaki, MD,
Amir S. Jadidi, MD, Daniel Scherr, MD,
Stephen B. Wilton, MD, PhD, Laurent Roten, MD,
Patrizio Pascale, MD, Michala Pedersen, MD,
Nicolas Derval, MD, Sebastien Knecht, MD, PhD,
Frederic Sacher, MD, Pierre Jais, MD,
Michel Haissaguerre, MD*, Meleze Hocini, MD

**KEYWORDS**
- Ventricular tachycardia • Catheter ablation
- Ventricular fibrillation • Defibrillation

Ventricular arrhythmias (ventricular tachycardia [VT] and ventricular fibrillation [VF]) are important causes of morbidity and sudden death.[1,2] Polymorphic VT and VF, the most life-threatening and complex ventricular rhythm disorders, are responsible for 80% of the 700,000 sudden cardiac deaths occurring every year in the United States and Europe (the remaining 20% are primary arrest of cardiac activity). Coronary heart disease is the most frequent cause of clinically documented ventricular arrhythmia (76%–82% of patients).[3–6] Other common causes of ventricular arrhythmias are nonischemic cardiomyopathy, hypertrophic cardiomyopathy (HCM), arrhythmogenic right ventricular cardiomyopathy (ARVC), congenital heart disease, and primary electrical disorders, such as long QT syndrome (LQTS), short QT syndrome (SQTS), Brugada syndrome, and catecholaminergic polymorphic ventricular tachycardia (CPVT). In a limited number of patients with ventricular arrhythmias (~5%) no known cardiac abnormalities (idiopathic) can be identified.

Therapeutic options for the treatment of these lethal arrhythmias include antiarrhythmic drugs, implantable cardioverter-defibrillators (ICDs), and surgical and catheter ablation.[1,2,7] Antiarrhythmic drugs have limited efficacy and adverse side effects that may outweigh benefits. ICDs effectively terminate VT/VF episodes and have been established as the frontline therapy in prevention of sudden arrhythmogenic death in a wide range of heart diseases. Although ICDs represent the mainstay of VF therapy, ICD interventions are often painful, reduce quality of life, provoke psychological distress, and predict increased risk of death and heart failure. Electrical storm is a class III indication for implantation of an ICD.[1,7] Moreover, these devices may not always prevent clinical arrhythmia recurrence. Ablation started as a surgical procedure as therapeutic option for ventricular arrhythmias.[8] Progressive developments in mapping technology and ablation tools allowed for percutaneous catheter-based procedures. The most relevant developments include the

Conflicts of interest: None.
Disclosures: None.
Hôpital Haut Lévêque and Université Bordeaux II, Bordeaux, France
* Corresponding author. Hôpital Cardiologique du Haut-Lévêque, 33604 Bordeaux-Pessac, France.
*E-mail address:* michel.haissaguerre@chu-bordeaux.fr

use of radiofrequency (RF) energy, introduction of steerable, large-tip, and irrigated catheters, activation and entrainment mapping, electroanatomic mapping with the possibility of performing substrate-based ablation during sinus rhythm, multielectrode mapping with the possibility of ablating hemodynamically unstable VT, and epicardial mapping and ablation. Improved safety and better outcomes have contributed to substantial expansion in the indications of ablation and extension of percutaneous catheter-based ablative therapy to the most complex and lethal ventricular arrhythmia: VF.

## VF STORM
### Definition

The syndrome of very frequent episodes of VT/VF requiring cardioversion/defibrillation has been termed VT/VF storm.[1] Three or more separate episodes of sustained VT/VF within 24 hours, each requiring termination by an intervention, is known as an electrical storm.[2,7]

### Clinicopathogenesis Regarding Therapeutic Targets

Polymorphic VT/VF underlies most preventable sudden death events from a wide range of cardiac causes. Because of lethal characteristics and momentary presence, polymorphic VT/VF have mostly been mapped and studied in animal hearts or models of coronary ischemia, the most common disorder associated with this form of arrhythmia.[9–11] In comparison with the sustained, monomorphic, reentrant, substrate-dependent VTs, the polymorphic VT and VF are mechanistically varied and more complex. Reentry involving the myocardial substrate and the Purkinje-myocardium junction and the migratory propagation of vortices emerged as the likely mechanism of the maintenance of this arrhythmia.[11–13] Various therapeutic drugs chronically alter the electrical properties (eg, conduction velocity, refractoriness) of the myocardial substrate to prevent recurrence of lethal clinical arrhythmia with variable efficacy limited by adverse effects from undesirable pharmacodynamics. Because of variable and limited efficacy, antiarrhythmic drugs do not play a primary role in the chronic management of polymorphic VT/VF.

Most of those who survive the episode respond to correction of the acutely provocative arrhythmogenic factor (eg, ischemia, metabolic and electrolyte disorder, compensated heart failure). Thereafter, ICD implantation is undertaken as a secondary prevention measure in patients with residual threat who continue to receive chronic optimal medical therapy and who have reasonable

expectation of survival with a good functional status for more than 1 year.[1]

Recently, distal Purkinje arborization was described as the trigger in initiating these arrhythmias in structurally normal and diseased hearts.[14–16] The discovery helped cultivate new insights into the mechanism and therapy for these arrhythmias and defined specific clinical therapeutic targets in the management of these arrhythmias. Fixed focal source arrhythmia can be more precisely and specifically targeted than rapidly migratory propagation of reentrant vortices.

## MANAGEMENT OF VF STORM
### Current Status of Defibrillators

#### Automated external defibrillator

The automated external defibrillator (AED) saves lives when external defibrillation can be rendered within minutes of onset of VF. The AED represents an efficient method of delivering defibrillation to persons experiencing out-of-hospital cardiac arrest, and its use by both traditional and nontraditional first responders seems to be safe and effective.[17,18] Appropriate device location to reduce the time delay after onset of cardiac arrest is critical. Efforts have been effective in placing AEDs in schools, sporting events, high-density residential sites, and airports as well as on airplanes and in police and fire department vehicles.[19–21]

#### Implantable defibrillators

Several prospective multicenter clinical trials, both primary and secondary prevention, have documented improved survival with ICD therapy in high-risk patients with left ventricular dysfunction caused by prior myocardial infarction and non-ischemic cardiomyopathy (**Fig. 1**).[5,22–28] ICD therapy compared with conventional or traditional antiarrhythmic drug therapy has been associated with mortality reductions from 23% to 55% depending on the risk group participating in the trial, with the improvement in survival almost exclusively the result of a reduction in sudden death from ventricular arrhythmias. ICD therapy enjoys an undisputed class I indication in the prevention and management of aborted cardiac arrest from the wide spectrum of structural and electrical cardiac disorders cited earlier.

### Catheter-Based Ablative Therapy for Refractory VF Storm

Polymorphic VT and VF may present as an arrhythmia storm in 20% of patients with ICDs,[29] whereas idiopathic VF is estimated to represent 5% to 10% of sudden cardiac death cases.[30–32] Patients with structural heart disease and storms

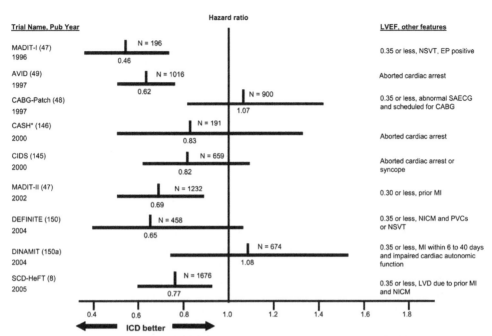

**Fig. 1.** Major implantable cardioverter-defibrillator (ICD) trials. CABG, coronary artery bypass graft; EP, electrophysiologic test; LVD, left ventricular dysfunction; LVEF, left ventricular ejection fraction; MI, myocardial infarction; NICM, nonischemic cardiomyopathy; NSVT, nonsustained ventricular tachycardia; PVC, premature ventricular complex; SAECG, signal-averaged electrocardiogram). (*From* Zipes DP, Camm AJ, Borggrefe M, et al. ACC/AHA/ESC 2006 guidelines for management of patients with ventricular arrhythmias and the prevention of sudden cardiac death. J Am Coll Cardiol 2006;48:1064–108; with permission. Copyright © 2006 American College of Cardiology Foundation.)

of lethal arrhythmias not responding to medical therapy are critically ill and likely to die without further intervention. In our experience, patients with ICDs or in intensive care units could have received up to 100 shocks in a period of less than 24 hours and be unresponsive to various drugs like β-blockers, isoprenaline, amiodarone, procainamide, quinidine, mexiletine, and lidocaine. General anesthesia may be effective. Hemodynamic support in the form of extracorporeal membrane oxygenation or a left ventricular assist device is often necessary to sustain life. Heart transplant is often the only therapeutic alternative. When the discussions of ending life-sustaining measures are initiated, many physicians do not realize that ablation could be a potential therapy. Ablation therapy for polymorphic VT/VF has recently been described.[33–35] Focal ventricular sites generating ectopy-initiating VT/VF offer specific ablation targets. In most cases, VF seems to originate from the distal Purkinje arborization, although some cases have focal triggers in the myocardium distinct from the cardiac conduction system.[14–16,36] Catheter ablation of the ectopy generating lethal arrhythmias has been successfully attempted as a bailout procedure after failure of optimum medical management in structural

heart diseases (ischemic heart disease, nonischemic dilated cardiomyopathy, after valvular cardiac surgery, myocarditis, infiltrative amyloid heart disease) and primary cardiac electrical disorders (LQTS, Brugada syndrome, early repolarization syndrome, and idiopathic VF).

Patients with idiopathic VF typically have isolated premature ventricular beats, best appreciated immediately following resuscitation and up to 2 to 3 days thereafter. These beats are the culprit ectopies initiating VF or polymorphic VT. The ectopies arising from the distal left Purkinje system have more morphologic variation and shorter QRS duration than those arising from the right Purkinje network, which often has more subtle changes. This difference can be explained by the small arborial mass of the right Purkinje network compared with that of the left (anterior, septal, and intermediate). Mapping requires frequent ventricular ectopy and is best performed at the time of arrhythmia storm. Ablation is not feasible when the triggering ectopic sources cannot be identified. In the absence of arrhythmia storm, provocative maneuvers including the use of isoproterenol or extra stimuli are not usually helpful. Pace mapping can be used in cases of monomorphic ventricular ectopy where a clear 12-lead recording of the ectopic beat has been recorded. To facilitate identification of ectopies before ablation, 12-lead electrocardiogram (ECG) is continuously undertaken in hospital before invasive mapping. At our center, we also mark the position of precordial electrodes on the patient torso to perfectly reproduce the same ECG pattern in the electrophysiologic laboratory during invasive mapping to prevent alteration in the morphology of clinical ectopies, especially in the precordial leads caused by a change in the position of body surface electrodes. Targeting ectopy from the Purkinje system, a low-amplitude and high-frequency signal (Purkinje potential) that precedes and is closely coupled to the ventricular signal is recorded at the successful site in sinus rhythm and ectopy. The end point of ablation is the abolition of the local Purkinje potentials and suppression of the targeted ventricular ectopic beats including during provocation with isoprenaline and pacing. Mapping and ablation of triggers in the right ventricular outflow tract, which is the most likely site in the patients of Brugada syndrome, is conventionally based on targeting the earliest myocardial activation site. Purkinje potential is not identified in this subset of patients.

### Guidelines

Catheter ablation of monomorphic VT has a different set of indications than polymorphic VT/VF. Catheter ablation is recommended as a potential bailout procedure for recurrent polymorphic ventricular tachycardia and VF that is refractory to optimized medical management including antiarrhythmic therapy (class IIa/b) in critically sick patients and when there is a suspected trigger that can be targeted for ablation. Ablation is also indicated as adjunctive therapy in patients with an ICD who are receiving multiple shocks from polymorphic VT/VF as a manifestation of a primary cardiac electrical disorder that is not manageable medically or by drug therapy or who do not want long-term drug therapy. This procedure is challenging and should be performed only in experienced centers. Success is facilitated by frequent ventricular ectopy to facilitate mapping, often necessitating that the procedure be performed emergently when the arrhythmia is active.

### Limitations

Catheter ablation of VF is intended to selectively eliminate distal His-Purkinje arborization triggers, which generate ectopic beats initiating the VF. In the absence of well-defined clinical targets, the likelihood of acute procedural success is low and that of the recurrent arrhythmia is high. Conduction block in the right bundle branch during catheter manipulation could adversely affect the ablation of triggers arising from the right Purkinje arborization. In the absence of normal His-Purkinje conduction, the frequency of the occurrence of the clinical ectopic beat reduces during the procedure. Often it completely disappears, which hampers the mapping and ablation of relevant foci. In patients with multiple morphologies of VF-triggering ectopies, the acute procedural success rates remain lower than in patients with fewer target beat morphologies.[15,37]

## CAN ABLATION SUBSTITUTE FOR ICD?

As mentioned earlier, the distal Purkinje network is the most frequent site of initiation of VF. Because the ablation procedure is carried out in patients who fail to recover from the arrhythmia storm despite optimum medical management, the number of patients in each of the series is small (**Table 1**). However, the acute procedural success rates are in the range of 88% to 100% without any serious complications. The Purkinje network is present on the superficial endocardium and tends to respond to ablation quickly and without the need for prolonged ablation times or high power. Medium-term arrhythmia freedom in survivors is also in a similar range. These findings suggest promising acute and medium-term efficacy of an ablation procedure in patients who could not have survived otherwise. In contrast, there were about 20% of patients who required more than 1 procedure in the idiopathic VF group for a recurrent device-recorded arrhythmic event without any clinical symptoms or therapy triggered from the device.[38] Thus, ICDs that were previously implanted for primary/secondary prevention of sudden death served as monitoring devices in patients with successful ablation procedures. This finding implies that the severity of the arrhythmia in terms of duration and frequency of episode were effectively modified by ablation precluding any further therapy from the device. In some, the antiarrhythmic drug that was previously ineffective could exercise arrhythmia control in patients with recurrence after ablation.

The device logs (see **Table 1**, last column) in the series of patients with successful ablation of VF storm show that none of these patients had recurrent VF-triggering device therapy during a variable period of follow-up. If the device delivered therapy, it was for monomorphic VT. In 1 patient in the series by Peichl and colleagues,[45] newly observed morphology of ectopy caused recurrence from a distinct site, necessitating reablation. Thus, if new arrhythmogenic triggers develop and cause VF storm from a distinct source, ICD will provide the necessary secondary prevention.

**Table 1**
**VF ablation case series**

| Series | Clinical Disorder | Number of Patients | ICD (%) | Acute Success (%) | Mean Follow-Up (mo) | Follow-Up Deaths (Cause) | Freedom from VF in Survivors (%) | Recurrence on ICD (Type/Therapy) |
|---|---|---|---|---|---|---|---|---|
| Haissaguerre et al[15] Knecht et al[38] | Idiopathic VF | 38 | 97 | 100 | 52 ± 28 | 00 | 95[a] | Polymorphic VT/none |
| Haissaguerre et al[36] | Long QT and Br syndromes | 7 | 71 | 100 | 17 ± 17 | 00 | 100[b] | None/none |
| Bansch et al[39] | Acute MI | 4 | 100 | 100 | Median 10 | 00 | 100 | None/none |
| Marrouche et al[40] | Ischemic cardiomyopathy | 8 | 88 | 88[c] | 10 ± 6 | 00 | 100 | VT/shock NSVT/none |
| Szumowski et al[41] | Ischemic cardiomyopathy | 5 | 100 | 100 | 16 ± 5 | 00 | 100[d] | None/none |
| Mlcochova et al[42] | Amyloid heart disease | 2 | 100 | 100 | 8 | 1 (Ischemic Colitis) | 100 | None/none |
| Bode et al[43] | Structural heart disease[e] | 7 | 43 | 100 | Median 10 | 2 (heart failure) | 100 | None/none |
| Sinha et al[44] | Nonischemic cardiomyopathy | 4 | 100 | 100 | 12 ± 5 | 00 | 100 | NSVF/none |
| Peichl et al[45] | Ischemic cardiomyopathy | 9 | 100 | 89 | 13 ± 7 | 1 (heart failure) | 88[f] | VT/shock VF/shock |

*Abbreviations*: Br, Brugada; MI, myocardial infarction; NS, nonsustained.
[a] Mean 1.28 ± 0.6 procedures/patient and 13% patients also took antiarrhythmic drugs.
[b] Two patients continued drug therapy.
[c] One patient experienced recurrent VF after ablation, and needed a left ventricular assist device but succumbed later to septic shock.
[d] All patients were on either amiodarone or sotalol.
[e] Ischemia in 4, remote myocarditis in 2, and aortic valve replacement in 1.
[f] Three of the 7 patients were on amiodarone therapy.

The procedural success rate is high in centers with high volume and expertise and the data support the feasibility of ablation in VF in such centers, at present. The number of case series in VF storm ablation is limited, which reflects low disease burden. Most patients with VF storm respond to optimization of medical management. Moreover, medically unresponsive VF storm is not always the presenting feature in patients with structural or electrical cardiac disorder surviving sudden death. Thus, many of these patients who experience VF storm later in the course of the disease have already received an ICD after the index event. More usually, an ICD is implanted for primary prevention in contemporary practice.

In contrast, ICD implantation is indicated in patients who are receiving chronic optimal medical therapy and who have a reasonable expectation of survival with a good functional status for more than 1 year. Many patients with structural heart disease are critically ill at the time of acute arrhythmic event. Within a short period of time after successful catheter ablation of VF storm, they often succumb to heart failure or severe noncardiac ailments. Because ICD implantation is guided by overall expected survival, these cases may not be suitable for device implantation for other reasons mentioned earlier.

## SUMMARY

Ablation data are currently limited to a small, select population of patients with refractory VF storm with medium duration of follow-up. It might be too early to recommend against the implantation of ICDs in patients with successfully ablated medically refractory index VF storm. Further study is needed to define the role of ablation in cases that are not medically refractory.

## REFERENCES

1. Zipes DP, Camm AJ, Borggrefe M, et al. ACC/AHA/ESC 2006 guidelines for management of patients with ventricular arrhythmias and the prevention of sudden cardiac death. J Am Coll Cardiol 2006;48: 1064–108.
2. Natale A, Raviele A, Al-Ahmad A, et al. Venice Chart International Consensus Document on ventricular tachycardia/ventricular fibrillation ablation. J Cardiovasc Electrophysiol 2010;21(3): 339–79.
3. Investigators TC. Randomized antiarrhythmic drug therapy in survivors of cardiac arrest (the CASCADE Study). Am J Cardiol 1993;72:280–7.
4. Kuck KH, Cappato R, Siebels J, et al. Randomized comparison of antiarrhythmic drug therapy with implantable defibrillators in patients resuscitated from cardiac arrest: the Cardiac Arrest Study Hamburg (CASH). Circulation 2000;102:748–54.
5. Anonymous A comparison of antiarrhythmic-drug therapy with implantable defibrillators in patients resuscitated from near-fatal ventricular arrhythmias. The Antiarrhythmics Versus Implantable Defibrillators (AVID) Investigators. N Engl J Med 1997;337: 1576–83.
6. Connolly SJ, Gent M, Roberts RS, et al. Canadian Implantable Defibrillator Study (CIDS): a randomized trial of the implantable cardioverter defibrillator against amiodarone. Circulation 2000;101:1297–302.
7. Aliot EM, Stevenson WG, Almendral-Garrote JM, et al. EHRA/HRS expert consensus on catheter ablation of ventricular arrhythmias. Heart Rhythm 2009; 6(6):886–933.
8. Couch OA Jr. Cardiac aneurysm with ventricular tachycardia and subsequent excision of aneurysm; case report. Circulation 1959;20(2):251–3.
9. Friedman PL, Stewart JR, Wit AL. Spontaneous and induced cardiac arrhythmias in subendocardial Purkinje fibers surviving extensive myocardial infarction in dogs. Circ Res 1973;33:612–26.
10. Myerburg RJ, Stewart JW, Hoffman BF. Electrophysiological properties of the canine peripheral conducting system. Circ Res 1970;26:361–72.
11. Berenfeld O, Jalife J. Arrhythmias in a 3-dimensional model of the ventricles Purkinje-muscle reentry as a mechanism of polymorphic ventricular. Circ Res 1998;82:1063–77.
12. Overholt ED, Joyner RW, Veenstra RD, et al. Unidirectional block between Purkinje and ventricular layers of papillary muscles. Am J Physiol 1984; 247:H584–95.
13. Pak HN, Kim YH, Lim HE, et al. Role of the posterior papillary muscle and Purkinje potentials in the mechanism of ventricular fibrillation in open chest dogs and swine: effects of catheter ablation. J Cardiovasc Electrophysiol 2006;17:777–83.
14. Saliba W, Abul Karim A, Tchou P, et al. Ventricular fibrillation: ablation of a trigger? J Cardiovasc Electrophysiol 2002;13:1296–9.
15. Haissaguerre M, Shoda M, Jais P, et al. Mapping and ablation of idiopathic ventricular fibrillation. Circulation 2002;106:962–7.
16. Haissaguerre M, Shah DC, Jais P, et al. Role of Purkinje conducting system in triggering idiopathic sudden cardiac death. Lancet 2002;359:677–8.
17. Marenco JP, Wang PJ, Link MS, et al. Improving survival from sudden cardiac arrest: the role of the automated external defibrillator. JAMA 2001;285: 1193–200.
18. Priori SG, Bossaert LL, Chamberlain DA, et al. ESC-ERC recommendations for the use of automated external defibrillators (AEDs) in Europe. Eur Heart J 2004;25:437–45.

19. Koster RW. Automatic external defibrillator key link in the chain of survival. J Cardiovasc Electrophysiol 2002;13:S92–5.

20. Valenzuela TD, Roe DJ, Nichol G, et al. Outcomes of rapid defibrillation by security officers after cardiac arrest in casinos. N Engl J Med 2000; 343:1206–9.

21. Caffrey SL, Willoughby PJ, Pepe PE, et al. Public use of automated external defibrillators. N Engl J Med 2002;347:1242–7.

22. Bardy GH, Lee KL, Mark DB, et al. Amiodarone or an implantable cardioverter-defibrillator for congestive heart failure. N Engl J Med 2005;352:225–37.

23. Moss AJ, Hall WJ, Cannom DS, et al. Improved survival with an implanted defibrillator in patients with coronary disease at high risk for ventricular arrhythmia. Multicenter Automatic Defibrillator Implantation Trial Investigators. N Engl J Med 1996;335:1933–40.

24. Bigger JT Jr. Prophylactic use of implanted cardiac defibrillators in patients at high risk for ventricular arrhythmias after coronary-artery bypass graft surgery. Coronary Artery Bypass Graft (CABG) Patch Trial Investigators. N Engl J Med 1997;337: 1569–75.

25. Buxton AE, Lee KL, Fisher JD, et al. A randomized study of the prevention of sudden death in patients with coronary artery disease. Multicenter Unsustained Tachycardia Trial Investigators. N Engl J Med 1999;341:1882–90.

26. Moss AJ, Zareba W, Hall WJ, et al. Prophylactic implantation of a defibrillator in patients with myocardial infarction and reduced ejection fraction. N Engl J Med 2002;346:877–83.

27. Lee DS, Green LD, Liu PP, et al. Effectiveness of implantable defibrillators for preventing arrhythmic events and deaths meta-analysis. J Am Coll Cardiol 2003;41:1573–82.

28. Ezekowitz JA, Armstrong PW, McAlister FA. Implantable cardioverter defibrillators in primary and secondary prevention: systematic review of randomized, controlled trials. Ann Intern Med 2003;138: 445–52.

29. Verma A, Kilicaslan F, Marrouche NF, et al. Prevalence, predictors, and mortality significance of the causative arrhythmia in patients with electrical storm. J Cardiovasc Electrophysiol 2004;15:1265–70.

30. Survivors of out-of-hospital cardiac arrest with apparently normal heart: need for definition and standardized clinical evaluation. Consensus Statement of the Joint Steering Committees of the Unexplained Cardiac Arrest Registry of Europe and of the Idiopathic Ventricular Fibrillation Registry of the United States. Circulation 1997;95:265–72.

31. Belhassen B, Viskin S. Idiopathic ventricular tachycardia and fibrillation. J Cardiovasc Electrophysiol 1993;4:356–68.

32. Meissner MD, Lehmann MH, Steinman RT, et al. Ventricular fibrillation in patients without significant structural heart disease: a multicenter experience with implantable cardioverter-defibrillator therapy. J Am Coll Cardiol 1993;21:1406–12.

33. Ashida K, Kaji Y, Sasaki Y. Abolition of torsade de pointes after radiofrequency catheter ablation at right ventricular outflow tract. Int J Cardiol 1997; 59(2):171–5.

34. Kusano KF, Yamamoto M, Emori T, et al. Successful catheter ablation in a patient with polymorphic ventricular tachycardia. J Cardiovasc Electrophysiol 2000;11:682–5.

35. Takatsuki S, Mitamura H, Ogawa S. Catheter ablation of a monofocal premature ventricular complex triggering idiopathic ventricular fibrillation. Heart 2001;86:E3.

36. Haissaguerre M, Extramiana F, Hocini M, et al. Mapping and ablation of ventricular fibrillation associated with long-QT and Brugada syndromes. Circulation 2003;108:925–8.

37. Haïssaguerre M, Derval N, Sacher F, et al. Sudden cardiac arrest associated with early repolarization. N Engl J Med 2008;358:2016–23.

38. Knecht S, Sacher F, Wright M, et al. Long-term follow-up of idiopathic ventricular fibrillation ablation: a multicenter study. J Am Coll Cardiol 2009;54(6): 522–8.

39. Bansch D, Oyang F, Antz M, et al. Successful catheter ablation of electrical storm after myocardial infarction. Circulation 2003;108:3011–6.

40. Marrouche NF, Verma A, Wazni O, et al. Mode of initiation and ablation of ventricular fibrillation storms in patients with ischemic cardiomyopathy. J Am Coll Cardiol 2004;43(9):1715–20.

41. Szumowski L, Sanders P, Walczak F, et al. Mapping and ablation of polymorphic ventricular tachycardia after myocardial infarction. J Am Coll Cardiol 2004; 44(8):1700–6.

42. Mlcochova H, Saliba WI, Burkhardt DJ, et al. Catheter ablation of ventricular fibrillation storm in patients with infiltrative amyloidosis of the heart. J Cardiovasc Electrophysiol 2006;17(4):426–30.

43. Bode K, Hindricks G, Piorkowski C, et al. Ablation of polymorphic ventricular tachycardias in patients with structural heart disease. Pacing Clin Electrophysiol 2008;31(12):1585–91.

44. Sinha AM, Schmidt M, Marschang H, et al. Role of left ventricular scar and Purkinje-like potentials during mapping and ablation of ventricular fibrillation in dilated cardiomyopathy. Pacing Clin Electrophysiol 2009;32(3):286–90.

45. Peichl P, Cihák R, Kozeluhová M, et al. Catheter ablation of arrhythmic storm triggered by monomorphic ectopic beats in patients with coronary artery disease. J Interv Card Electrophysiol 2010;27(1): 51–9.

# Index

# Moving?

## Make sure your subscription moves with you!

To notify us of your new address, find your **Clinics Account Number** (located on your mailing label above your name), and contact customer service at:

**Email: journalscustomerservice-usa@elsevier.com**

**800-654-2452** (subscribers in the U.S. & Canada)
**314-447-8871** (subscribers outside of the U.S. & Canada)

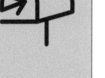

**Fax number: 314-447-8029**

**Elsevier Health Sciences Division**
**Subscription Customer Service**
**3251 Riverport Lane**
**Maryland Heights, MO 63043**

*To ensure uninterrupted delivery of your subscription, please notify us at least 4 weeks in advance of move.

ELSEVIER